The Madness of Fear

The Madness of Fear

A History of Catatonia

Edward Shorter, PhD, FRSC

Jason A. Hannah Professor of the History of Medicine
Professor of Psychiatry
Faculty of Medicine
University of Toronto
Toronto, Ontario, Canada

Max Fink, MD

Professor of Psychiatry and Neurology, Emeritus
Stony Brook University School of Medicine
Stony Brook, New York, USA

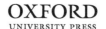

OXFORD
UNIVERSITY PRESS

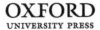

OXFORD
UNIVERSITY PRESS

Oxford University Press is a department of the University of Oxford. It furthers
the University's objective of excellence in research, scholarship, and education
by publishing worldwide. Oxford is a registered trade mark of Oxford University
Press in the UK and certain other countries.

Published in the United States of America by Oxford University Press
198 Madison Avenue, New York, NY 10016, United States of America.

Library of Congress Cataloging-in-Publication Data
Names: Shorter, Edward, author. | Fink, Max, 1923– author.
Title: The madness of fear : a history of catatonia / Edward Shorter, Max Fink.
Description: New York, NY : Oxford University Press, [2018] |
Includes bibliographical references.
Identifiers: LCCN 2017047176 | ISBN 9780190881191 (pbk.)
Subjects: | MESH: Catatonia—history | Psychiatry—history
Classification: LCC RC514 | NLM WL 11.1 | DDC 616.89/8—dc23
LC record available at https://lccn.loc.gov/2017047176

3 5 7 9 8 6 4

Printed by Webcom, Inc., Canada

In memory of Martha Gross Fink

CONTENTS

PREFACE

Sometimes my body becomes demented.
Male, 19, at West Park Hospital in Surrey, 1939.[1]

What are the real disease entities in psychiatry? This question has bedeviled psychological medicine for a hundred years or more. Now, you'd think that this would be high on the research agenda of psychiatry. But it is low, and such basic science fields as neuroimaging, neurochemistry, and genetics carry the day instead. Not that there is anything wrong with laboratory science. But before you can study the role of brain circuits or cerebral chemistry, you have to be able to specify how the various diseases present clinically, meaning what the patients actually look like, and then identify homogeneous cohorts for study.

This brings us to catatonia. Unlike schizophrenia, we know what symptoms count as catatonic. Some are serious, with patients dying as their temperatures accelerate; they become dehydrated because they refuse to drink, and they risk inanition because they refuse to eat or move. Autistic children with catatonia may repeatedly hit themselves in the head. We don't really know what catatonia is or its causes, in the sense that we know what pneumonia is. But we can identify it and recognize its many forms, with the added benefit that catatonia is eminently treatable. We can make these patients better on a reliable basis. The same can be said of few other disease entities in psychiatry.

But why has there been so little psychiatric interest in catatonia? Why is it simply not on the radar of most clinicians? Actually, catatonia occurs in many medical illnesses, but it certainly doesn't leap to mind among internists or emergency room specialists. Why this ignorance? That's why we're writing this book. It is a remarkable story about how medicine flounders and then finds its way. And it will help doctors, their patients, and the public to recognize catatonia as a core illness in psychiatry and in medicine in general.

Psychologically, catatonia seems associated with fear. It is not clear if fear causes it or if fearful images surge from the inner mind during stupor and sustain it. Patients' faces are often filled with fear, and afterward they say they thought a catastrophe had occurred. In a catatonic stupor, they are usually motionless, their muscles rigid, as animals are in a fearful response to a predator. Maybe, in the long haul of evolution, Nature has built these fearful responses into us—and we still have them.

ACKNOWLEDGMENTS

Interest in catatonia came full forward with my assumption of clinical responsibility for the ECT Service and the treatment of acutely ill patients admitted to the Psychiatric Services of the University Hospital at Stony Brook University in 1980. Gregory Fricchione, then in charge of consultations, brought the wealth of case material to my attention and encouraged effective treatment protocols. Collaboration with Michael Alan Taylor, who challenged the Kraepelin delineation of catatonia as schizophrenia in the 1970s, led to our review of the place of catatonia in the classifications of the *Diagnostic and Statistical Manual of Mental Disorders* (DSM) and to the publication of our texts on catatonia in 2003 and on melancholia in 2006. Collaborations with Andrew Francis, Georgios Petrides, and George Bush, among other Stony Brook staff members, led to the catatonia rating scale, the sedation test, and the optimized treatment protocols with benzodiazepines and induced seizures. David Healy's tests of the incidence of catatonia in Wales and India reinforced our studies. My acquaintance with Edward Shorter began with his history of the shock therapies, written with David Healy; our clarifications of the types of catatonia; and our collaboration on the history of melancholia and now catatonia. I am also indebted to Krysten Nyitray, archivist of the Stony Brook University Special Library collections for her support of the Max Fink Archives.

—Max Fink

It was Max who interested me in catatonia, and I wrote the historical part of this book with a real sense of, "here, we are reviving psychiatry's ancient wisdom for the benefit of a contemporary world that has largely forgotten it." Catatonia is a disease concept that is simply unfamiliar to many, and we hope that *The Madness of Fear: A History of Catatonia* will increase its recognition among clinicians and the general public. Susan Bélanger, the administrator of our history of medicine program in Toronto, helped immeasurably with this task, as did Esther Atkinson and Hannah Johnston. Our agent, Beverly Slopen, was a kind and immensely well-informed ally. We are grateful to Andrea Knobloch at Oxford University Press for her assistance.

—Edward Shorter

1

INTRODUCTION

Yes, this rigidity of his, his fits of perspiration, that periodic twitching of the eyes, he observes us intently, but won't talk or eat, all that looks like catatonic trouble.[1]
—A description of Franz Biberkopf, in Alfred Döblin, *Berlin Alexanderplatz* (1929)

"Our son is an athlete, a college recruited athlete," said one mother of a lad of 21 who lapsed into catatonic mutism and staring. "At the hospital, the nurses would seek to draw out speech by asking him about his sports. Always, no response."

Then one day, a nurse handed him a "ball" that she had made from the Play Doh at the craft center.

"He reached for the ball, got out of bed, went into the hall, and started pitching."
The mother went to catch his throws. He would respond to her commands.

"I'd say: 'full wind-up.' He'd pitch full wind-up.

"I'd say, 'now, out of the stretch.'" He'd switch to stretch position.

"I'd say, 'runner's going.' " He'd do his pivot and throw to 'first base' to stop the steal."

Finally, the nurse said they couldn't throw balls on the unit, and he went back to bed, and was silent again.[2]

THIS IS CATATONIA

This is catatonia. It is quite common. About 10 percent of the patients in a psychiatric intensive care facility are found to have it. Here also is good news: three-quarters have a full remission within 2–4 days when recognized and properly treated.[3] Yet, for many physicians, to say nothing of the patients and their families, catatonia has been a mystery. "The structure of catatonia remains to be discovered," said Jo Ellen Wilson and Stephan Heckers at Vanderbilt University in 2015.[4] We have the skills to find it and to treat it successfully (better than almost all other disorders labeled in the *Diagnostic and Statistical Manual of Mental Disorders* [DSM-5]). But first it must be diagnosed.

Catatonia is a behavior syndrome of movement and mood, classically marked by stupor, mutism, posturing, rigidity, and repetitive speech and acts. Usually acute in onset, its signs are recognizable, and, when recognized, it can be successfully treated.

What is it? Not an infection, nor a specific tissue pathology, nor a posttraumatic consequence. Like schizophrenia and personality disorder and melancholia, we know it when we see it. But what is it in Nature?

We wonder whether catatonia has been put into a very weak part of medical neuroscience among pill-prescribing psychiatrists because it is more often seen on acute medical services. These clinicians are best enabled to treat the syndrome successfully.

"I assume," says Max Fink, "that I had been shown catatonic patients during my days in the 1940s in medical school and residency training. Indeed, I recall walking through hospital wards, dressed in the short white coat of the student, with two vials of the barbiturate Amytal sodium, each of 500 mg in one pocket, a metal box with sterile syringe and needles, tourniquet and bottled water in the other, to sedate the excited and the manic and to relax the negativistic and the mute.[5] But during the decades of clinical practice as a research physician in New York and St. Louis hospitals, I cannot recall recognizing catatonia as a distinct syndrome. In my research positions, I had little front-line responsibility to examine and treat the acutely ill.

"It was during a visit to the Bakirköy Hospital in Istanbul in 1965 that I saw nude women, standing in Christ-like postures, in hospital windows and rows of posturing men. Turan Itil, my research colleague, and I were visiting to supervise a study of a new neuroleptic, butaperazine. When we arrived we were welcomed by a patient band, dressed in nineteenth-century Turkish pantaloons and multicolored shirts, an image of the mental hospital before the psychopharmacology era.

"My interest in catatonia was aroused when I became responsible for the teaching of students and the care of patients on the in-patient unit at University Hospital at Stony Brook. My experience with a fully restrained delirious woman, sick with lupus, referred for ECT, and the resolution of her illness pointed me on the road taken."[6]

CATATONIA IS IDENTIFIED

Catatonia today is a syndrome that is identifiable, verifiable, and eminently treatable, a circumstance existing in the armamentarium of psychiatry only for melancholia and neurosyphilis. And like melancholia and neurosyphilis, catatonia is a disease of the brain. Karl Kahlbaum, who coined the term in 1874, said flatly, "Catatonia is a brain disease with a cyclically variable course."[7] There is a psychological component, yet the main symptoms of catatonia—stupor, agitation, "waxy" flexibility of the limbs, mutism, and negativism—seem brain-driven. The attacks often come suddenly.

Stupor is very common. Stupor does not mean a clouding of consciousness just a peg above coma. It means being shut off from communication with the outside world while remaining mentally awake. The patients' eyes dart about freely, and patients later remember most of what occurred around them during the stupor even though they were silent, motionless, and unresponsive to communication or pain. This book has one piece of news about what happens in stupor, and it is news that gives the book its title: these patients are frequently overwhelmed by fear, dread, and anxiety. They imagine that their house has burned down or that the hussars are coming. These are psychotic symptoms, out of touch with reality, and we therefore speak of "the madness of fear."[8] Catatonic stupor is a terrifying experience, not a gentle oblivion.

We recognize degrees of stupor going from the marble-like rigidity of apparent death to a transitory fixing of gaze on a spot on the wall. Catatonia is more than a movement disorder, although it differs from other psychoses in embedding movement in its core definition. It entails negativistic behavior and psychotic ideation as well as rigidity, immobility, posturing, muscle tension, stupor, agitation, tics, echolalia (repeating others' words), echopraxia (imitating others' movements), and mannerisms.

There are two forms. The catatonic symptoms that are present in other diseases might be termed "*catatonic syndrome*," as they adhere in a recognizable syndrome rather than just occurring as isolated "features." Then there is the full-fledged form of "*Kahlbaum's disease,*" which Kahlbaum described in 1874. Kahlbaum's catatonia and the catatonic syndrome are part of the same underlying condition, all parts of which are responsive to benzodiazepines and to electroconvulsive therapy (ECT). Parkinson's disease offer an interesting parallel, as we speak of Parkinson's disease, which is a disease *sui generis*, and a row of other diseases with parkinsonian symptoms.[9]

Kahlbaum's catatonia and the catatonic syndrome are related manifestations. Their basic unity is the commonality of their response to the anticatatonic treatments.[10] Among the guidelines in modern psychopharmacology is the belief that the common response of a population to a single treatment identifies their biological commonality. It is useful to insist on Kahlbaum's catatonia as a separate presentation to counteract the field's century-long tradition of diagnosing catatonia as "schizophrenia" when psychotic symptoms appear. This "schizophrenia" tradition in the interpretation of catatonic symptoms has been a barrier to effective care. Calling attention to Kahlbaum's catatonia is a start on breaking the stranglehold of "schizophrenia" on catatonia in its psychotic manifestations. The test of treatment responsiveness is also a metric of other diagnoses that have sprung up as supposedly independent clinical entities, such as neuroleptic malignant syndrome and pediatric "stereotypic movement disorder." These respond to ECT and to the benzodiazepine lorazepam, and current evidence suggests that these, too, are forms of catatonia.

Fed up with the DSM and its contrived categories, a group of investigators led by Max Fink has been trying to get back to the basic illness entities in psychiatry as they exist in Nature. Members of this group have written about three such entities— hebephrenia, catatonia, and melancholia—which we have called elsewhere "the Three Ugly Stepsisters." The group has produced monographs about two of the stepsisters— melancholia and catatonia.[11] Here, we take on catatonia again, but this time its history. The history of catatonia demonstrates clearly that the symptoms of catatonia are among the most fundamental clinical pictures in psychiatry and, as such, deserve wide attention.

While at the University of Michigan in the first decade of the twenty-first century, Michael Alan Taylor, formerly the chairperson of psychiatry and psychology at Chicago's Rosalind Franklin University, described patients in various intensive care units of the large academic hospital as "Lazarus patients." "With lorazepam and ECT we raised them from the dead and they walked out of the hospital back to baseline. Some literally had hospice papers on their bed stands."[12] With lorazepam and ECT, the Consultation and Liaison psychiatrists were able to give these patients—many of whom were in long-term catatonic stupors—new lives.

Today, the situation is quite different: patients are being more readily diagnosed with catatonia, treated effectively, and returned well to the community. Often they do not relapse, nor do they have residual symptoms. It is a kind of miracle. This book is about that miracle.

A HISTORY OF CONFUSION

Anyone who thinks that medicine is one brick of knowledge carefully laid upon the next will despair at reading the history of catatonia. In 1873, David Skae, professor of psychiatry in Edinburgh, described a typical case of "adolescent insanity" caused, he thought, by masturbation: "The boy was sometimes preternaturally excited, but more often dull, and sullen—he wept, and said he had committed the unpardonable sin [masturbation], and tried to tear off his clothes and throw them into the fire. Sometimes he appeared to be in a cataleptic fit, falling down and appearing to be in a trance. He had a silly and stupid look, refused to take his food, and would not answer questions when spoken to. Sometimes he would suddenly throw himself on the floor, but whether voluntarily or involuntarily could not be made out. . . . He occasionally practiced some curious movements. He would stand for more than an hour at a time working his hands backwards and forwards. . . . On other occasions he would devote as long a period to twitching the corners of his mouth up and down, and jerking his body backwards and forwards. If any one went up to him and shook him gently he immediately stopped these movements." The boy recovered within "three or four months."[13]

The patient had an array of catatonic symptoms: alternation of stupor and agitation, posturing, negativism (food refusal, refusing to answer), and stereotypical movements. Skae's article was published in the very year that Kahlbaum's classic German work appeared, 1874, yet it is unlikely that Skae would have diagnosed the patient with catatonia because the term was slow to catch on in Britain[14]

The Paris of the celebrated neurologist Jean-Martin Charcot was full of catatonia in the 1870s and '80s, although it was called "hysteria" or "catalepsy." Charcot positively cultivated it at the vast women's hospice, the Salpêtrière, where he was the medical director. Under the term "hysteria," many of the young female patients went into stupors at a signal such as the clanging of a bell. Jules Claretie, a boulevardier who frequented the hospital, reported in 1881, "The ringing of a gong, an overly bright light, or staring fixedly at an object—suffices to set off catalepsy. During a religious holiday at the Salpêtrière, someone forgot to stand down the brasses and the cymbals in the military music that accompanied the parades through the courtyards of the hospital. The music played, the cymbals resounded, and—suddenly—a whole column of patients remained in place, in catalepsy, their eyes turned upward, their limbs stiff as a statue. This won't happen again. There'll be no more parades at the Salpêtrière."

Out on the streets of Paris as well, there was catalepsy, continued Claretie. "One fine day she'll give a sudden laugh, penetrating, nervous: and a fit happens! There's a tremor, and what one calls choreiform movements appear. The woman, seized suddenly, emits a prolonged scream, holds out her arms and falls backwards, almost gently. Then, her jaw locked, her neck tensed and swollen and the sounds of digestion in her gullet [stertor]: she's fixed there, her eyes wide open, pupils dilated, looking upwards, arms rigid, spread out like a cross, literally crucified—her legs extended, next to each other, stiff. . . . There are fits that can last up to five hours."[15]

US psychiatry, by contrast, had definitely not been accustomed to thinking about catatonia, and it was simply not on the radar of many clinicians. William T. McKinney Jr., later a distinguished figure in psychosis research, was a medical student at Vanderbilt in the early 1960s. "I'll never forget my first patient in my clinical psychiatry rotation," he said in a later interview. "I was out at Central State Hospital near Nashville. The patient didn't talk and was mute; the diagnosis was catatonic schizophrenia. Frank [Luton] and Bill Orr [McKinney's teachers] taught us to respect the patient's need for distance and predictability. You're respectful, not too demanding, but just there. They had their space and you don't encroach on it." McKinney would return to the patient week after week, to see if he was ready to talk. But he wasn't, not for a long time.[16] The anecdote is heartwarming as an expression of humanism in medicine, yet rather chilling as an illustration of inadequate care. Whether the patient had "schizophrenia" is impossible for us to know now, but he certainly had catatonia, a serious and potentially fatal disease. In the early 1960s, catatonia was eminently treatable with barbiturates and ECT, as it had been since the 1930s. So, out of respect for his "space," the patient, in the grips of a major illness, was not treated.

Today, we are much occupied with psychiatric diagnosis. Commissions appointed by the American Psychiatric Association produce the fat volumes of the DSM. In the famous third edition in 1980, the commissioners invented such diagnoses as "major depression" or "posttraumatic stress disorder (PTSD)," more or less on the spot, either to solve a political problem within the Association (as with major depression—to get approval by the psychoanalysts) or in response to an outside pressure group (as with the Vietnam veterans, who foisted PTSD upon the disease-designers in a strong-arm political play). Diagnoses tended to be someone's bright idea that then became heavily politicized and acquired lobbies on their behalf.[17]

Things used to be different in psychiatry. Diagnoses would percolate for decades before crystallizing and taking a place in the manuals. There would be a vast input from individual clinicians in many lands that would finally turn into a river of certainty as one of the principal figures, such as Emil Kraepelin or Sigmund Freud, incorporated the diagnosis in a definitive system. Delirious mania percolated in this manner in mainline psychiatry and "neurosis" within psychoanalysis. Such broad streams were the opposite of the horse trading that goes on around a DSM table: "I'll give you your diagnosis if you give me mine." Catatonia came together in one of these broad-stream stories, beginning as a wide variety of different terms—"stupidity," "catalepsy," "*Starrsucht*"—then coming together in the work of a central figure, Karl Ludwig Kahlbaum, who owned a small, private mental hospital in Görlitz, Germany, and who, in 1874, coined the term "catatonia." (Not that it was immediately accepted, anything but.)

Which system is better, the slow convergence or the sudden inspiration from heaven? Hard to say. "Hysteria" was the product of the slow convergence of many minds, and it turned out to be a disaster, especially for women. "Major depression" was the bright idea of Robert Spitzer, head of the DSM Task Force, in 1980. The takeaway lesson from this book is that we learn valuable lessons about psychiatric diagnosis from the storied past, and this has been forgotten in a psychiatry that today is highly presentist.

2

CATATONIA BEFORE KAHLBAUM

A girl of five, having been quite shocked at mealtime that her sister had taken for herself some choice morsel that the girl desired, all of a sudden became stiff. The hand holding the spoon remained in the same position stretched out towards the platter; she looked at her sister sideways, with an indignant expression; although people called out loudly to her, and shook her firmly, she understood nothing; she moved neither her mouth nor her lips; she walked when she was pushed or taken by the hand; her arms, whether they were raised, lowered or placed transversally, remained in the same position; you would have thought you were looking at a statue of wax; after this fit, she remained stiff and cold, as though of marble; after an hour she started to warm up little by little, stretching out her limbs with deep sighs. . . . Finally, after a lot of sweating, she returned to normal.[1]
—Samuel-Auguste Tissot, physician in Lausanne, mid-eighteenth century

One often encounters the statement, "Catatonia was first identified by Karl Kahlbaum in 1874."[2] The statement is technically correct but historically wrong. For centuries, physicians have described the symptoms of catatonia, although it was indeed Kahlbaum who assembled them into a neat package bearing the label "catatonia." Before Kahlbaum catatonia was called different things, and the commonest term was "catalepsy."

CATALEPSY

Catalepsy meant stupor plus waxy rigidity, the limbs holding the new position in which they had been placed. The earliest descriptions are in Hippocrates' writings, with the first careful account appearing in the work of Galen in the second century AD. Thereafter, descriptions of stiff limbs and stupor appear sporadically.[3] One scholar tabulated 150 cases in the medical literature from Galen to Madame D in 1855.[4] In Toulouse, in 1415, a monk saying Mass, on the moment of raising the chalice, "became stiff and immobile, his eyes open and turned upwards. The Brother who was serving Mass, saw that the monk remained overlong in this state, approached him, and. having shaken him several times by the robe, found him in this same immobility." There was a murmur among the congregation. Perhaps a miracle? A physician examined the stricken monk and said there had been no miracle, but that it was "a very dangerous malady and difficult to cure." Thereupon, a second monk began the continuance of the Mass, raised the chalice, and was stricken by the same symptoms! There was now a great tumult in the city. But the opinion of the physicians was that the first monk "had been surprised at that moment by a malady that they call *caroche* or *catalepsy*, and that this had an effect on the second monk of 'fear' together with his 'wounded imagination.'"[5]

In 1737, Madame AA left her home in Vesoul to be judged in a criminal affair in Besançon, the regional capital. But a medical problem developed. The physicians who rushed to her bedside found

> the lady seated on a chair, immobile, her eyes fixed upwards and glistening, her pupils wide open and motionless, her arms and hands raised together, as if she were in ecstasy. . . . Her limbs were supple, light and let themselves be positioned wherever one wanted without resistance, but—and this is what characterized her illness—they were too obedient; they didn't leave the position in which they were placed. . . . We raised one arm, then the other; they did not drop down again. . . . We raised them so high that even the strongest man would not have been able to keep them in that position; they remained up of their own.

Samuel-Auguste Tissot, the Lausanne physician who gave us this account in 1789, went on at length about how one could reposition Madame AA's limbs at will and see them retain their new positions.[6] It was as though one were molding a candle of soft wax, hence the term "waxy flexibility." That plus stupor were the essential features of catalepsy.

In the view of Paris surgeon Ambroise Paré in 1628, "catalepsie" eventuated when "putrid vapors" rose from the uterus to affect the brain. "The body becomes rigid and cold. . . . The eyes are open, without seeing, without hearing; lethargy, apoplexy follow, and frequently death."[7] Here, we have some key elements of catalepsy as seen in the Paris of Louis XIII—the stupor in which vision and hearing are lost, the body rigid—and, indeed, death may follow in a lethal version of catalepsy discussed later.

Catalepsy may not have been frequent, but it was not infrequent either. References to it dot the medical publications of the day. In his account of "periodic illnesses" in 1764, Mannheim physician Friedrich Casimir Medicus—who actually is better known as a botanist than a medical writer—described "periodic catalepsy" (*periodischer Starrsucht*) as a "repeated obtunding of the senses occurring at certain times, with a distinctive cramping [or tonic stiffening (*Krampf*)] of the body." Several authors, he said, had described the symptom in its recurrent form. "I myself previously knew a woman who was therewith afflicted."[8]

Catalepsy was called "*Starrsucht*" in German, the patients turned into "blocks of marble" yet displaying waxy rigidity. "Persons afflicted with it," said Leon Hirschel, a physician in Berlin, in 1769, "after a previous headache become . . . rigid and immobile, like a poster-pillar, lose their awareness, see nothing even with open eyes, neither hearing nor feeling anything, but they are able to get their breath, although weakly, and the pulse is natural. . . . The limbs may be moved, but remain in the position that is given them, so that, for example, if you flex or extend an arm or a finger, it remains flexed or extended until the attack is over."[9]

François-Xavier Mezler was a court physician to the prince of Hohenzollern-Sigmaringen. One of his young patients, a pregnant woman, was subject to loss of consciousness plus muscular rigidity. "When I visited her," he reported in 1794, "I thought she was sleeping. . . . I wanted to awaken her, but she was rigid, like wood, when I wanted to move her hand. This lasted for several more minutes and then she came to herself." She remembered only that she thought "something had climbed in her throat" (*globus hystericus*). In other attacks, Dr. Mezler reported, "It took a great deal of slow and steady pressure to move her arm, e.g. to give it another position." (This would later be known as *gegenhalten*.) Dr. Mezler apparently became a frequent caller. "I once saw, as she kissed her husband, that she got an attack; [her husband] was thus obliged to hold her in his arms until she came to her senses again."[10]

Around 1800, catalepsy was sidetracked into a near-fatal byway, as "magnetizers" associated with Franz Friedrich Anton Mesmer, first of Vienna, then of Paris, latched on to it as evidence of the action of the body's "animal electricity." This was the beginning of hypnotism—but hypnotism more as a psychodrama of suggestion rather than a medical tool. An entire hypnotic circus flourished for around 20 years, in which physicians imagined that their patients' hearing, for example, had been transferred to their abdomen or to the tips of their fingers, and "cataleptic" trances became common for highly suggestible individuals. All this had nothing to do with catalepsy as a symptom of catatonia; one of us has discussed this elsewhere, and the subject will not be reviewed here.[11] But this is why Paris psychiatrist Claude-Etienne Bourdin wrote a big book on catalepsy in 1841: to save the concept from being abducted by "the magnetizers." (Bourdin, anticipating Kahlbaum, thought catalepsy a unique disease entity.[12])

The first modern description of catalepsy comes from Philippe Pinel, the founder of psychiatric nosology. In his *Nosographie Philosophique* in 1803, Pinel defined catalepsy as "the sudden privation of sensory function and muscular movement." There may be posturing, he said, and waxy flexibility of the limbs as well. He reproached his predecessors for attaching the term "catalepsy" to all manner of conditions (this would be "symptomatic catalepsy" meaning not primary but caused by other diseases), and he argued for the existence of a single cataleptic disease. (Kahlbaum would pick up this thread.) The core symptom, said Pinel, was muscular tonic contraction, which permitted waxy flexibility to take place. But stupor, the eyes generally open, was also part of the core picture, with the patients unresponsive to external stimulation. (There was also an ecstatic catalepsy, with the patients frozen in place in religious enthusiasm.)[13] Pinel's authority sufficed to center catalepsy in the nineteenth-century pantheon of distinct diseases.

The English have always been parsimonious with diagnoses, shunning many of the fads that drifted over from the Continent, such as "hysteria." Many of the patients described by English asylum alienists early in the nineteenth century as in the grips of "insanity" or "madness" exhibited catatonic symptoms that, in France or Germany, would have been deemed catalepsy. Here is James W, 29, admitted to the New Bethlem Hospital ("Bedlam") in 1821:

> When the paroxysm came on, however he happened to be situated, his whole frame from head to foot became stiff, as if all his joints and muscles were ossified. His eyes, though staring open, became fixed, and he foamed at the mouth. If sitting or walking when his fit came on, he would instantly fall to the ground, generally extended at full length on his back, with the same symptoms of rigid stiffness and insensibility: his eyes, open and inclined upward [oculogyric crisis], were insensible to the touch of

a hand passed over them, which did not produce the slightest wink. No symptom of animation remained, with the exception of breathing, but this so faintly as to be scarcely perceptible. His condition in all other respects resembled death; and in this state he would sometimes continue for one, two, three, and even four days. . . . On being roused from his stupor, he recollected nothing of what had passed.

In a previous admission, he had been violent and seriously injured one of the attendants.[14]

By 1856, Henry Monro, chief psychiatrist ("physician") of the St. Luke's Hospital in London, reported that the British had become more accepting of the diagnosis of catalepsy. Monro had "half-a-dozen cases" of "cataleptoid" patients on his service, including some "who stand in apparently profound sopor; their eyes are glued down or else staring open in a fixed manner, so immovable that you do not observe the least twinkle of the eyelid. . . . You speak to them, they will not answer; you offer them food, they will not eat. They indeed are most unwilling to move from the spot which they have taken up," and if "you try to cross their will then you often find a most resolute resistance." Monro's patients were negativistic, mute, posturing, and agitated.

Were they "demented"? Not at all. Monro said, in a passage that today would leave the hospital ethics committee open-mouthed, "Sometimes when you lay hold suddenly of such a patient, you may shake him out of the stupor, and you find that his mind is by no means lost; that he has a clear perception of all that has been going on even during the trance; and he will argue about it as about an incubus which he could fully appreciate but could not control." Monro thus described the range of symptoms in catalepsy that anticipates Kahlbaum. "I am in the habit of pointing them out as specimens of the cataleptoid class, and the term has, I am happy to say, gained some approval."[15] Some might feel that Monro has the priority over Kahlbaum in that the "cataleptoid class" could easily qualify as catatonia. Yet Kahlbaum described the syndrome so much more comprehensively—with movement disorders, negativism, a sequence of stages, and so forth—that his priority remains intact.

Stupor, of course, was part of catalepsy, but English clinicians seemed more comfortable with it, often using stupor to describe incoherent symptoms. John B, 26, for example, fell ill on his honeymoon, "suffer[ing] pains in his head followed by mental depression." He was admitted to the Holloway Sanatorium outside of London in September 1894, discharged six weeks later. It was not quite clear what was wrong with him. His clinicians' diagnosis: "connubial stupor."[16]

Catalepsy appeared in the New World just as in the Old. In 1839, in Philadelphia, Isaac Parrish was called to the bedside of a lad of 15, whom he found "lying upon his back, motionless, and in a state of partial insensibility. . . . The eye balls were fixed in a wild stare." He had taken fright at a great fire at the Chestnut Street Wharf several months previously, and since then, "as soon as he closed his eyes, the scene of the fire would come before him, causing him to cry out with alarm." For several days prior to calling Dr. Parrish, the boy had been "unusually despondent and sat down during the greater part of the day with his head bent toward his chest; it appeared difficult for him to look up. Now at the bedside, Dr. Parrish elicited waxy flexibility: "I succeeded on several occasions in forcing his jaws open with the handle of a spoon; this appeared to cause him great pain; and so great was the tendency to remain open, that I was obliged to assist him in closing them."

The young patient became increasingly insensible and

"the most powerful efforts failed to produce consciousness. . . . The statue-like expression of the countenance was now still more remarkable, which, with the pallid face, the immovable position of the body, the dilated pupil and fixed eyes presented a most singular appearance. . . . I discovered for the first time a rigidity in the muscles of the upper extremity . . . I found that in raising the head, the muscles of the neck were completely rigid, drawing the head back." A colleague, summoned to the bedside, then made a further discovery: "Dr. [John C] Otto discovered an unusual rigidity of the limb, and in elevating it from under the bed clothes, and raising it up, it remained in the position in which it was placed. . . . After the limbs were flexed they maintained the bent position, until altered by an attendant. During these motions, the fixed statue-like countenance, and inanimate stare of the patient remained unaltered.

A week later: "Patient cataleptic; lying with his arms folded across the breast; his hands firmly clenching the wrists; so firm was his hold, that it required considerable force to disengage them." (This would be termed *gegenhalten*.)

Writings on catalepsy by the patients themselves are sparse. St. Theresa of Avila, however, who in the sixteenth century reformed the Carmelite Order, had more presence of mind in recalling the episodes that plagued her during her novitiate as a nun, which were seen by subsequent commentators as "hysterical" attacks:

In the night [of Assumption] there erupted such a terrible crisis that I remained almost four days without any feeling. I was given the Last Rites in this condition. . . . I felt that all my limbs were dislocated and perceived great dizziness in my head. . . . Without help, I was unable to move either the arm or the foot, neither the hand nor the head; I was so immobile as if death had frozen my limbs to ice; I had only the strength to move one finger of the right hand. . . . This condition lasted over eight months, and it took three years before I recovered from the paralysis.[17]

Yet even though few patients penned memoirs, the subject of catalepsy gripped the popular imagination. André De Lorde's 1901 play *La Dormeuse* (The Sleeper) featured a woman who'd been asleep for six years; it was apparently based on a case reported by Paris neurologist Georges Gilles de la Tourette (to whom De Lorde dedicates the play; De Lorde dramatized several psychiatric themes from the Salpêtrière, the great women's hospice in Paris). Madame goes to sleep, scarcely twitches for 6 years, and is fed by a physician who was intrigued by the case and has taken up residence nearby. Finally, she awakens, learns from a blabby servant that her two children are dead, and goes back to sleep.[18] The play, which opened at the Odéon Theater, was a critical success.

Catalepsy had many flavors, and one, known as "ecstasy"—a sturdy term meaning a variety of trances, visions, and the like—involved stupor and catatonic symptoms. In 1833, Joseph Guislain, the psychiatrist of the Ghent Asylum, said that, in ecstasy:

[The disorder] begins with immobility of the body. The patient is constantly seated on a chair, standing upright against a wall, or stretched out in his bed. From his immobility, his fixed gaze, one has the impression of a statue in a state of muscular rigidity. If one pinches his skin, the patient scarcely moves the affected part, or withdraws it only slowly. Movements of the arms are difficult, and all the muscles offer strong resistance to being moved. These patients may go for months without offering a single word; and whatever instructions you might give, the immobility of their features shows that they understand nothing at all.

Guislain said that a tenth of the patients at the Ghent Asylum were afflicted with ecstasy, and that 17 of 20 recovered.[19]

Stupor in catatonia does not necessarily mean a lowered level of consciousness, one step above coma. The patients may be fully alert, although unresponsive. We rocket forward momentarily in time to 1955, when Erwin Straus, an émigré psychiatrist from Berlin then at the Veterans Administration Hospital in Lexington, Kentucky, described stupor in his patients: "Catatonic stupor should not be interpreted as a sleep-like condition; the patient, though stuporous, is really alert. He keeps his eyes on the scene of events. While he permits a fly to crawl over his face without so much as twitching a muscle, he responds with a suppressed smile to some remark of a passerby. . . . His rigid gaze finally yields to excessive blinking."[20]

The authorities agreed that prognosis was good in catalepsy. Timothée Puel, who tabulated outcomes in the 150 cases in the literature from Galen to the 1850s, said "Catalepsy ends most commonly with the return to good health. . . . Prognosis in catalepsy is in general favorable."[21] We will shortly see Emil Kraepelin disagree.

DISORDERED MOVEMENT: STEREOTYPIES, MANNERISMS, TICS, AND CHOREA

A capital achievement of nineteenth-century psychiatry was the discovery of movement disorders, along with "madness," as a psychiatric symptom. Impoverished is a psychiatry that depends for information based solely on what patients say. Their movements tell part of the story, too. Michael Trimble, a noted English neuropsychiatrist, told the authors much later than the events described in this chapter, "I have been a considerable advocate for the reintroduction of movement into psychiatric understanding. And to understand the somatic-neuromuscular basis for all our expressions and the associations with psychopathology, it just became too simple to classify psychiatric disorders on what people said, not what they did." More learned that most, he went on confidently, "I'm sure you know your Goethe."

Trimble proceeded to quote in German some of the classic lines of poet and playwright Johann von Goethe's play *Faust* (1831). Faust says, of the Bible,

It's written here: "In the Beginning was the Word!"
Here I stick already! Who can help me? It's absurd,
Impossible, for me to rate the word so highly
I must try to say it differently.

. . . .

The Spirit helps me! I have it now, intact.
And firmly write: "In the Beginning was the Act!"[22]

In the beginning was movement. Classical Kraepelinian psychiatry of the late nineteenth century differentiated between stereotypies, or ceaselessly repeated movements, and mannerisms, or odd purposeful movements.[23] John Charles Bucknill, superintendent of the Devon County Lunatic Asylum and well-known medical editor, described in 1858 disordered movements that occur in mania but seem to be intrinsically catatonic: "Sometimes the head, or some other part of the body, is twitched convulsively; sometimes the hands are rubbed together perpetually, or the patient stands on one foot at a time, or in walking he slithers his feet, or he crouches or kneels, or indulges in some other bizarre movement."[24] Here, stereotypies and mannerisms converge.

Jean-Pierre Falret, chief psychiatrist at the Salpêtrière Hospice, in 1864 introduced the term *stéréotypés* to mental medicine (also written *stéréotypies*): "With some patients, words, gestures and actions, in a word all the phenomena of madness [*délire*], are *stéréotypés*, which means they are constantly repeated in exactly the same way and with the same characteristics."[25]

Tics are close enough to stereotypies to be synonymous. Paris psychiatrist Étienne Esquirol, the godparent of modern psychiatric classification, said in 1814 of patients with "dementia" (meaning cognitive disorders):

> Almost all the patients who fall into dementia have a tic or mania; some walk constantly, as though searching for something they haven't yet found; others move slowly in a labored pace; some pass days, even months or years, seated in the same spot, drawn up in bed, or stretched out on the floor; this one writes perpetually, but what he writes is disconnected, without meaning.... One person may persist in incomprehensible babble, repeating loudly the same expressions; another, ceaselessly moving his lips, offers in a very low voice a few poorly articulated sounds, or begins a phrase without ending it. This one speaks not at all; that one claps his hands day and night, while his neighbor rocks his body in a monotonous movement that is fatiguing even for the observer to look at.[26]

Thus, Esquirol describes practically the entire gamut of catatonic movement disorder as a "tic."[27]

Chorea, or jerky, involuntary, arrhythmic movements, might be seen by neurologists as Huntington chorea (a disorder centered in the caudate nucleus) or as Sydenham chorea (associated with a streptococcal infection). Indeed, some observers—such as Moriz Rosenthal, who taught neurology and psychiatry at the Vienna University—dismissed catalepsy in 1869 as just another form of "chorea magna," and, when it was not, thought it a kind of hysteria.[28] Yet choreiform movements may also resemble the motor disorders of catatonia. But caution here: the chorea of a modern neurologist may not be what Berlin professor Wilhelm Christoph Hufeland described in 1836 as chorea: "Movements that compel patients to the most extreme muscular exertions and contortions against their will, such as dancing for hours on end until falling over with exhaustion, spinning around on one leg, and forcefully flipping the body up in the air or across the room. There are also running attacks [*Laufkrampf*], where the feet simply run away with the patient, and he is obliged to run involuntarily for hours, until he falls over." Moreover, Hufeland noted that chorea could spread epidemically in crowds. But the patients, usually teenage females, tended to recover.[29]

Under the pen of David Skae in 1873, superintendent of the Royal Edinburgh Asylum, rheumatism might entail "rheumatic Insanity," in which delirious excitement would give way to "depression of mental condition, with suspiciousness, taciturnity, and languor." What is of interest, however, is Skae's account of the motor symptoms in this condition: "At the same time choreic movements of almost all the voluntary muscles in the body commence, and sometimes are so violent that the patient cannot remain still for a moment. His features are contorted, his head jerks from side to side, his limbs are thrown about, and his body is raised up and down."[30] This would be a description of alternation of agitation and stupor, stereotypies and grimacing. For years, catatonia in Edinburgh would be conceived as "rheumatic insanity."

OTHER SYMPTOMS OF MOVEMENT

Repetitive often nonsensical speech was a hallmark that Kahlbaum later called "verbigeration." In the context of catalepsy, Johann Christian Reil, professor of medicine in Halle, said in 1803, "I know a distinguished lady, who in an attack of mental disorder would say a single word, for example, 'my cousin' or 'Louis the Sixteenth,' continuously, for days, repeating it with great rapidity." Posturing was also present. "Then, when the catalepsy of the imagination had spread as well to the organs of movement, she would place herself for long periods in one spot in her room, like a statue, without changing the position of her body in the slightest."[31] Here, Reil is describing catatonic immobility or stupor together with verbigeration.

Many patients struck statue-like postures, maintaining them for days and months on end, the stereotypic movements frozen. "How does one know that mental illness [Seelenstörung] is about to strike?" asked Johann Baptiste Friedrich, an academic psychiatrist in Würzburg, in 1829. "The next thing is that there is senselessness and confusion of the ideas, manifest through senseless gestures, strange postures and positions of the body."[32]

The grimacing of catatonia has been distinctive enough to be seen as a separate symptom, even though it is part of the muscular cramps and spasms of the motor side of the disorder. As Joseph Guislain told medical students in 1852, "I'm going to present some subjects who execute without letup the most bizarre movements of the mouth, the tongue, and the face. I call these insane patients 'les grimaciers.'"[33] Among the patients who voiced their personal dramas, Guislain found four different kinds: "the orators, the declaimers, the monologists, the dialoguers."[34] Today, this kind of dramatization rarely finds a place on lists of "catatonic" symptoms, yet past physicians were well aware of it.

Rather than parceling out all the stereotypies, mannerisms, and cramps of the catatonic movement disorders, Guislain lumped them all together as "psychotic automatism" (l'automatisme fantastique). He thought it an antechamber to dementia.[35]

The theme of self-mutilation, today self-injurious behavior (SIB), was never far. At the Stéphansfeld asylum in Strasbourg, Henri Dagonet, the chief psychiatrist, described "Mlle Eugénie X," admitted in 1858 in a cataleptic state, who demonstrated a "repellent" negligence to grooming. "Saliva runs continually from her mouth, her hair is in disorder and her face has been lacerated by her nails." As she began to recover, the facial mutilation stopped.[36] This theme would be reactivated a century later as SIB observed in children with autism and intellectual disability (see Chapter 12).

STUPIDITÉ AND DEMENTIA

The terms catalepsy and stupor were often used synonymously. Yet, to be precise, catalepsy was a motor sign: the patient was immobile, and one could reposition his or her limbs. Even though many cataleptic patients also went into stupor, the focus in catalepsy was on movement and its blockage. Stupor was more a mental symptom and, over the years, was called by many names. In France, the term *stupidité* figured prominently. In 1759, for example, "*stupidité*" was among the first prodromes of a looming cataleptic illness in a shepherd lad, 17, who soon developed the staring, mutism, and other symptoms of catalepsy.[37] François Boissier de Sauvages, the Montpellier nosologist, mentioned it briefly in his *Nosologia Methodica* of 1763, and, in a dissertation for Göttingen University in 1764, Rudolph Augustin Vogel touched on "*Stupidität*" as part of his nosology, classifying it under the "*Paranoiae*."[38]

With Boissier's and Vogel's academic imprimatur, the term *stupidité* became widely used. In 1794, in his textbook, Vincenzo Chiarugi, who founded in Florence the first modern asylum, employed "*stupidità*" several times to mean "defective mentation" (*amenza defettiva [stupidità]*).[39]

Prompted by Esquirol in 1814, there was a vogue for calling catalepsy and stupor "dementia." In one of the earliest descriptions of young men and women with what was later called schizophrenia, Ésquirol qualified as "*démence aigüe,*" or acute dementia, the adolescents and young adults whom he was seeing in his private asylum and at the state asylum Charenton: they suddenly veered dramatically off course and deteriorated in cognitive terms. But some of them also had symptoms of catatonia. "PJD," 29, "spent the winter and part of the spring in these alternations of agitation and stupor." He had been discharged to the care of his family but returned two months later "in a state of complete stupor." "This is not a case of simple dementia," Esquirol noted, "because this patient, although apparently insensible to what was going on around him, was not deprived of intelligence. . . . I have seen a number of insane patients who, finding themselves in a similar state, were very dangerous, and it was necessary to supervise them closely, because, intermittently departing from their habitual torpor, they tried to commit the most dire acts."[40]

In 1820, Étienne-Jean Georget, 25, a staff psychiatrist at the Salpêtrière hospice, in his book *De la Folie* (On Madness), popularized the familiar term "*stupidité*" for the abolition of intellectual function in a previously well adult, "either because the patient doesn't have any ideas or cannot express them." Georget told the story of Adèle F, 36, who entered the psychiatric service of the Salpêtrière in 1817, "for the fifth time in ten years. . . . She had generalized insensibility; she was quite unresponsive to questions put to her; she didn't even seem to hear them, and remained in the place and the position she was put in [waxy flexibility]." She was quite insensitive to pain (and they inflicted on her some of the horrors of traditional medicine, such as inserting a "seton" under the skin of her neck to create pus).[41] Adèle recovered in three months' time, a straightforward case of what later generations would view as "stupor" but which Georget launched as a new diagnosis.

Mlle R's path to *stupidité* in the Salpêtrière, said Gustave-François Étoc-Demazy, in a Paris medical dissertation, began in 1831 when her fiancé jilted her. She had a "violent attack of rage . . . breaking furniture, tearing her clothes." She said that, "She was not the kind that a man could play with, that she was as good as a man and she will jolly well prove it. . . . This idea dominated her mind, and she proceeded to make the [gender] change, taking on the clothing of her new sex." In the Paris of the early 1830s, such transgendering would mean admission to the Salpêtrière. At admission, with a diagnosis of *stupidité*, "She was extremely weak, mute, seemed not to see nor hear. . . . She was incontinent of urine. . . . Her general sensory functions diminished with every passing day; needles stuck into different areas of her skin seemed to cause no pain. . . . She was immobile, her eyes fixed, dull, the iris without movement . . . . " But then improvement set in: "Her physiognomy lost its stupid aspect; her general sensory abilities returned." But she continued to believe that she was a man.[42]

Yet the worker who put *stupidité* on the map was not Georget, but the Parisian psychiatrist Jules Baillarger, a staff member of the psychiatry division of the Salpêtrière and co-founder in 1843 of the main French psychiatry journal the *Annales Médico-Psychologiques*.[43] In 1843, Baillarger dissertated on "*stupidité*," a stuporous disorder (with staring, waxy rigidity, and so forth), yet in which the stupor resembled more a dream-like state that he considered part of melancholia than suspension of thought. Contrary to Georget and other authors, he said, "I have seen no patient in whom intelligence has been suspended."[44]

The *stupidité* vogue in France reached its acme in 1851, with Louis Delasiauve at the Bicêtre, who said that the disorder was a disease of its own involving a suspension of thought.[45] Thus, *stupidité* was the diagnosis that leapt to mind when "D," a laborer, 23, was admitted in April 1852 to the Asile Saint-Pierre of Marseille. Frightened by a mugging, he had fallen silent at home, failed to answer his mother's questions, and, on admission to the asylum, had stopped eating. D's state worsened. He continued to refuse food, taking on a haggard appearance. He was incontinent of urine and stool. He became insensitive to pain and seemed not to hear, see, or feel anything. By July, D's physical recovery was well under way, yet he remained mute for months to come. "The case confirms our view," said his clinician, Jehan-Victor-Alfred Sauze, "of the psychological nature of *stupidité*. One cannot in good faith consider it to be a variety of *lypémanie* [depression]. It is rather a more or less complete suspension of the intellectual facilities."[46]

Outside of France, *stupidité* struggled on a while longer. In the hands of American psychiatrists, *stupidité* became "amentia," "the most abject state of mental imbecility," said Pliny Earle of the Friends' (Quaker) Asylum in Frankford, Pennsylvania, in 1841. He was describing stupor. "Many patients in this state remain motionless, perchance, during the day, their eyes fixed upon the ground, as if unconscious of the things or persons around them, or even of their own existence. They would not retire to bed nor rise were they not forced to do it by their attendants."[47]

Georget's *stupidité* turned into "acute dementia" at the West Riding Lunatic Asylum in Yorkshire, England. "Acute or primary [dementia] has also been called apathetic dementia," said James Crichton-Browne, superintendent, "an allusion to the complete torpor of feeling by which it is marked, and the same mental condition is described by Georget as *stupidité*." In addition to stuporous retardation, Crichton described echo phenomena: "The patient will slowly repeat any question that is asked of him. . . . He never attempts to answer the question, he simply echoes it. Occasionally he will feebly echo any sound that he may hear, or will clumsily reproduce any gesture that he may witness." Crichton described "automatic crises," "certain automatic muscular movements that are sometimes seen in cases of this kind. . . . Thus if the patient is made to run, he will run on, when left to himself, steadily and rhythmically, until he is stopped by some obstacle."[48]

In Germany, Friedrich Hoffmann, superintendent of the Siegburg Asylum near Bonn, deemed "*Stupidität*" in 1862 "one of the most important forms of serious psychiatric illness [the *Vesanie*] because, more than the others, it points to material changes in the brain and demands an active therapy."[49] German brides went into *Stupidität* on their wedding nights! Yet *Stupidität* would soon vanish from German psychiatry as well. (It goes unmentioned in the first edition of Emil Kraepelin's famous 1883 textbook.)[50]

Of interest is Crichton's description of the alternation of "profound stupidity" and bursts of excitement: "There are sharp but transient attacks, displayed in restlessness, incoherence, mischief, and destructive violence. . . . It subsides in a few days, and gives place again to dullness and passivity." The moments of stupidity, on the other hand, were better described as "complete lethargy." "The patient will sit or stand for hours in one position, lacking spontaneity to change it. . . . He is as inane and helpless as a statue. And now it is that a species of catalepsy is observed. The limbs remain for a time in any position in which they may be placed. . . . If the arms be raised above the head they will be held there for perhaps an hour." Yet the muscles, said Crichton, were not rigid. "The limbs are flaccid and are readily flexed and extended."[51] Here, Crichton has described almost the full range of catatonic phenomena—including stereotypies, echoing, and the alternation of stupor and agitation—and his accounts of the patients' toileting and eating would amount as well to negativism. The year was 1874. Here, the essential point is that under such terms as "*stupidité*" and "stupor" the world of psychiatry was struggling slowly toward the concept that Kahlbaum unified in 1874 as "catatonia."[52]

NEGATIVISM

Negativism may be defined as doing exactly the opposite of what one is told, or expected, to do. It involves direct disobedience of staff; it may incorporate such antisocial behavior as retaining one's feces and then letting go in bed; at the motor level, it entails resisting efforts to reposition one's limbs (the resistance is called *gegenhalten*).

Negativism was long known, though not under that name. Guislain described it in 1833 as "*l'humeur contrariante*" (contrary disposition):

Not wishing to conform with the wishes of others, the patients affected with delusional egoism [*"l'egoïsme fantastique"*] are opposed to everything; they do not want, they do not desire anything that someone else wants them to do. Such a patient refuses to remain in the bed assigned to him, and stays standing all night, or seated, or stretched out on the floor. If you give in to his wishes, then he no longer wants to leave the bed assigned to him; you bring him his dinner, and he objects to consuming it;

doesn't want tea, doesn't want coffee when it's offered. He stubbornly stays out in the cold and doesn't want to put on warm clothing; he likes to run around bare-headed; in summer, he stations himself in the boiling sun and puts on warm clothes.[53]

Kraepelin considered negativism the single most important symptom of cata-tonia: "compulsive, purely passive resistance."[54] Such patients refused all food, all or-ders and suggestions, all efforts to make the patient compliant with the staff or with fellow patients. Negativism also included resisting attempts to reposition a limb, mutism, and proper toileting (including a positive pleasure in soiling the bedding). As Guislain told medical students in 1852, "Certain insane patients put up an opposition that you cannot imagine if you have not seen it close up. To the maximum, they resist efforts to change their bedding. They refuse to lie down in their bed and spread out on the floor, on the tiles. They don't want to wash themselves. They go out bareheaded in a driving rain [a no-no in the medical lights of the day]. They oppose doing everything one asks them to do. . . . It is the madness of opposition [la folie d'opposition]." [55]

The madness of opposition was a mental, not a motor symptom, one of the few mental symptoms in catatonia. But that these authorities made it more or less the core symptom tells us that, in catatonia, much more is involved than disorders of movement.

MADNESS

Today, many authors report the majority of catatonic patients to be psychotic.[56] Catatonia is no longer considered a subtype of schizophrenia, yet some of the patients historically did anticipate what would later be called "dementia praecox" and, after 1908, "schizophrenia." English psychiatrist William Perfect, of Westmalling in Kent, saw "a young gentleman of family and fortune" who in 1777 had contracted an unnamed disorder and was treated with the full therapeutic palette of the day, which included the liberal ingestion of mercury. Whether from the mercury (as Perfect believed) or for other reasons, by the time the fellow reached Perfect, he had "sunk into a state of torpid insensibility, and must have perished for want of food, had he not been nursed and fed with the same care as is shewn to a baby; he often slavered from his mouth, stood like a statue with his eyes immovably riveted to the ground, and could not easily be roused." What is of interest, aside from the young man's catalepsy, is that he was mute, a cardinal symptom of catatonia. Within a few months, Perfect "was just able, by repeated interrogations now and then, to extract from him a word or two, by way of answer." And now, said Perfect a decade later in 1787, "he still continues pretty nearly in the same state," except that he was able to feed himself and walk about. The lad had, in other words, undergone an apparently terminal decline: "From being a sensible, accomplished and well-educated young man, of a lively imagination and the most acute and promising parts . . . he is now reduced to a melancholy spectacle of half-animated human existence, nor has he the most forlorn hope of ever again being capable of tolerably well fulfilling the ordinary duties of life."[57] This account matches closely the later descriptions of decline and disorder in young men and women who received the diagnoses of "dementia praecox" and "schizophrenia."

Some of these young patients, with their mix of catatonic symptoms and in-sanity, would have been poster-perfect for Emil Kraepelin writing decades later about "dementia praecox." At the Maréville asylum in eastern France in the early 1850s, Morel saw a young woman, 18, who, in addition to depression, "had some strange tics. Her stupid attitude was increased by her stubbornness in widening her eyes and in arching her eyebrows. . . . She stays immobile in a corner, adopts cataleptic poses and is incontinent of feces." When staff were finally able to motivate her to undertake some activity, "her style of walking resembles very closely that of certain spring-powered dolls [*certains automates mus par un ressort*]. This patient has been here for three years and all of our efforts have not been able to prevent her transition to imbecility."[58]

A young man, 20, was admitted to the Oldenburg asylum at Wehnen in 1862:

> His restlessness increases so greatly, that he has to be transferred to the agitated ward, where he dirties his bed, stuffs his socks into the toilet. He shows flight of ideas; the patient speaks of a woman whom he has shot, repeats the words, *"Schuss, Nuss, Nuss, Nuss"* [shot, nut, nut, nut]. He tears up his clothes, eats little, is restless in sleep. Sometimes he sings, rhymes and is very voluble. After two months, this condition of agitation passed into depression: The patient becomes silent, dreamy, his movements are slow, he cannot be motivated to tasks, answers only after repeated questioning, and then very slowly; demonstrates a complete lack of interest in everything.[59]

This sounds like catatonia overlaid on psychotic manic-depressive illness (the imagined murder).

ALTERNATION

On July 24, 1803, a 26-year-old woman was sitting of an afternoon in her chair happily sewing. Her previous life had been entirely normal aside from the occasional headache. Her husband was said to love her, her children were growing strong, the family was economically well situated. "Suddenly," said a local doctor, "and without the slightest occasion, she leapt up and cried, 'I must drown myself, I must drown myself.' She ran down to the moat of the town, not far from her home, and without hesitation plunged into it. She was immediately retrieved from the water, to all appearances dead, and carried back to her house. A doctor was quickly called who restored her to life, but she remained mute, with staring eyes fixed on a point in front of her, paying no attention to what was going on around her." The physician who gave us this account in 1821 saw her three days later. In the meantime, she had not spoken a word, nor eaten nor drunk anything; she had not slept, nor had she demonstrated interest in anything. "As I came to her in the evening, she lay in bed sighing continuously. At my greeting she seemed totally shocked and called out my name. Light was brought, and as she saw me, she asked, 'My God, where am I, and what has happened to me?' She began sobbing heavily." After ascertaining that her family was well, she fell asleep soundly and awakened cheerfully the following morning.[60] The patient clearly had an episode of delirious agitation, followed by an episode of stupor. Of interest is that one followed the other immediately. They alternated.

In one of the earliest descriptions of the apparent alternation of stupor and agitation, in 1818, Esquirol—in an essay on a very broadly conceived notion of "mania"—said, "[There are patients] who fall into a profound stupor, seemingly deprived of all sensation, of all thought. They are motionless, they remain however one poses them, it's necessary to clothe them, hand-feed them; their facial features are tensed.... Suddenly mania erupts with all of its delirium, with all of its agitation."[61] If one substitutes agitation for "mania" in this account, one has a description of alternation in catalepsy. "It happens," said Louis Calmeil in 1839, at the time a public health official in psychiatry, "that a state of profound *stupidité* suddenly gives way to paroxysms of manic delirium and fury."[62]

Thus, many authorities were struck not just by individual symptoms such as muteness, but by *patterns* of symptoms. One pattern was the alternation of agitation with stupor, something that occurs in no other form of psychiatric illness and is virtually pathognomonic for catatonia.

Other patterns of alternation occur in catatonia. Tonic rigidity of the muscles may alternate with clonus (cramps). As Robert Whyte, among the founders of neurophysiology, noted in Edinburgh in 1765, "Of all the nervous or spasmodic disorders, there is none more surprising than the catalepsis, or stupor vigilans.... In this the patient becomes either wholly, or in great measure, insensible of what is doing about him, and remains exactly in the same posture in which he was first seized. His joints are sometimes so stiff, that they can scarcely be bent, or, if they are, they remain in whatever situation they are placed." And then he commented on what was for him (and remains for us) a scientific puzzle: "All we know is that whatever irritates, or disagreeably affects the brain, nerves, or any of the more sensible parts, occasions continued spasms or convulsive motions ... and that, when the nervous system is delicate, or the irritation great, almost all the muscles will be sometimes agitated with alternate contractions, or affected with tetanus or general rigidity."[63]

Thus, it is not just the occurrence of stupor and agitation but their alternation that forms a steady theme in catatonia. In 1853, Morel commented,

> We observe some patients who are not imbeciles nor idiots but for the most part individuals with limited intelligence and in whom the development of psychological sensitivity has never really occurred. They may spend weeks or months, gloomy and silent, having no initiative and apparently bereft of any intellectual activity. Then it happens that at periodic intervals they suddenly leap out of this state and precipitate themselves upon those around, striking, tearing, biting. Some are motivated to these acts by exterior events. Others find in their own pathological disposition the making of an agitation so powerful as to bring them to commit the most dangerous acts imaginable.[64]

For Louis Delasiauve at Bicêtre, the men's hospice, writing a year later in 1854, this alternation supplied a dramatic counterpoint: "In a word, on one side, violent agitation, frightening, irresistible; on the other, more or less complete immobility, a rigidity that one might almost call cadaveric: The contrast could not be more clearly delineated nor more striking."[65] On another occasion Delasiauve commented on patients in "*stupidité*" (stupor), "A number of them pass frequently from torpor to a violent manic delirium."[66]

These nineteenth-century alienists considered alternation a part of the clinical picture in catalepsy—later in catatonia—and one of the mysteries of this story is how this evident clinical pattern was lost from view. (We revisit this subject in Chapter 10.)

IS CATALEPTIC (CATATONIC) STUPOR DIFFERENT
FROM DEPRESSIVE (MELANCHOLIC) STUPOR?

A big question today in neuroscience is the overlap between catatonia and melancholic depression: Both have stupor as a main symptom. Both respond to convulsive theray.[67] Do they share a common neurophysiological substrate?

Clinicians in the past were more intent upon separating catatonia and melancholia than in finding common ground. In 1778, Viennese physician Leopold Auenbrugger—who is remembered for describing percussion as a diagnostic technique in 1761—was called to the bedside of a well-to-do woman, 40, whose husband had just been imprisoned; she had fallen into "such a melancholia that she was left unmoved by all attempted performances and amusements." She lay rigidly in bed, and Auenbrugger was unable to obtain any utterance from her. Her friends told him she had been in this state for several days, refusing to take even "a drop of water." Auenbrugger diagnosed severe melancholia at great risk of suicide. The patient obligingly consumed a complicated prescription that Auenbrugger ordered but remained "depressed, mute and continually disinclined to look at other people." The next day, "she sat quite motionless on her sofa. That night she was put to bed, midst heavy sighing and sobbing, and seemed not to sleep at all." She developed a fever. Thereupon, she cunningly took advantage of the temporary absence of one of her servants (two others assigned to her were asleep) to quietly steal from the drawer a dull knife and slit her throat, thus committing suicide.[68] The evidence is incontrovertible that this well-situated lady had a melancholic depression. Rigid, mute, negativistic, and suddenly febrile, did she also have catatonia?

Morel in his various writings had a good deal to say about catalepsy and *stupidité*. Yet, in discussing serious depression (*lypémanie*), his thoughts were so fixed on mood that he missed an abundance of cataleptic symptoms. A lypemaniac, he said in 1851, "might adopt the most bizarre and fatiguing postures, repeat ceaselessly the most painful acts. . . . One of our patients spends hours on end jumping up and down on one leg from his bench to the ground, jumps about some more, then interrupts these monotonous exercises by kneeling and kissing the ground. Some run rapidly, suddenly stop, seem to reflect, their index finger resting on their lips or brow, then start up running again." [69] A catatonic overlay on depression, or just catatonia?

In his 1861 textbook, which included much biological psychiatry in the nineteenth century, Zurich psychiatry professor Wilhelm Griesinger, shortly bound for Berlin, said that "Melancholia with hebetude" (*Stumpfsinn*) was a form of depressive illness. Yet patients often, in addition to deep sadness and anxiety, were characterized as follows, "They are entirely mute, completely inactive, almost immobile without a powerful stimulus; their appearance is stupid; their facial expression one of a generally deep psychic oppression. . . . They have cutaneous sensory anesthesia as well." And motor symptoms: "The voluntary muscles are sometimes rigid, sometimes flaccid; it is not unusual that complete cataleptic pictures appear, retaining a given position, and many observations about catalepsy, in fact belong to this [melancholic] illness. Invariably, the will greatly reduces the mobility of the limbs, sometimes almost abolishing it. There is a kind of blocking of the entire motor side of cerebral processing."

When interrogated later, continued Griesinger, "the patient is often unable to say why he was incapable of the least volitional act, why he didn't answer, not even cry out."[70] What is Griesinger describing? Severe depression, severe catatonia, or a mixture?

A whole nineteenth-century literature argues this differentiation. In 1867, Henry Maudsley, a psychiatrist at the West London Hospital and later benefactor of the Maudsley Hospital, commented on the atonic form of melancholia as "melancholia with stupor . . . where the mind is entirely possessed with some terrible delusion, the patient sits or stands like a statue, and must be moved from place to place; the muscles are generally lax, or some of them are fixed in a cataleptic rigidity; the patient, as if in a trance or as one only partially awake, scarcely seems to see or hear; consciousness of time, place, and person is lost; and the bodily wants and necessities are alike unheeded."[71] As with Griesinger, is Maudsley describing psychotic depression, melancholic depression with a catatonic overlay, or catatonia?

A most thoughtful differentiation of melancholic stupor from catatonic stupor was written in 1886, by Heinrich Schüle, the last great representative of asylum psychiatry. Schüle said that what differentiated an "organic" (catatonic) stupor from the "psychically motivated inhibition" of melancholia was: (1) in organic stupor, acute onset, as opposed to "the gradual development from the melancholia"; (2) in organic stupor, a "stupid, flaccid facial mask with half-opened mouth and usually profuse salivation," opposed to "being rigid and anxious, with features distorted with pain" of melancholia; (3) in organic stupor, incapacity to take food because of dementia and lack of will, in melancholia deliberate refusal of food from delusive beliefs; (4) in organic stupor, cutaneous anesthesia, in melancholia, "the silent toleration of correctly perceived pain from melancholic feelings of guilt"; (5) in organic stupor, no memory of "the time of the actual vacuity of consciousness," in melancholia "painfully exact recollection of a time that flooded consciousness with threatening horrors."[72] Subsequent observers might disagree with the contents of this list as patients in catatonic stupor seem to have experienced plenty of terror and fear of their own (see Chapter 7). Yet Schüle's list shows that contemporary clinicians were indeed mindful of the difference between melancholia and catatonia.[73]

APPARENT DEATH

Early in the eighteenth century, a drama transpired in the Rue St. Honoré in Paris. A local merchant had promised his daughter to a young man, also a merchant in the same street. A wealthy financier appeared on the scene and won permission to marry the daughter. She, however, apparently resisted and "fell sick and was held for dead, enshrouded, and buried. But the first suitor suspected that she had fallen into lethargy or syncope [catalepsy], and disinterred her body that night. Physicians revived her and he married her." The Benedictine monk who gave us this account in 1746 concluded with a paean to medical science and scorned the superstitious of the day with their beliefs in "demons and spirits": "Persons who have . . . fallen into syncope, into lethargy or ecstasy, or held for dead in whatever manner, may be cured and brought back to life, to their normal routines, to their original health without any miracle."[74] Apparent death, often of a catatonic nature, was thus a familiar problem.

On July 10, 1730, in London, Ann Bullard, a servant, 21, "very much afflicted for the loss of a friend," complained of a headache and upset stomach. "Next morning, July 11, about 9," said Richard Reynell, an "apothecary" (the equivalent of a family doctor), "she was found in bed, senseless, stiff, and void of feeling, with her eyes shut; and upon the first surprise, it was thought she was dead. When I came," continued Reynell, "I found her in a true cataleptic fit, senseless, without motion, her limbs very stiff, but warm, and not easy to be bent; but in whatever posture any limb was put, it continued in the same."[75] Catalepsy had been long known, but of interest here is that she was considered dead. This was the most dramatic form of catatonic stupor: apparent death, called "lethargy," "*Schlafsucht*," or "trance."

The late sixteenth-century statesman and philosopher Francis Bacon related similar stories. "There have been many instances of men who have been left for dead, laid out, and carried forth to burial; nay, of some who have been actually buried; that have yet come to life again. In the case of those who have been buried, this has been ascertained, on opening the grave, from the wounded and bruised states of the head, by reason of the body striving and tossing in the coffin. The most recent and memorable instance thereof was the subtle schoolmaster Duns Scotus, who having been buried in the absence of his servant (who appears to have known the symptoms of these fits), was by him afterwards disinterred and found in this state."[76]

How to tell if they were dead or just cataleptic? One physician suggested that in death, waxy rigidity disappears. You can hold up the arm, and it falls back down.[77] In 1724, London physician John Maubray confronted this same question: how to "distinguish a patient in the extreme fit of this [hysteric] passion [stupor], from a person actually dead: such as lint, feathers, or burnt paper being held to the mouth; if moved, the patient breathes. A glass of water being set upon the breast. . . . Or, a looking-glass well wiped, being held to their mouths; if infected, the patient is still and certainly alive." However, there was one test, he said, that was infallible: "When the body begins to send forth a cadaverous odor."[78] The point is interesting because it shows how unaccustomed these physicians were to actually touching their patients.[79]

Among the people there was a fixation about mistakenly being buried alive because a physician had confused stupor with death. This confusion could betray the most skillful practitioner. In Vienna, in 1821, George Pfendler was called to the bedside of a 15-year-old girl, who had had a long string of catatonic incidents such as tetanic rigidity and inability to swallow; this time, she went into a stupor. In the stupor, she approached death, and, in one terminal moment, she was able to rouse herself sufficiently to embrace Dr. Pfendler to say goodbye, then collapsed back in bed, "as though stricken by death." There she lay motionless for 28 hours, without apparent respiration (the stethoscope had not yet reached Vienna), or evident movement. Her body was believed to give off the odor of putrefaction. The Viennese clinician Johann-Peter Frank was called to the bedside and judged her dead. The death knell was sounded. Her girlfriends came to clothe her in white for burial and to place a crown of flowers upon her head. "To convince myself of the progress of the putrefaction," said Pfendler, "I returned to the bedroom, but the odor was not more advanced than previously; to the contrary, how great was my surprise when I thought I detected a small movement of respiration! I observed her more closely, and I saw that I was not mistaken." Pfendler began a frenzied bout of rubbing, medications, and so forth, and "she recovered consciousness and smiled at me, 'I am too young to die.' "[80]

Another young Viennese woman with catalepsy, Rachel N, 28, actually was buried alive. Her "lethargy," or profound sleep, had extended off and on for several months. But in her most recent attack, which lasted several days, "she was declared dead: After her burial the gravedigger, wishing to purloin her gown, opened the coffin at night; but during this operation, she suddenly returned to life. The gravedigger, horrified, wanted to flee. Rachel called to him and told him to take her to the physician who had looked after her. The latter informed the husband of the resurrection of his wife. . . . She is called *la belle Juive ressuscitée* [the beautiful Jewess brought back to life]."[81]

When Michel-Augustin Thouret, Dean of the Faculty of Medicine in Paris, supervised the exhumations of the graves in the cemetery of the Innocent Saints in the 1780s, he was surprised to see in some of the coffins "bones in a position indicating that the unfortunates, buried too precipitously, had returned to life." Alarmed, Thouret is said to have indicated specifically in his will that measures be taken to avert a similar fate for him.[82]

Clinicians in the early nineteenth century were not unmindful of this risk. "Some cataleptics have been taken for cadavers and buried alive," said Louis Calmeil in 1834. "In very severe attacks, respiration and circulation are imperceptible, the body is almost cold, the skin has taken on the pallor of death, the joints are stiff." How could one avoid being buried alive? Calmeil gave a kind of textual shrug: maybe something in "the expression of the physiognomy" would be revealing.[83]

Very reassuring. As late as 1900, a young Parisian woman, 18 at the time, began her career of anxiety with "the obsessive idea that she could be buried alive."[84]

Lethargy was a Snow White syndrome that would later merge into stupor; the danger of being buried alive faded with the diffusion of the stethoscope and clinical thermometer (if there were any doubt: the body cools in death). Yet not all the Snow Whites were young females. In 1833, John Conolly, at the time the inspecting physician of the county asylums in Warwick (he was later famous for introducing the "no-restraint" system), told the story of Lady Russell—evidently the grandmother of his friend Lord John Russell—who had died. "[Her] funeral having been postponed for a longer period than usual, afforded time for her happy recovery, which took place while the bells were ringing for prayers; the supposed dead person exclaiming that it was time to go to church." Conolly considered such cases evidence of "hysteria."[85]

Folkloric beliefs about trances and stupors are held worldwide. Folklorist J. A. Macculloch wrote in 1971, "Among the Bantu peoples of South Africa it is firmly believed that wizards and doctors can send people into a trance and then torment or mutilate them without their feeling any pain." There were, in other cultures, said to be "wizards who reduce people's wills to a state of abject slavery, and send men into the forest to eat grass, and in other ways show their mastery over them."[86] In Europe, apparent-death phenomena were adjacent to the issue of "episodic hypersomnia," or patients who sleep for extended periods of time, known also as Kleine-Levin syndrome.[87] These are the Snow White tales of yore, and they must have had a popular experiential root to become the gist of fairy tales. A female patient with the diagnosis "lethargy" at the Salpêtrière is said to have "slept," at intervals from a month to a year, off and on for more than 20 years; she was fed by a nasogastric tube.[88] This *belle-au-bois* (the French version of Snow White) story comes from that psycho-circus of suggestion at the Salpêtrière under Charcot, yet there are other "*dormeuse*" stories as well of a possibly catatonic-stuporous nature.

Almost all the phenomena that Kahlbaum drew together in 1874 under the term "catatonia" had long traditions of medical and folkloric description. But with the exception of Heinrich Schüle's perceptive essay in 1867 (see earlier discussion), people believed they were separate, discrete phenomena, conditions as disparate as mumps and tuberculosis. Kahlbaum's genius was to see all this as a single disorder.

3

KARL KAHLBAUM

The voyage of discovery lies not in seeking new horizons, but in seeing with new eyes.
—Marcel Proust[1]

Next to Emil Kraepelin, Karl Kahlbaum is arguably the second most towering psychiatrist in late nineteenth-century central Europe, then the world epicenter of psychiatry. Even though it was Kraepelin who originated the modern classification of diseases, it was Kahlbaum who, in 1863, conceived a clinical science in psychiatry. Catatonia came 11 years later, in 1874. "Clinical science" is a concept with which psychiatry, beset with waves of faddishness, has struggled ever since. It means knowledge gained at the bedside rather than in the "laboratory," and, even today, the field—beset with drug company marketing, faddish novelties, and emphasis on scales rather than observations—finds the concept of clinical science difficult.

Kahlbaum was born in 1828—of humble origins, his father was a coachman—in the small town of Driesen (Drezdenko), then in German Pomerania, now in Poland. He gained his MD degree in 1854, from the University of Berlin, and, two years later, in 1856 accepted a post as assistant psychiatrist in the East Prussian provincial asylum of Allenberg.[2] Kahlbaum was drawn to clinical science. His careful case notes are models of the genre. He lived at the asylum, came to know the patients well, and, in 1863, submitted his postdoctoral thesis (*Habilitation*) to Königsberg University, in the capital of East Prussia. (The German system is characterized by two doctoral theses: the basic dissertation [which Kahlbaum wrote on mammalian anatomy] and the much more ambitious Habilitation, acceptance of which is necessary if one wishes to teach at a university.) In 1863, Kahlbaum began lecturing on psychiatry at Königsberg and, in these lectures, in 1866, made the first mention of catatonia.[3]

DIE GRUPPIRUNG, 1863

His 1863 Habilitation, entitled *Die Gruppirung der psychischen Krankheiten und die Eintheilung der Seelenstörungen* (The Grouping of Psychiatric Diseases and the Classification of Disturbances of the Mind)[4] is a key document of the new psychiatry that was just emerging from the moralizing, speculative bog of previous generations of writers. It laid out a rational classification of diseases of the mind, classified by course and outcome, not on the basis of the current clinical picture. Impatient with the riot of older terms for psychiatric afflictions, Kahlbaum coined a number of neologisms in his new classification. Medicine is highly resistant to neologisms, especially from 35-year-old junior clinicians, and the new classification did not catch on.

Diseases arising from a "biological" development he called "paraphrenias," among which most notably was "hebephrenia," a subclass of "paraphrenia hebetica," arising in puberty. Diseases with a chronic course that changed in character over time were called "vesanias," an old term for madness, and diseases that did not change in character and seemed less chronic were called "vecordias."[5]

Among the dysthymic (mood) vecordias were the familiar *melancholia attonita*, meaning stupor, and *dysthymia maläna*, or melancholic depression. Another vecordia was *dysthymia elata*, or euphoric mania. And there were the paranoid vecordias, with various subcategories.

Finally came the more serious diseases, the "vesanias," the modern use of a term going back to the Swedish classifier Carolus Linnaeus in 1759.[6] At the core of the entire system were the "vesania typicas," which later would be called schizophrenia. The vesanias came with and without accompanying mood disorders (the former would anticipate psychotic depression).

Kahlbaum was highly mindful of neurosyphilis, called "progressive paralysis," because the asylums were full of dying patients with this invariably fatal disease. He made "vesania progressiva," which included mainly neurosyphilis, one of the subclasses of general vesanias; he made the other big vesania, "vesania typica," another stage-like illness that became the template for catatonia.

The four stages of vesania typica were melancholia, mania, confusion, and dementia. These stages were, at the time, entirely conventional in psychiatry. The notion that psychiatric illness progressed through stages had been introduced in the Francophone world by Joseph Guislain in 1833 as "morbid intellectual associations"[7] and in the German-speaking world by Ernst Albert Zeller, superintendent of the Winnenthal Asylum in southwest Germany, in 1844. The stage concept was developed more fully by Zeller's student Wilhelm Griesinger in a psychiatric textbook that appeared in 1845.[8] (Contemporaries often used the term "cyclical," which implies to modern ears "up-and-down," as in manic-depression. But Kahlbaum's catatonia, as Kahlbaum defined it, progressed in a straight line forward, hence in "stages.") So we now find Kahlbaum applying his predecessors' concepts of staging to core insanity and envisioning staging in which categories of illnesses—the vesanias—changed their clinical pictures, or stages, throughout the course of the illness.

The term "catatonia" does not appear in *Die Gruppirung*. The importance of this text lies in Kahlbaum being the first clinician to differentiate the momentary clinical picture—how the patient appeared at that point in time—from the underlying progressive disease. The shift from symptoms to diseases was a capital one for psychiatry, and it begins with Kahlbaum in 1863.

GÖRLITZ

Increasingly frustrated by the fussy narrow-mindedness of Allenberg Superintendent Carl Reinhold Bernhardi and the refusal of the Königsberg faculty to grant him academic status, Kahlbaum accepted Hermann Reimer's offer in 1866 to become an associate physician at Reimer's private nervous clinic in Görlitz, on the banks of the Neisse River (now on the Polish border). Reimer had founded the facility in 1855 for the treatment of patients with epilepsy. When they proved too few in number, he repositioned it as a private hospital for nervous diseases. In 1867, Kahlbaum bought the Görlitz clinic from Reimer and proceeded to greatly enlarge it. It must have been at some point in the transition from *Die Gruppirung* to getting to know the nervous patients at Görlitz that the importance of motor symptoms dawned on Kahlbaum.

At a meeting of the psychiatric section of the Natural Scientists' Society at Innsbruck in September 1869, Kahlbaum first publicly aired his new concept of catatonia, reporting "two cases of so-called melancholia attonita, complicated with great muscular tension, constructing on this basis a new disease entity of 'tension insanity' [*das Spannungsirresein*]." In the following discussion, the participants were little inclined to expand the nomenclature of psychiatry in this manner.[9] Another journal reported that Kahlbaum had presented "a special form of insanity that arises from other forms, and which manifests itself early in motor phenomena with tension; paralyses are not observed."[10]

The tension insanity concept began to circulate. In March 1872, Kahlbaum gave a brief talk at the meeting of the German Psychiatric Society in Berlin "on the clinical disease, Tension Insanity or Catatonia." (This marks the second time that the term "catatonia" had been used in public; the first time was in Hecker's two articles in 1871.) Hermann Reimer, the former owner of the Görlitz clinic, stood up to pooh-pooh catatonia as nothing more than melancholia attonita. Kahlbaum responded strongly. "The muscular symptoms that catatonia patients show, in combination with their singular patterns of speech and the prognostic significance of this disease, thoroughly justify giving it a special name."[11]

The dueling continued. In August 1872, Rudolph Gottfried Arndt, who had just accepted a lectureship in psychiatry at Greifswald University, presented at a Leipzig meeting of the psychiatric section of the Natural Scientists, the same group where Kahlbaum had held forth in 1869, his ideas about "tetany" (severe muscular twitching and cramping) as a motor disturbance in psychiatry. Thereupon, young Ewald Hecker, an associate of Kahlbaum at Görlitz, stood up and said there was nothing new about Arndt's ideas and that such tension was part of Kahlbaum's "Katatonie," the disease that Kahlbaum had introduced at Innsbruck and that would be the object of a forthcoming book. Hecker's intervention led to a furious back-and-forth between him and Arndt.[12]

HECKER'S HEBEPHRENIA, 1871

It is actually quite extraordinary that two of the major diseases in psychiatry—hebephrenia (which is core schizophrenia) and catatonia—should have been described within three years of each other by two obscure physicians in a private clinic with no academic affiliation in eastern Germany.

Ewald Hecker was born in 1843, 15 years after Kahlbaum, in Halle, Saxony, his father a municipal official. He graduated with an MD in 1866 from Königsberg University and took up a trainee post at Allenberg, where he met Kahlbaum. As Hecker's biographer Karl Wilmanns, a Heidelberg chief, later put it, "Between the serious, mature Kahlbaum, who already was standing on firm scientific ground, and the younger Hecker, who radiated fresh energy and thirst for knowledge . . . there soon developed a close relationship resting on personal affinity and common interests, a relationship that would be important for the development of psychiatry."[13]

In 1866, Kahlbaum had accepted Reimer's invitation to come to Görlitz, and the following year, 1867, Hecker followed him. In 1871, Kahlbaum made Hecker an astonishing scientific gift, letting him write up a new disease that Kahlbaum had adumbrated in his *Gruppirung* in 1863. The disease was hebephrenia, and it became known, naturally, as "Hecker's hebephrenia." Why Kahlbaum would proffer such great scientific generosity is explicable only in the fact that the two men had become quasi-relatives: in 1868, Kahlbaum married Hecker's aunt, and, in 1871, Hecker married a friend of Kahlbaum's wife.[14] Neither man lost sight of Hecker's intellectual indebtedness. Kahlbaum later noted that Hecker's work was based "upon my material and my ideas."[15] And Hecker, in his obituary of Kahlbaum in 1899, readily acknowledged that "[Kahlbaum] left the describing of hebephrenia to me."[16]

In his 1871 article, Hecker said that "Kahlbaum first pointed out in his lectures that hebephrenia unfolded in stages," like the stages of neurosyphilis. It began in the pubertal years and occurred "in connection with the great transformation of physical and mental development of these years." Of the 14 cases that Hecker himself had seen in Allenberg and Görlitz, in addition to the other cases that Kahlbaum had placed at his disposition, the common denominator was "the quick transition to dementia [*Blödsinn*]." True to stage theory, Hecker maintained that these cases began as melancholia, then turned into mania, transitioning to full psychosis in such forms as "Kahlbaum's confabulation," or as major delusional systems, and thence to dementia. As with neurosyphilis, there was great variability in the clinical picture at any given moment. But, said Hecker, "The invariable distinctiveness of the course, and above all the early onset and the later dementia—which it is impossible to overlook—circumscribe with confidence [this disease entity]."

How was hebephrenia different from Kahlbaum's catatonia? Hecker said that in catatonia there was no quick transition to dementia. "In all the cases [of hebephrenia] that I have seen, feeble-mindedness usually sets in within the first three months and at the latest (very rarely) a year."[17]

What Hecker did, that Kahlbaum had previously neglected, was to present six careful case histories. In *Gruppirung*, there are no case histories, and the text, unconvincingly to the medical mind of the day, spills forth one bright idea after another. Hecker nailed hebephrenia with his detailed descriptions of the patients, all of whom were admitted in terminal stages from outside facilities or directly from the community. Patient Xaver E, 23, was admitted directly from Danzig with a note from the medical officer of health that he was fully psychotic (our term): "He frequently grimaces, gesticulates in doing so, and looks about uncertainly in the interview." Admitted to Görlitz in April 1868, "The patient makes a decidedly stupid impression. His eyes have a staring, expressionless quality. He grimaces often, laughs stupidly without reason, and closes his eyes while speaking. . . . Instead of answering the questions directed at him, the patient repeats them . . . throws himself flat on the ground, does somersaults, climbs about on the tables and benches, crawls around the garden under the bushes—all without manic excitement. Sometimes he speaks a great deal and rapidly, but it is difficult to follow his logic, in which he discusses quite remote subjects, then turns to the interviewer with a sudden 'ach so.'" Soon the patient was in a state of "pronounced hebephrenic dementia."[18] (The continued somersaults could have deadly results. Georg Ilberg, a staff psychiatrist at the Sonnenstein asylum in 1898, recalled from his training days at Heidelberg under Kraepelin a female patient with catatonia "who ceaselessly did somersaults for weeks on end until, weakened to the utmost, she died of the injuries she had sustained."[19])

Kahlbaum stayed the rest of his life in Görlitz, dying there in 1899. He never received an academic appointment, not even an honorary one. But the intensity of his commitment to science was communicated to his assistant physicians, many of whom became significant figures in history. Theodor Ziehen, later himself a major academic figure, said in his obituary of Kahlbaum, "At the human level Kahlbaum had the basic quality of an absolute commitment to his ideals. For people who had no such commitment, he was incomprehensible and inaccessible. But those who were capable of this commitment—no matter whether to Kahlbaum's own ideal or some another— found in him a dear friend and helper."[20]

KAHLBAUM'S CATATONIA, 1874

Kahlbaum's catatonia is essentially a motor syndrome together with psychosis. The main motor symptom was stupor. Stupor plus psychosis would be the commonest presentation of the full catatonic clinical picture, as opposed to catatonia syndrome, meaning motor symptoms that may be present in a wide variety of medical and psychiatric illnesses.

For the first time, Kahlbaum, in his 1874 book on *Catatonia*, or *Tension Insanity*, defined a major psychiatric disorder on the basis of motor symptoms. (To be sure, in 1867, Heinrich Schüle, then an assistant physician at the Illenau asylum, in an essay on "delirium acutum" did assemble some of the major pieces of catatonia. Yet he did not give motor symptoms the centrality one finds in Kahlbaum.[21])

Kahlbaum had the view that catatonia was a disease of its own, like neurosyphilis. The basic symptoms of catatonia—stupor, rigidity, muteness, food refusal, waxy flexibility, and so forth—were long well-known. It was this emphasis on the unity of the motor side, on movement and its blockage, that created a new entity and took attention from the field's previous preoccupation with "insanity." Kahlbaum was not the first worker to notice motor symptoms,[22] but he was the first to make them the basis of a big, independent disease entity.

In his book, he said he was using the clinical method, not the anatomical. "Clinical" means at the bedside. "We have now come to the insight, that only the comprehensive clinical study of cases of disease [permits us] to array and explicate the empirical material [of the patients] according to the methods of clinical pathology, and thus to prepare the psychiatric ground for the further use of anatomical detail." (Today, we would say it is important to identify the phenotypes of psychiatric illness before we can study them in the laboratory.) This process would make new discoveries possible. "One such discovery is the proposal of a quite new variety of psychiatric disease, on the basis of a previously unused method of delineating, which we may indicate as the clinical method." He had already used this method to delineate hebephrenia. Now this method would serve for catatonia.[23]

The catatonia book is important not just because he described a new disease entity but because, for the first time, he clearly contrasted the previous "syndrome" ("*Symptomenkomplex*") approach to psychiatry, with the "underlying disease" ("*Krankheitsprozess*") approach that Bénédict-Augustin Morel in France and Kahlbaum himself and Hecker had been elaborating: "We have now realized that it is a doomed attempt to search for an anatomy of melancholia or mania, because each of these forms occurs under the most varied circumstances and combinations with other clinical pictures, and in and of itself is no more to be seen as the essential expression of an underlying disease process than, let us say, fever."[24]

The parallel with neurosyphilis dominated his thinking. "In this work I want to show a disease picture in which certain somatic and muscular symptoms accompany certain psychiatric symptoms in exactly the same way as in paralytic mental illness [neurosyphilis]." A still better comparison would be melancholia attonita, which also went through stages, as Zeller, Griesinger, and Guislain had pointed out in the case of "simple melancholia, mania, and dementia." Attonita wasn't a disease of its own, Kahlbaum continued, but the picture was familiar: "The patient sits there silent, or fully mute, with a rigid expression, unmovable, and a gaze fixed on the distance, without movement nor will, without reaction to sensory impressions, and sometimes with a fully developed symptom of *flexibilitas cerea* [waxy rigidity], as in catalepsy." But unlike melancholia attonita, there are patients with these symptoms who show epileptiform attacks at the beginning or other spasm-like conditions (*krampfartig*). These would be the catatonics.

He returned to neurosyphilis, a well-defined psychiatric disease associated with changes in muscle tension. "I now want to attempt in this work to demonstrate a clinical picture, in which certain somatic and, just as in progressive paralysis, muscular symptoms accompany certain psychic phenomena and thus in both cases take on a central significance for the formation of the entire disease process."[25] The main difference was in regard to course and outcome.[26] As Kahlbaum later pointed out, progressive paralysis was fatal, catatonia recoverable.

Thus, a new disease: "From these [spastic symptoms of neurosyphilis] one might derive the naming of a similar form of disease, because in every case a change occurs in the tension-state of the muscles.... I thus want to name this disease tension-insanity, or *vesania katatonica (Katatonia)*."[27] For Kahlbaum, catatonia was "primary," meaning arising de novo instead of piggybacking on some other disease. When other psychiatric symptoms, such as depression, mania, or psychosis, appeared, they were secondary. These other psychiatric symptoms usually involved psychosis, and so, in Kahlbaum's view, the main form of psychosis plus motor symptoms would be catatonia. Later scholarship reversed this, with schizophrenia, depression, or other symptoms becoming the primary disease and catatonic symptoms the secondary overlay.

The first case of catatonia in the volume, Benjamin L, 27, was initially admitted to the district hospital in Königsberg suffering from "convulsive contractures of the muscles of the face and neck" and extremities. On admission to Allenberg, he was "completely immobile. Sits or stands in one spot.... Gaze rigid ... upper extremities hang slackly. He does not answer, either during the physical investigation of his body or to questions." No reaction to needle pricks. Ate very little. Had to be dressed and undressed. Every few days convulsive twitches of his arms and the corner of his mouth were observed.

Months passed. "When sitting, he is the prototype of one of those colossal Egyptian statues: for hours and days holding his upper body upright, forearms upon his thighs, staring rigidly straight ahead. Facial expression ... empty and cold."

Suddenly, after nine months, there was an episode of agitation. "He attacked one of the attendants around the neck, laughed and cried and wandered about for an hour in the corridor." There were several more such episodes of agitation, alternating with stupor.

In the next two years in the asylum, he acquired a bit of speech. His body remained rigid, his gait clumsy and slow. After three years, he was sent home because of lack of space.[28]

Kahlbaum presented 26 cases, in 21 with enough detail to make possible a tabulation of symptoms. In 1992, Daniel M Rogers at Queen Square in London, the main English neurological hospital, noted the motor symptoms: 20 had abnormal speech, including 11 with mutism; 17 had disorders of posture; 16 had decreased activity, including 13 with motionlessness; 7 had outbursts; 6 destructiveness; 6 fixed gaze.[29] Each became the classic symptoms of catatonia, and it was in 1874 that Kahlbaum brought them all together under one roof.

In retrospect, some of these patients had a unitary disease called Kahlbaum's catatonia without any other disease that would explain their motor symptoms and psychosis; others had a catatonic syndrome, which may overlay many other diseases, including neurosyphilis (of whom there were at least 4 among the 26). As noted earlier, this would be much like the difference between Parkinson's disease and the various illnesses that compose parkinsonism.

To emphasize the psychosis component alongside the motor, in 1878, Kahlbaum referred to "Spannungs-Totalirresein (Katatonia)" (Tension-Total Insanity [Catatonia]).[30] It was thus madness plus motor deficits.

KAHLBAUM AND STAGE THEORY

Now, Kahlbaum's analysis had a second dimension, one generally overlooked today but that loomed large for him: Following the tradition of Zeller, Griesinger, and his own pupil Hecker (and faithful to *Gruppirung* in 1863), Kahlbaum said that the unitary disease of catatonia moved progressively and irreversibly through stages: "Most cases of this psychiatric illness [catatonia] begin with depression . . . which should be designated as melancholia . . . transition then to mania, in which symptoms may become very dramatic, then offer the picture of confusion, in which, with the disappearance of the maniacal symptoms of agitation, one psychic function after the other is extinguished, and end then in dementia, in which the disease process itself ceases and only the defect of the mind is apparent." If, however, the disease train did not progress to dementia, the prognosis of catatonia, he said, was "not bad."[31] It was this stage theory to which many of his contemporaries objected, more so than to his sketch of the symptom picture as such.

Stage theory, for example, precluded John Warnock at Peckham House asylum in Camberwell, Surrey, from diagnosing catatonia in 1895 in a patient who otherwise offered a veritable smorgasbord of symptoms—with mutism alternating with verbigeration, catalepsy alternating with agitation, stereotypies, and general cutaneous anesthesia—but who did not march systematically through the "stages." (The patient did not start with melancholia.) This couldn't possibly be catatonia, Dr. Warnock concluded.[32]

It was this hypothesis of stages that led Kraepelin, in 1893, to put a swift end to the whole staging business. Kraepelin, who had just become professor of psychiatry in Heidelberg, said in the fourth edition of his 1893 textbook that he simply did not believe that illnesses evolved in stages. Kraepelin wrote, "Drawing upon his teacher Zeller, Griesinger conceived the course of psychiatric illness as unitary, the individual stages of which were supposed to correspond to the various clinical forms of insanity (melancholia, mania, psychosis, confusion, dementia). Yet experience alone has failed to confirm the assumption of a clockwork-like course of "the mental illness" in determined stages, and the artificially constructed schema has recently been challenged with the demonstration of "primary" psychosis. In fact, even the simple observation of the forms of psychiatric disorder does not recognize the hypothesized unitary course but instead many various courses."[33] Thus, Kraepelin extinguished stage theory in the German-speaking world.

KAHLBAUM AND THE SYMPTOMS OF CATATONIA

Kahlbaum saw the core of the illness as stupor, which he called "atonicity" (*Attonität*), a term that conventionally had been used in connection with depressive stupor. And he made frequent reference to "mania" as well, as though catatonia were just a kind of mood disorder.[34] But other authorities quickly substituted "stupor" for "atonicity" and "agitation" for "mania" because catatonic stupor did not entail a mood disorder, and agitation was not mania. Stupor and agitation were not moods but behavioral opposites, and in Kahlbaum's catatonia they frequently alternated with each other.

Although many of the symptoms of catatonia had been well described under "catalepsy," "stupidity," and others, Kahlbaum fixed several new ones in place.

Making theatrical declamations, or "pathological pathos," for example, he ranked among typical symptoms. He described "something singularly dramatic ["pathetic"] in the comportment of the patients, a symptom that sometimes seems like the exaltation of the thespian, sometimes more as tragic-religious ecstasy, and to some extent constitutes the expansive coloration of mood, that many catatonics demonstrate in their speech, actions, and gestures."[35] St. Petersburg psychiatrist Victor Kandinsky warned in 1883: "The thespian-style exaltations of the catatonics, their dramatic posturing, their constant declaiming and reciting midst animated gesticulations, can occasionally lead to misdiagnoses, to the suspicion that hallucinations are present when in reality there are none, and where we are in fact dealing with voluntary, or involuntary 'theatrical performances.' "[36]

The frequent repetition of a given phrase counted as catatonic. Peter U repeatedly uttered single words, for example, "*Hund, Hund, Hund*" (dog, dog, dog). Or the patients might enunciate nonsense sentences, repeating "*Schmorbraten ist meine Sach*" (Pot roast is my thing; "Sache" in correct German). He proposed the term "verbigeration" for this behavior.

Mutism, of course, was well known, but Kahlbaum suggested a scale of symptoms, ranging from slight murmuring and moving the lips to "utter silence, for months, even years." Afterward, the patients explained that "They had not spoken because an inner voice commanded them not to; while in other cases, the patients complained about the lack of any thought and about their incapability of voicing it."

"Negation," also negativism, entered the Kahlbaum repertoire. Other authorities had previously reported the behavior, yet Kahlbaum gave it a name. "It is specially frequent as a resistance to changing place. The patients remain in bed, not from a . . . need, but from resistance to movement, or even from pleasure in contrariness. Once out of bed, they don't want to get dressed, or let themselves be dressed. Out of bed they stay firmly in one spot, don't want to sit down, or don't want to leave the most remote corner." And food refusal! It didn't result from fear of being poisoned or an effort to commit suicide: "It is without question only the result of resistance to any activity that might be deemed useful for the patient." An English physician later amplified this account of negativism: "No one who has not experienced the exaggerated obstinacy of such patients can have the least understanding of what it means to have to nurse them."[37]

The opposite of negativism is "automatic obedience," but, rather than Kahlbaum, it was Kraepelin who, in the first edition of his 1883 textbook, transferred this term (*Befehlsautomatie*) from the world of stage hypnotism to the psychiatric vocabulary.[38] In any event, it quickly became seen as a characteristic sign of catatonia.[39] In 1896, Kraepelin coined the term "stereotypies" for "the frequent repetition of the same muscular activity."[40] Various authorities before Kahlbaum had noted the resistance of catatonic patients to having their limbs or bodies moved. But it was in 1927 that Karl Kleist, professor of psychiatry in Frankfurt am Main (see later discussion), named it "*Gegenhalten*," a sign of negativism found not just in catatonia but in many neurological disorders.[41]

Kahlbaum noted mannerisms and bizarre gestures "in the movement and posture of the body." Here, he described what became known as *stereotypies* as well as the manneristic execution of routine actions. "One patient grabs himself every few minutes at the tip of his nose; another periodically swings his arm about his head and ends the movement by flinging away the hand . . . Patient Adolf L . . . had the mannerism of walking with the soles of his feet inverted and simultaneously keeping his knees bent." (Tics amount to the same thing as stereotypies.) Posturing was well-known, but Kahlbaum described what became known as "psychological pillow," the patient lying in bed with his head raised up off the pillow.

Pressing the lips firmly together Kahlbaum called "*Schnauzkrampf*." He included cutaneous anesthesias in the package, as well as sensory hyperesthesias, especially pain in the occiput of the skull.

Finally, he thought that catatonics had a special predisposition to pulmonary tuberculosis, more likely the result of contagion in the close living conditions in the asylum and the poor physical status of the food-refusing patients.[42] (In these years, of those patients who died in asylum, in 40 percent the cause was thought to be tuberculosis.[43])

Of this package of catatonic symptoms, only self-dramatization and tuberculosis have not withstood the test of time, though many others have been added. Kahlbaum's 1874 book was the seedbed of two of the great psychiatric syntheses of the twentieth century: Kraepelin's dementia praecox (see next chapter) and Karl Wernicke's "motility psychosis," including catatonia, which anchored movement disorders firmly in psychiatric waters.

Yet whatever the symptoms, Kahlbaum described a disease *sui generis*, not just a clinical syndrome that could be present in a number of diseases (though he admitted this possibility as well). And it is this distinction between disease and syndrome that has dogged catatonia over the years. If the patients are psychotic as well as negativistic and stuporous, do they have Kahlbaum's catatonia as their main diagnosis? Or do they have schizophrenia, manic-depression, or whatever? The field has been reluctant to let catatonia lap up too much "madness," preferring to delegate that task to "schizophrenia." Yet perhaps restoring madness to Kahlbaum's catatonia is appropriate? Maybe it is catatonia and not "schizophrenia" that is the core psychosis? Heinrich Schüle, by now superintendent of the Illenau asylum in Baden and the doyen of mental hospital psychiatry, said in 1901: "We must recognize that the so-called catatonic syndrome [*Zeichenverband*] may appear independently as a special form of primary dementia, as well as episodically in the course of other psychic diseases."[44]

THE RECEPTION OF KAHLBAUM'S CATATONIA

After *Catatonia* appeared in 1874, a small corps of acolytes greeted it because it described their own clinical experiences well; they recognized their patients in Kahlbaum's account. On the subject of negativism, Caspar Max Brosius at the private nervous clinic in Bendorf on the Rhine, said in 1877: "In fact, mute, motionless patients sunken into themselves, quite without will and appearing stupid, often react quite forcefully—less to painful impressions—but to efforts to change their momentary position. Appealing to them, asking them, severe words and demands, are usually in vain. But as soon as you touch or grab hold of them in order to move them from their spot, from the sofa or the bed, you feel the opposing tonic contraction of the muscles, the weight of their inert bodies; and if you go at this seriously, they cling convulsively to almost all the objects within reach, to all the corners, to the last handhold, screaming, cursing, pleading, physically resisting in various ways, but sometimes as well in uninterrupted muteness."[45] Brosius, a senior figure and editor of a mainline psychiatry journal, was a catatonia fan.

Julius Jensen, who was to die tragically in 1891 in Berlin at 49 of neurosyphilis, had succeeded Kahlbaum at Allenberg. In 1883, he became an impassioned defender of his friend. He called attention to the historic importance of Kahlbaum's attention to course, first in the 1863 book then in his catatonia book. Jensen added of his own experience that the illness might begin with stupor, not just with melancholia: "The patients then truly appear thunderstruck."[46]

In German-speaking Europe, Kahlbaum had no more enthusiastic supporter than young Clemens Neisser, at 26 a trainee at a provincial asylum in Leubus, when in 1887 he produced a doctoral dissertation on *Catatonia: A Contribution to Clinical Psychiatry*. It was an intellectual effort that, Neisser later said, "sought to achieve recognition for the disease of catatonia, which then in Germany counted partly as passé or partly was forgotten."[47] Neisser said in 1887: "It is the helpful and even brilliant accomplishment of Kahlbaum to have understood that scientific analysis means delineating clearly key symptoms and syndromes . . . which are so characteristic of a mental illness that their very presence points to the diagnosis." Neisser had the contempt of an eager young man for the hoary diagnoses of his seniors and their emphasis on "the fictional constituents of mental life: perception, ideas, will." But with Kahlbaum it was different, Neisser said. "In one word: for Kahlbaum, the entire sick person is the scientific object. And it is here that—in the impartial consideration of the condition of the entire sick individual from the beginning to the conclusion of the illness—are found the root and the apex of clinical science."[48] Bravo, and words to gladden the scientific heart even today!

In 1899, Georg Ilberg, 36, a staff psychiatrist at the Sonnenstein asylum, seconded Kahlbaum in almost every respect and emphasized several new features in catatonia that Kahlbaum had not mentioned, such as the "echo" phenomena, "repeating everything that a nearby person says, sometimes entire sentences, sometimes mere phrases ripped from context." (The term today is "echolalia," a familiar phrase in psychopathology.[49]) Imitating another's gestures is "echopraxia." "We observed and photographed in Sonnenstein three catatonics, who, with the same stupid facial expression, always goose-step in unison the same path. Here the second and third patients combine stereotypies with mutism and echopraxia."[50]

A bit of foreshadowing: Ilberg also made the point that the delusions of the catatonics that Kahlbaum emphasized were not really "fully developed systematized delusions" because they lacked content. "If you attempt to get to the bottom of this delusional system, the emptiness and desolation of their minds becomes quickly clear. However much you explore this, you will find nothing new or else just stereotypies." He remarked that if these patients did have a full delusional system, they would not be catatonics but "paranoiacs." Ilberg's thoughts here are of particular interest because, as we see in the next chapter, Kraepelin's dementia praecox was just starting to percolate. People were asking, are hebephrenia and catatonia the same disease? Are they subforms of dementia praecox? Is hebephrenia a subform of catatonia? Ilberg maintained that "The disease of catatonia should be maintained as an independent psychosis."[51]

The biggest supporter of Kahlbaum, in the sense of most influential, was Robert Sommer, professor of psychiatry at Giessen University. Sommer was among the leaders to introduce a motor component into psychiatry, and catatonia came to him as heaven-sent. Here was a clinical diagnosis that let him emphasize the motor side. He said in 1899: "In the study of psychopathic conditions my attention has been ever more drawn to one point . . . namely, how certain postures and movements, which completely deviate from normal, take on increasingly clear diagnostic significance. From the symptomatic concepts of stupor, catalepsy, negativism, the automatic repetition of certain patterns of movement and so forth—thus essentially from motor components—arose the clinical picture of catatonia, the core of which represented abnormal muscle innervation."[52]

GERMANY

Among German workers, the response was less enthusiastic. Carl Westphal, professor of psychiatry in Berlin and among the elite figures, said flatly in 1878 that catatonia was not a disease of its own, but rather a variant of delusional disorder ("*Verrücktheit*"). As for Kahlbaum's famous tonic contractions, Westphal saw them as secondary.[53]

Before Kraepelin, one of the most influential figures in German psychiatry was Heinrich Schüle, the superintendent of the Ilenau asylum in Baden and inveterate author. In 1867, he had given German wings to the French "delirium acutum," and, in noting that it had such motor symptoms as grimacing and a large psychotic component, it might be argued that Schüle more or less anticipated Kahlbaum's catatonia, though he never received credit for it—he was only 27 at the time. In the first edition of his textbook in 1878,[54] it was perhaps with a touch of sour grapes that Schüle applauded Kahlbaum's attention to motor symptoms because Schüle himself, in 1867, had dissertated upon "dysphrenia neuralgica," a supposed combination of pain and motor symptoms.[55] The diagnosis sank immediately from sight. So Schüle may have found it irritating in 1880 that Kahlbaum was back at this particular stand. In any event, psychiatry for him meant mental disorder. He didn't think that catatonia was a special disease *sui generis* and disagreed with lumping all forms of *Attonität*, or stupor, under catatonia.[56]

In 1881, Hecker and Kahlbaum ran into a wall of opposition at a meeting of the German Psychiatric Society. Wilhelm Sander, who had just taken over the chronic division of the newly opened Berlin City Asylum Dalldorf, doubted the existence of hebephrenia and found in the list of supposed symptoms "nothing special." (The quotes are not direct but stem from the transcriptionist's account.)

Emanuel Ernst Mendel, another member of the Berlin elite (who in that year, 1881, described hypomania[57]), "spoke out decisively against catatonia. He can find no justification at all for it and did not find the invention of new names helpful."

This intervention prompted Sander to seize the podium again. "Since catatonia has come up, he wanted to say he found the construction of catatonia even worse than hebephrenia for the classification of mental disorders and the formal nosology."

Franz von Rinecker, who led the Juliusspital at Würzburg, closed the discussion by saying he agreed with everything that had been said about catatonia (but gave hebephrenia a passing mark).[58] No one rose in catatonia's defense.

Carl Wernicke, one of the top names in German psychiatry at the turn of the century (and remembered for a special encephalopathy and an aphasia), had absolutely no time for Kahlbaum's diagnosis. He acknowledged Kahlbaum's importance as the first to explore the psychiatric significance of motor symptoms, but said that "catatonic" symptoms were found in many disorders and that an independent disease of catatonia did not exist.[59] Confronted in 1899 with a mute patient with stereotypies, grimacing, stupor, posturing, and negativism, he diagnosed "motility psychosis."[60] Wernicke gets credit for pivoting psychiatry further toward motor symptoms but low marks for the ability to see past the diagnoses that he himself originated. (At a psychiatric meeting in 1887, Wernicke was explaining that verbigeration was found in many disorders, whereupon young Neisser stood up and doubted that the examples were true verbigeration. Then Kahlbaum entered the room; Wernicke called upon him for a definitive judgment, and Kahlbaum said that Neisser was right.[61])

Many clinicians didn't believe. In 1886. Christian Roller, superintendent of the Brake asylum and, at mid-nineteenth century, the dean of German asylum psychiatry, was able to write on "motor disturbances in uncomplicated insanity," without even mentioning Kahlbaum and catatonia. Roller invoked authorities from hither and yon; a number of his patients clearly met the diagnostic criteria for catatonia. Yet Roller was silent on catatonia.[62] Adolf Freusberg, who had just taken over the direction of a private nervous clinic in Bonn, didn't believe it either, and, in a major article in 1886 on motor disorders in psychiatry, gave Kahlbaum the back of his hand: "so-called catatonia is typical," said Freusberg, "of many chronic mental diseases."[63]

Against these clouds of dubiety there were a few advocates, not really acolytes of Kahlbaum, who kept catatonia alive. Eugen Bleuler was one, and, in 1897, was just about to become professor of psychiatry at Zurich's prestigious Burghölzli university psychiatric hospital. Bleuler was then at the Cantonal Insane Asylum at the Rheinau, which housed mainly chronic young patients. "Every conceivable psychosis name was applied to them," he told a meeting in 1897. "It was only catatonia that was never diagnosed."

So, Bleuler went to work at the Rheinau and diagnosed his patients correctly. He found that "probably a third of the patient population were catatonics." To be sure, Bleuler had not seen any patients going through the stages that Kahlbaum described, yet the prognosis was poor. The cause? Usually masturbation.[64]

Now, Bleuler's presentation at the above-mentioned 1897 meeting of the Southwest German Psychiatric Society provoked interesting discussions, and here we can see these disease forms, later as solid as concrete, being shifted uncertainly about as people tried to find firm scientific ground. In 1897, Kraepelin was just elaborating his own dementia praecox concept (see next chapter), and a decade later, in 1908, Bleuler would follow with "schizophrenia." At the meeting, Heinrich Kreuser, who had spent most of his career at Zeller's Winnenthal asylum (where stage theory in Germany began), expressed astonishment that the prognosis of Kahlbaum's once positive catatonia had now become so negative. Kraepelin, who was at the meeting, agreed that there could be a variety of outcomes and that "Dementia praecox, just as progressive paralysis, represented a collective basin for a row of different disease processes."[65] (Kraepelin, as far as we know, never again made such a concession and would always portray dementia praecox as a unitary disease. Ironically, progressive paralysis did turn out to be a unitary disease caused by a spirochete.)

In any event, Kreuser had jumped on the key point: "The variety of illness courses must point to the fact that we are dealing with catatonic symptoms in a number of different diseases, and not with a unitary form of illness."[66] Kreuser's comment was echoed over the years by many other observers. There was general agreement that Kahlbaum's concept of catatonia as a single disease didn't exist, and that catatonia as a clinical syndrome could be present in many different diseases.

FRANCE

National traditions had a big impact on the willingness to invoke Kahlbaum's new disease. In the 1880s, Albert Mairet, at an asylum in the Hérault department in France, was arguing for the existence of a special kind of "madness of puberty" (*folie de la puberté*). One form involved stupor, "what the Germans call catatonia." But Mairet preferred his own denomination "*stupeur lypémanique*," on the grounds that the patients were often depressed (lypemania stemmed from Esquirol); Mairet was willing also to accept Jules Baillarger's "*mélancolie avec stupeur*."[67] Thus, familiar French diagnoses are always better.

In French psychiatry, the sentinel commentators were, in 1888, Jules Séglas at the Salpêtrière hospice and his friend Philippe Chaslin, at Bicêtre. (These were the two classical Parisian hospices, the former for women, the latter for men.) The authors balked at Kahlbaum's catatonia, refusing to subordinate all stupors, as Kahlbaum had proposed, to catatonic stupor. They accepted some of Kahlbaum's symptoms, such as verbigeration. Yet, on the whole, there was nothing new here, they said. "We thus see that katatonic phenomena taken singly have nothing to characterize them, for they are found in a multitude of mental afflictions." Accordingly, "the insanity of tonicity is not a disease, but may develop upon the most diverse grounds and under the most varied conditions."[68]

In much of French psychiatry, Kahlbaum's catatonia remained a dead letter. Some of the important Parisian figures—for French psychiatry was Paris—either continued to use catalepsy or had little interest in motor symptoms.

Pierre Janet was a leading light in French psychological medicine. Just before Charcot died in 1893, he created for Janet, then age 34, a laboratory for experimental psychology—to which Janet could admit patients. Under Charcot's successor, Fulgence Raymond, Janet developed his theories about "psychasthenia" that involved either too much psychic energy (leading to anxiety) or too little (leading to aboulia). So Janet led French psychiatry away from motor symptoms and frequently misrecognized those he encountered.

In 1903, Janet reported as "stubbornness" a young woman, 16, who, indeed, was so stubborn that she spent 39 hours standing in a corner (or at least that's why they thought she was standing there). As well, "She smashes the things she is given, she masturbates, and above all, she seeks ways to inflict self-harm. In little crises of agitation, she violently bangs her head, and tears out handfuls of hair." Janet suspected that her diagnosis was the hebephrenia of dementia praecox, but he was silent about catatonia, of which the young lady had ample signs.

On another occasion, Janet presented a young woman of 27 to the medical students. "You can see immediately what's going on. This young woman . . . is seated in front of you, her eyes fixed, her face inert and she remains motionless. She responds to no questions. She makes just a little grimace of discomfort if one pinches her hard. . . . These symptoms are thus what is called a state of stupor." Her illness had begun with an episode of psychotic self-accusation surrounding the death of her mother. "Little by little, she refused to move, to respond and now it's been ten days that she's in stupor." Refusing to eat, she was fed with a nasogastric tube. Janet made no effort to test for waxy rigidity or other diagnostic signs of catalepsy and catatonia, and he weighed most actively the diagnosis "hysteria."

Among Janet's 236 patients, there was one with "cataleptic posturing," a familiar diagnosis from the days of Charcot. She was a young woman from the province of Alsace—how old they didn't know because she spoke only a German "patois." "For a year this young woman has experienced periods of immobility. . . . Then these periods grew closer together and became prolonged, causing the present crisis that has lasted for three months. During these periods, she wishes to do nothing, she refuses to eat, she appears to dream because from time to time she smiles or she cries. It is evidently one of those states of stupor that today are classified in the large group of mental confusions." For Janet, catalepsy was mental confusion, and catatonia was not recognized.[69]

In France, catatonia became a nonentity. When Maurice Dide, chief of the Braqueville asylum, and his deputy Paul Guiraud wrote *Psychiatry for the Medical*

Practitioner in 1922, all of Kahlbaum's symptoms were there—verbigeration, negativism, and so forth. But Kahlbaum himself and the word catatonia were "missing at muster," as they say in France.[70]

UNITED KINGDOM

The English demonstrated little interest in Kahlbaum's new diagnosis of catatonia. In 1883, Thomas Clouston, superintendent of the Royal Edinburgh Asylum for the Insane and lecturer at the university, dismissed catatonia as "simply a variety of the diseases in which the functions of the motor and trophic centres are specially involved," a variant of what the Germans would soon be calling "psychomotor disorder."[71]

Yet many English patients displayed catatonic symptoms, which the medical people ascribed to "acute mania," "depression," and similar diagnoses (the patients may have had these disorders as well, yet the catatonic symptoms were generally not singled out of the mix). Holloway House, a semi-public sanatorium to the west of London, had "closed" units for males and females. In 1889, in the female wing, 66 patients were admitted for serious disorders. At least five had striking symptoms of catatonia, including Constance L, 27, who was mute and delusional on admission. On the ward, "she will sit for hours in a semi-stupor; she absolutely refuses to answer questions, in fact does not take the slightest notice when spoken to." Some months into her admission, she "at times will kick violently at anyone passing in front of her." She was usually mute, picked constantly at her face, and displayed an affected limping gate "although there is nothing wrong with her feet." Later, "She has a habit of beating her head with the heel of her shoe."[72] Her muteness and stupor, manneristic gait, rhythmic beating of her head, and face-picking (now called self-injurious behavior) are considered signs of Kahlbaum's catatonia.

Louisa S, 35, sat continuously "with her hands folded. . . . Occasionally when pressed to do a little work she becomes violent and attempts to strike an attendant." She was incontinent of urine and evidently stool ("dirty in her habits"). "She will remain standing or sitting in one position for hours at a time, entirely unoccupied, allowing her nasal mucus to drip into her lap. If questioned she takes no notice. . . . Although silent and unoccupied it is apparent from her manner that she notices and takes in what happens around her."[73] Here stupor leaps to the eye, but it alternates with agitation as she tries to kick the nurse. She is not demented; she pays close attention to what is going on, but she is entirely withdrawn from her surroundings.

Laura I, 31, came in grossly manic and psychotic, believing that she was "the Virgin Mary, or Cardinal Manning." Yet, two months later, she "has passed into a condition of perfect catalepsy; arm, hand, or leg placed in any position remains fixed for several minutes. She appears not to be affected by any form of external stimuli, and requires feeding by the nurses."[74] Catalepsy was an ancient diagnosis, and the clinicians of Holloway House were familiar with waxy flexibility. But Laura's other symptoms were ascribed to her depression—as perhaps they should properly have been, as catatonia is often an overlay on depressive illness.

Thus, the British psychiatric profession resisted "catatonia" as a diagnosis. As Edwin Goodall, a psychiatrist at the West Riding Asylum in Wakefield, Yorkshire, said in 1892, 18 years after Kahlbaum's book, "At no time does there appear to have been any widespread enthusiasm in alienist circles about this affection. . . . Probably it may be said with justice that katatonia, for the majority of medical men in asylums in this country (at any rate), was but a name up to quite recent times; having a doubtful significance for some, for many quite without meaning."[75]

UNITED STATES

Kahlbaum described his patients so well that, within three years, in 1877, James G. Kiernan, at the New York City Asylum for the Insane on Ward's Island, had seen 30 patients, concluding that "in reality the cases are frequent, but pass unrecognized." He thought it a disease *sui generis*, like general paresis. As well, "The prognosis according to Kahlbaum is good; as far as my experience goes, it is bad. Three cases only out of thirty have recovered, and of the permanence of the recovery of two of these I have my doubts."[76] Kiernan thus gets the credit for landing catatonia in the United States, although it was a Kraepelinian poor-prognosis version.

In 1883, catatonia reached the office of William A. Hammond, former Surgeon General of the Army and professor of psychiatry at the New York Post-Graduate Medical School. A merchant came to consult him, who kept repeating "And the Lord spoke unto Moses, saying." A week previously, the man had passed into a melancholic stupor and was silent and almost completely immobile. "On my taking hold of his arm and extending it at right angles with his body and leaving it there, it remained outstretched for thirteen minutes, and then slowly descended to his side. All the time that I was making this and other examinations of his muscular system, he was saying in a loud voice, 'And the Lord spoke unto Moses, saying.'"

Hammond wanted to take him into the next room to perform an eye examination. "I raised him from his chair to lead him into the apartment [and] he made himself rigid as a bar of iron, so that we had to carry him. Arrived there he would not sit down, but stood as erect as a statue."

When Hammond saw him again five days later, "He was then in a state of high excitement." He started declaiming about the solar system, and ended every sentence with the phrase "And there shall be no night there." The patient further exhibited violence and maneristic speech.[77] Hammond's patient embodied the main characteristics of Kahlbaum's catatonia: verbigeration, negativism, declaiming, alternation of excitement and stupor, and muscular rigidity.

Yet catatonia did not flourish in the New World. In 1897, Frederick Peterson, who had several clinical appointments in Manhattan, and Charles Langdon at the Hudson River Hospital for the Insane in Poughkeepsie, reached the somewhat dispiriting conclusion that "Katatonia is not a distinct form of insanity, not a clinical entity. There is no true cyclical character in its manifestations." (They thus revealed that they had completely misunderstood Kahlbaum's concept of "cyclical.") They found that "It is simply a type of melancholia" and that, furthermore, "It is not desirable . . . to retain the name katatonia."[78]

The great panjandrum of American psychiatry, Adolf Meyer, professor of psychiatry at Johns Hopkins University, set his face against catatonia and procured thereby its definitive burial. As Meyer said with pseudo-pity apropos Kahlbaum at a meeting in 1929, "I cannot help but feel that it was, in a way, one of the saddest things that happened to Kahlbaum when he had the impression that the disease entity of paresis [neurosyphilis] . . . could be paralleled by a similar entity or psychosis."[79]

Oh, poor Kahlbaum! The irony of Meyer's position was that, in the most venal and self-serving manner possible, he attached himself as an advisor to the wealthy McCormick family of Chicago as they struggled with the illness of an affected member, Stanley McCormick. Stanley met the criteria for catatonia (which after 1930 was treatable), yet not once did the word catatonia pass Meyer's lips, and, while Meyer collected fat consulting fees, Stanley languished in a prison-like private residence in California until he died in 1947.[80]

4

EMIL KRAEPELIN

Kraepelin founded an epoch as no other German had done, indeed as no one else at all.[1]
—Kurt Schneider, 1956

Psychiatry took Kahlbaum's diagnosis of catatonia, which corresponded to a real clinical entity, and almost discarded it. Kraepelin (pronounced Krep-LEEN), however, picked up catatonia and eternalized it as a subform of dementia praecox; until recently, that is exactly how most clinicians knew catatonia.

The story develops in two lines.[2] One line is anatomical localization, seeking the roots of catatonia in specific areas of the brain and treating the clinical symptoms as neurological phenomena. Further chapters will introduce Carl Wernicke and Karl Kleist, who, with such concepts as "disordered motility," pursued this organic biological agenda.

In a second line, Kahlbaum saw catatonia as a mixture of neurology and psychiatry. Symptoms such as negativism were "phenomena of the disordered action of the will," meaning the mind. Thus, catatonia depended on psychological sources, on the mind and its derangements. Emil Kraepelin, who makes an appearance in this chapter, continued this psychological analysis and placed great emphasis upon "disorders of the will." By contrast, Kraepelin's interest in localizing catatonia in the brain or in neurophysiological fancies was close to zero.

DEMENTIA PRAECOX BEFORE KRAEPELIN

Although Kraepelin turned adolescent insanity into a disease of its own—one that represented 50 percent of all admissions to the Heidelberg University Psychiatric Hospital by 1901—he was not the first to come across the concept. It is possible that the incidence of schizophrenia had been rising steadily throughout the nineteenth century.[3] In this case, a number of clinicians would have appreciated that here was something new. Among the first to use the term "dementia praecox," or "*la démence précoce*," was French clinician Bénédict-Augustin Morel at the Maréville asylum in eastern France in 1852. "When the manic excitement is not terminated, as frequently happens, by *une démence précoce* or by death, it invariably results . . . in establishing a kind of order within this extreme disorder."[4] Here, he used the term not as a disease *sui generis* but as a condition.[5] In 1890, René Charpentier, a staff psychiatrist at the Bicêtre Hospice, dilated upon "*les démences précoces*,"[6] and, in 1891, Arnold Pick, at the medical school in Prague charted the "primary chronic dementia (so-called dementia praecox) of youth."[7]

When, in 1893, Kraepelin, described "dementia praecox" he could scarcely claim priority for the label. Yet what he recounted was a clear disease entity: "As dementia praecox we designate the subacute development of a distinctive, simple condition of mental weakness in the youthful years."[8] He devoted an extensive section to it, followed by another on catatonia. Catatonia and dementia praecox were, at this point, both distinctive and well-defined disease entities.

KRAEPELIN CHANGES HIS MIND

Between 1893 and the First World War, Emil Kraepelin gave us the disease structure of modern psychiatry. He originated three changes: first, proposing manic-depressive illness and dementia praecox as the basic diseases of psychiatry; second, creating a firewall between them so that, forever after, mood disorders would be quite distinct from "schizophrenia"; and third, creating schizophrenia subtypes, of which catatonia was one. There was no place for anxiety in Kraepelin's nosology, and, as anxiety later gained prominence, it was owing to the influence of Sigmund Freud. But otherwise the psychiatry of the American Psychiatric Association's *Diagnostic and Statistical Manual of Mental Disorders* (DSM) series is heavily indebted to the psychiatry of Heidelberg and Munich.

It may seem curious to dwell at such length on the various editions of a textbook—given that journal articles today are the fundamental vehicle for conveying new knowledge. Yet Kraepelin's textbooks did report new knowledge, and every fresh edition was eagerly awaited. The textbook offered the unity of a "clinical" system of diagnoses—not a system based on pathological anatomy or genetics—that pulled together the sprawl of previous classifications into two master diagnoses: dementia praecox and manic-depressive insanity. And such was the intellectual power of this division that, rightly or wrongly, it has remained with us to this day. In 1926, Swiss-born Adolph Meyer, professor of psychiatry at Johns Hopkins University, called the Kraepelin textbook "the most comprehensive presentation of psychiatry ever written by any one writer."[9]

Kraepelin was born in 1856—the same year as Freud—in the North German town of Neustrelitz, then in the Grand Duchy of Mecklenburg-Strelitz; this was before the German unification of 1871. His father was a musician and opera singer, much given to alcohol. Kraepelin was, say his biographers, "a child of the Founding Years of the German Empire. He grew up during the euphoria of the Unification that Bismarck had directed politically and pushed through militarily." Kraepelin, his biographers continue, "experienced his academic socialization in the medical schools of Würzburg, Munich and Leipzig in the late 1870s and early 80s, those halcyon years of scientific optimism and national self-assertion."[10] He graduated with an MD from Würzburg in 1878, after clerking in Franz von Rinecker's university psychiatric hospital, then trained in psychiatry for four years in Munich under Bernhard von Gudden (who notably was dragged to his death at the bottom of Lake Starnberg in 1886 by his crazed patient, King Ludwig II).

In the 1880s, a powerful surge began among German psychiatrists away from brain anatomy and toward psychology, and, as historian Eric Engstrom points out, Kraepelin was part of this trend.[11] Kraepelin's psychological interests began with a two-year stint with Wilhelm Wundt, the founder of measurement in experimental psychology, in his laboratory in Leipzig. Simultaneously in Leipzig, Kraepelin worked with neurologist Wilhelm Erb in the outpatient department of the psychiatric hospital. It was apparently on Wundt's advice that, in 1883, Kraepelin penned the first edition of his psychiatric textbook[12], which heavily emphasized the "psychological standpoint of psychiatry . . . as opposed to Berlin-style slicing up the spinal cord," as Kraepelin told Zurich psychiatrist August Forel.[13] The volume went on to become in its subsequent editions the standard world guide to the discipline, comparable to the status of the DSM today.

This first edition gave full measure to motor disorders in psychiatry but under the label of "catalepsy." Kraepelin, who by this time had accumulated in Würzburg, Munich, and Leipzig about seven years of clinical practice, described "stupor" as "a psychopathic condition in which the perception of the outside world is distorted with hallucinations and delusions, thought is slowed, while the mood is dominated by severe depressive feelings, and the transformation into actions is almost completely blocked." This was a conventional description of catalepsy, with its waxy flexibility and stupor. Kraepelin considered the prognosis of catalepsy guarded: "Not infrequently does it pass into incurability, and even to death. Seldom does a recovery occur quickly, within a few days, but rather as a rule slowly and with time." Death, he pointed out, might eventuate through suicide "or through exhaustion as a result of food refusal and the profound depression of all bodily functions." There was indeed a role for psychotherapy, "but only after the anxious tension begins to subside."[14] It is curious that Kraepelin should have used this phrase without mentioning Kahlbaum's catatonia. After Kraepelin's little *Compendium* appeared, a friend wrote to him in 1885 to ask, "Did you leave out the stupor of the insane . . . catatonia, on purpose, just because of Kahlbaum?"[15] Kraepelin's reply is unknown.

In this first edition, there surfaced a theme that would stay with Kraepelin for the rest of his days and that hallmarked much of the epoch's psychiatry as well: psychiatric pathology as disorders of the "will." It was assumed that weak people did insane things because they were lacking in willpower. As Kraepelin explained in 1883, "In fully developed normal people the capability exists, up to a certain extent, of dominating natural drives through a superior will, and of satisfying these drives only when no other rational considerations demand their suppression."[16]

In 1886, at 30, Kraepelin was called to the chair of psychiatry at the University of Dorpat (now Tartu), the capital of Estonia. There, at least the middle classes spoke German. In 1887, the second edition appeared, by now entitled *Psychiatry: A Short Textbook*. Kraepelin acknowledged the existence of Kahlbaum's catatonia, though only to pour cold water on it. Kraepelin called it "catatonic delusional disorder" (*die katatonische Verrücktheit*). He said that Kahlbaum had united the various disease pictures in which catatonic symptoms might appear into the single disease entity. "Because this effort appears to me to have had unsatisfactory results, in my own account I have treated separately these highly diverse forms of illness—melancholia attonita, ecstatic insanity—clinically different in course and prognosis." Kraepelin accepted catatonia as the main stupor diagnosis and left catalepsy behind.[17]

A third edition in 1889, written at Dorpat, moved even more explicitly to link "catatonic insanity" (*"katatonischer Wahnsinn"*) to motor disorders. "We are dealing essentially with the acute appearance of confused psychotic ideation and hallucinations having episodic depressive or expansive episodes of agitation, combined with the appearance of a singular psychomotor blocking that manifests itself as catalepsy and tonic cramping."[18] This is tantamount to announcing catatonic insanity as a distinctive psychomotor disease of its own, and the importance of this third edition in 1889 has often been overlooked. (In this edition, Kraepelin said the prognosis was "grim": "A large number of cases pass into incurable feeble-mindedness."[19] And some of the cases on which he based this judgment were truly grim: a medical student in Dorpat investigated two of the catatonic patients Kraepelin had seen to learn that they had serious brain lesions and had died.[20])

In June 1890, with Kahlbaum present in the audience, Kraepelin read a report to the Society of East German Alienists on what he persisted in calling "catalepsy." Yet the influence of the Wundt years was evident in Kraepelin's emphasis on "will" and "suggestion": "The phenomena of experimental catalepsy under hypnosis shine a light on [clinical catalepsy]. [Under hypnosis] catalepsy is obviously only an epiphenomenon of general suggestibility, a particular form of automatic obedience that manifests itself in the involuntary execution of all suggestions coming from outside."[21]

It was in these Dorpat years that the importance of clinical course started to dawn on Kraepelin. "[I began to realize] from these continual cases of more or less quickly dementing outcomes that this was hebephrenia as Hecker had conceived it."[22] Kraepelin's assistant at the time, Leon Daraszkiewicz, became especially interested in this question and wrote his 1891 doctoral dissertation on forms of catatonia that ended in dementia.[23] Once again, the theme of disorders that begin in youth and reach a grim end reared its head.

By this time, Kraepelin's textbook was arousing such interest that he was ready for one of the big psychiatry chairs and simultaneously the direction of a university psychiatric hospital in a main German center. In 1891, he accepted the chair at Heidelberg. He assembled about him residents and associates who would form a tight circle defending his thoughts. For better or worse, Kraepelin now concentrated on the major psychotic illnesses because lesser disorders at Heidelberg fell into the province of neurologist Wilhelm Erb. Aided by his ability to present patients to the students in lectures and get their feedback (which he could not do in Dorpat because he didn't speak Estonian), Kraepelin now began sorting out the principal disorders requiring institutional care.[24]

In the fourth edition of the textbook in 1893, Kraepelin changed his mind in two ways. First, he announced that catatonia was a definite disease of its own, adding the phrase "a distinct disease" (*eine eigenartige Krankheitsform*) to a discussion not otherwise much unchanged from 1889 except to ascribe it to "processes of psychic degeneration." (The word "degeneration" suggested a genetic express train that gathered speed over the generations in its downhill race.)

Second, in this 1893 edition, Kraepelin added the concept of dementia praecox to his nosology, which also counted as a form of psychic degeneration. Dementia praecox was an insanity occurring expressly in adolescence and young adulthood. The distinctive feature from other forms of youthful insanity was the trend to "feeble-mindedness [*Verblödung*], progressing sometimes quickly, sometimes more slowly, that may stop at various stages." He acknowledged Hecker's 1871 description of hebephrenia as an account of mild cases but noted that the dementia praecox diagnosis also included much more severe cases, described by other workers.[25] Why call it "dementia praecox"? Kraepelin later said he had selected the term because the French were using it and it was familiar.[26]

In 1893, to whittle paranoia down, Kraepelin introduced into the fourth edition "dementia paranoides" as a separate disease—delusions of rapid onset that quickly eventuate in dementia.

Now firmly ensconced in Heidelberg, with the entire *Klinik* reoriented toward research, Kraepelin was rapidly spinning off ideas. In 1894, he told a meeting of the Southwest German Psychiatrists that such huge concepts as "paranoia" were scientifically pointless. Said the stenographer, "He demanded the dissolution of this clinical population into small groups of truly homogenous cases that could be described monographically, under the most exact observation, not only of individual symptoms but of the entire illness picture, on the basis of etiology, course, duration and outcome."[27] This was Kraepelin's operational principle for originating new disease entities. (And even though we today have inherited Kraepelin's dementia praecox as "schizophrenia," it is precisely this principle that we do *not* follow in our own use of the term.)

By this time, Kraepelin had inserted into his schema all the concepts that would later constitute the dementia praecox subtypes—catatonia, dementia paranoides, and hebephrenia (which in this edition he described as core dementia praecox[28]).

The fifth edition, in 1896, stands as a landmark, ending the concern with momentary symptom pictures and shifting attention to underlying diseases, as defined by course and outcome. Kraepelin is thought to have changed his mind: going from symptoms to diseases. A kind of conventional wisdom, initially laid down by Kraepelin's colleague in Heidelberg, the neurohistologist and psychiatrist Franz Nissl, insisted that with the fifth edition of his textbook Kraepelin initiated a historic change, shifting the focus from current clinical pictures to underlying diseases.

Nissl claimed that "Kraepelin's views in the first four editions of his textbook corresponded to the conventional concepts of the day. In the fifth edition he abandoned the symptom viewpoint and, adopting Kahlbaum's research methods, went over to the clinical viewpoint. In delineating various diseases, he relegated symptoms to second place, and then took up concepts that arose from the course and outcome of individual disorders. Quite specifically, Kraepelin noted the practical significance of prognosis, a factor to which Hecker twenty years previously had called attention. Kraepelin emphasized the certainty with which one could forecast the future course of events if one used Kahlbaum's method of circumscribing the individual diseases." The impact of this change was enormous.

Nissl continued: "This was a new departure, a fresh wind for clinical psychiatry in its previous sterility. People started once again to think more of purely clinical problems. Therewith the period of brain-anatomical research came to an end."[29] Thus, as in neurosyphilis, the presentation of an illness at any particular moment was not meaningful. At a given point, a neurosyphilitic might exhibit symptoms of mania, depression, paralysis, or insanity. Thus it was in the mainline psychiatric diagnoses: what counted was the underlying disease, and determining its prognosis and outcome.

This interpretation of events, while not false, is incomplete. The problem with this "epochal" interpretation of Kraepelin's years at Heidelberg is that it doesn't work very well for dementia praecox and catatonia, which Kraepelin now considered as "metabolic diseases" rather than diseases of degeneration. He had already designated dementia praecox and catatonia as independent diseases, and his analysis of both in 1896 differs little from the previous edition. The "epochal" reading of Kraepelin's system may well be based on the insertion in 1896 of a new section on "constitutional predisposition," which attempted to take the long view on "paranoia," the "periodic insanities," epilepsy, hysteria, and the traumatic neuroses. Kraepelin did, however, announce with confidence that his diagnostic scheme permitted the future to be forecast: "What convinces me of the superiority of the clinical procedure I recommend here is the certainty with which we are in a position to forecast the future course of things."[30] Kraepelin had previously uttered similar sentiments, but never before with such confidence.

The issue of clinical course in catatonia is crucial, given that Kahlbaum in 1874 had adjudged the prognosis as "not bad." In addressing the Southwest German Psychiatric Association in November 1895, Kraepelin tried to pin down the prognosis of catatonia. Does it progress to dementia or not? He presented data on 63 patients from Heidelberg, of whom 39 were still symptomatic years later. Of interest are the 24 who experienced remissions. Fourteen of them later relapsed, most within five years. Even in remission, the relatives continued to view them as ill; the patients themselves lacked insight, and each new relapse carried the patients closer to dementia. Kraepelin concluded: "In catatonia we are dealing with an organic brain disease, which leads to a more or less deep dementia."[31] Kraepelin repeated this judgment, though not the data, in the fifth edition, in 1896: "Catatonia ends most commonly . . . in deep dementia."[32]

It was in this fifth edition in 1896 that Kraepelin laid down his first detailed description of dementia praecox, which, together with dementia paranoides—mentioned earlier as well—now replaced the "insanity" (Wahnsinn) of earlier editions. Here, we encounter such classic descriptions of dementia praecox as the supposed "silliness" of the patients, which has survived as a core trait: "Very conspicuous is the frequent humorless laughter, which lacks the slightest pretext and occurs uncounted times in every interview; entirely absent is any kind of euphoric mood. To the contrary, one learns from the patients that it comes over them automatically, even against their will." Kraepelin also described in these dementia praecox patients numerous catatonic symptoms, such as grimacing and stereotypies, though he makes no mention of catatonia. Onset is in youth, with a long prodrome involving fluctuating mood, followed by psychotic episodes, followed finally by dementia: "The common outcome of all severe forms of dementia praecox is dementia." As the cause, Kraepelin indicted not heredity but an as yet unidentified organic brain change, or "autotoxicity."[33]

In a talk in November 1898, at the Southwest German Psychiatric Society, Kraepelin summarized what he understood by "dementia praecox": Emotional blunting and the lack of interest and of intellectual activity, delusional systems in the absence of affect or agitation, mannerisms and stereotypies, and changes in mood or agitation in the absence of changes in affect.[34]

Much of Kahlbaum's ideas on the importance of course and outcome are embodied in these ideas of Kraepelin. Clemens Neisser later noted that Kahlbaum's original emphasis in 1874 on course had been on the verge of becoming lost, submerged in contemporary musing about "paranoia," until Kraepelin came along: "[It was Kahlbaum's idea] that the entirety of the symptoms, their existence alongside, before, and after one another, the course and the outcome—should all form the basis of the clinical diagnosis. In the meantime, this clinical viewpoint has become generally accepted, thanks not least to Kraepelin's own work, and it is from him that the towering doctrine of dementia praecox was conceived and executed."[35] Here, Hecker and Kahlbaum shine through clearly. Yet "dementia praecox" was ripe for a change.

BIG CHANGES

In 1899, in the sixth edition, Kraepelin created two new illness entities that are with us today: "manic-depressive insanity" that included mood disorders of whatever polarity, and an enlarged "dementia praecox" that included as subtypes several diseases previously held separate: catatonia, hebephrenia, and dementia paranoides. Thus, Kraepelin changed his mind again, but this time, the consequences for catatonia as an independent disease were catastrophic. By making catatonia a subtype of dementia praecox, he ensured that whenever clinicians encountered catatonia in obviously nonschizophrenic patients, they would either overlook the symptoms or make some other diagnosis. Catatonia, a previously well-recognized disease of its own, was to become clinically invisible save as a form of schizophrenia.

How did this dramatic fusing together of what had been three separate disease entities come about? For one thing, several members of the tight Heidelberg circle around Kraepelin had been urging him to consider hebephrenia and catatonia the same disease. In November 1897, Gustav Aschaffenburg, then a staffer at the Heidelberg *Klinik*, reported his study of 227 catatonic patients admitted from 1891 to 1897 who had since been discharged. Comparing this cohort with a group of hebephrenic patients, Aschaffenburg said that both diseases began in adolescence, that hebephrenia had many catatonic features, and that both ended in dementia. "Under these circumstances, we may reach no other conclusion than that the diseases of hebephrenia and catatonia form a unitary disease process. The name 'Dementia praecox' seems to me most suitable for it."[36] Thus, Aschaffenburg may deserve part of the credit for the subtypes that Kraepelin proposed in the sixth edition of his textbook in 1899.

At the above-mentioned meeting of the Southwest German Psychiatry Society in November 1898, Kraepelin himself presented data on almost 300 dementia praecox patients observed over four years: Of those with "pronounced catatonic signs," 59 percent ended in severe dementia, 27 percent in milder dementia, 13 percent in recovery. Of those with hebephrenic tendencies, 75 percent ended in severe dementia, 17 percent in milder dementia, 8 percent in recovery.[37] The differences were not great.

In this sixth edition in 1899, the subtypes were characterized as follows. First came hebephrenia, defined as "a mental disturbance that begins subacutely entailing a simple state of more or less severe weak-mindedness." This was close to Hecker's 1871 concept, and, in the future, hebephrenia would be regarded as "core schizophrenia."

Second, catatonia. Kraepelin invoked Kahlbaum as the originator of this form of dementia praecox with its initial mood disorder, followed by stupor, confusion, and dementia, and accompanied by motor symptoms of all kinds. "The end stage of catatonia in 59 percent of my cases is a distinctive, constitutionally predisposed [*erblicher*] dementia." Here, Kraepelin parted from the Kahlbaum model of catatonia as a mostly recoverable illness. Kraepelin attached great importance to negativism and automatic obedience as symptoms, and it is here that the notion of "negative symptoms" of schizophrenia was reinforced, although Kraepelin meant by the term patients' resistance to clinical care, mutism, food refusal, and misbehavior around toileting rather than flatness of affect.

Third, Kraepelin distinguished a "dementia paranoides" form, which, in contrast to the main diagnosis of paranoia (found elsewhere in the volume as *Verrücktheit*), ended in dementia. The main feature was delusions and hallucinations in the presence of otherwise preserved presence of mind (*Besonnenheit*).[38]

The Achilles heel of the entire dementia praecox construct is at once apparent: if one doesn't accept the notion that all three end almost inevitably in "dementia," they have little to do with one another. Hebephrenia is adolescent insanity, denoted by age at onset; catatonia had been well characterized by Kahlbaum, and, even though Kahlbaum thought all kinds of other mental symptoms accompanied it, motor symptoms nonetheless clinched the diagnosis, and the mental changes were accessory. Dementia paranoides seemed really a variant on "paranoia," on what became delusional disorder, and delusional disorder did not usually end in dementia.

Did all these disorders truly end in dementia? It is quite possible that Kraepelin and his acolytes confused episodes with end-stage conditions. Patients who relapsed in the Heidelberg University Psychiatric Hospital often recovered later. As well, it was difficult to follow many patients who'd been transferred from the overcrowded Heidelberg *Klinik* to other mental hospitals in Baden because the hospital superintendents were begrudging about cooperating with Kraepelin, who represented for them the threat of university academic psychiatry.[39] Then, too, patients discharged to the community as recovered were often lost completely from view.

The seventh edition in 1904, composed while Kraepelin was still in Heidelberg, changed little. It showed, perhaps inadvertently, how "catatonic" features easily come and go. Kraepelin pointed to the confused, nonsensical writings of catatonics as examples of "catatonic incoherence" (*katatonische Zerfahrenheit*).[40] In the eighth edition in 1913, he said that incoherence better characterized dementia praecox as a whole than catatonia in particular.[41] Such was Kraepelin's prestige by this time that, we may be sure, had he decided to maintain "catatonic incoherence," it would appear today in the symptom lists.

In the seventh edition, Kraepelin refined the markers of catatonic motor disturbances to include "eccentricity" (*Verschrobenheit*) and "the loss of graceful movement" (*der Verlust der Grazie*). Both terms addressed the idea that the movements of catatonic patients were often stiff, awkward, and ungainly. There isn't really a good English translation of the German term "*Verschrobenheit*," but by it Kraepelin meant movements that were clumsy and involved the loss of efficiency and purposefulness inherent in normal human movement. The term survived in German analyses for years but was not really accepted abroad. By "loss of graceful movement" Kraepelin again approached the same concept: "Graceful movement attains its goal with the least possible but sufficient expenditure of energy and movement. In contrast, catatonic movements are either stiff and wooden with excessive contraction of antagonistic muscles, or flaccid and slow as a result of an insufficient expenditure of energy. . . . The simple naturalness, which aspires directly to a goal, is lost through bizarre movements and derailments [*Verschnörkelungen und Entgleisungen*]."[42] Kraepelin singled out a marker of motor pathology that should have survived—the "awkwardness" marker—but somehow hasn't.

Where to situate catatonia in the diagnostic classification had a big influence on the apparent prevalence of "dementia praecox" or "manic-depressive insanity." At the Heidelberg University Psychiatric Hospital, the number of dementia praecox cases soared from zero to more than half of all admissions between 1893 and 1901. Kraepelin said, "This development is explained by the fact that, as people got accustomed to applying the diagnosis of dementia praecox, at first the pathognomonic significance of individual symptoms was overestimated. In particular, many cases of manic-depressive insanity with catatonic phenomena were incorrectly assigned to dementia praecox." This error was then realized and corrected, so that, at Heidelberg after 1901, the frequency of dementia praecox fell appreciably and that of manic-depressive insanity rose sharply.[43] Given such erratic shifts in diagnostic judgment at the very home of dementia praecox and manic-depressive illness themselves, it is difficult to take seriously the argument that these are two sharply delineated disease conditions. Such dramatic shifts, moreover, were reported from other venues. In 1959, Paul Hoch, at the New York State Psychiatric Institute, mentioned an (unnamed) US state where, "In the beginning they admitted about 45 to 50 percent manic depressives. In five years they admitted the same number of schizophrenics, and the manic depressives dropped down to only 5 percent, where before the schizophrenics represented about 5 percent."[44]

In 1903, Kraepelin assumed the professorship of psychiatry in Munich and held the position until his retirement in 1922; he died in 1926. He had begun to tower over the field. His Viennese colleague neurologist Constantin von Economo called him "[a] North German schoolteacher in giant format."[45] Kraepelin himself cut a formidable figure, as Edinburgh psychiatrist David Henderson, who trained for a year at the Munich *Klinik*, recalls. "He was thick-set, bullet-headed, intensely serious, a total abstainer from alcohol and tobacco, and very determined in his views. His appearance was more of a prosperous industrialist than that of a world-renowned professional man."[46]

THE LAST EDITION

The last edition of Kraepelin's work, the dementia-praecox volume which was published in 1913, bears the stamp of the Munich years, with its large and highly variegated patient population, as opposed to the Heidelberg period. By the time of the five-volume eighth edition in 1909–1915 (the last edition that Kraepelin himself completed), Kraepelin had become a little less absolute about whether dementia praecox always ended in dementia; he also conceded that catatonia could be found in other illnesses. "The supposition has been often expressed, that apparently recovered cases [of dementia praecox] probably belong to some other disease process than the dementing process. I am not going to dispute this possibility. Partly, some of these will be simple missed diagnoses, usually cases of manic-depressive insanity. But there may be other, recoverable diseases with catatonic phenomena, that we at present are not capable of differentiating from dementia praecox."[47]

Kraepelin went on to make a distinction, already adumbrated in 1901 by Schüle, between catatonic symptoms that could be found in various illnesses and "Kahlbaum's catatonia," a disease of its own, which is to say a subtype of the disease dementia praecox. . . . We may consider Kahlbaum's catatonia mainly as a distinctive kind of dementia praecox. And 'catatonic phenomena' are undoubtedly observed in many other disease processes . . . so that their occurrence alone does not permit the conclusion that catatonia in the narrow sense is present."[48]

The characteristic symptom of Kahlbaums' catatonia, for Kraepelin, was the alternation of agitation and stupor: "I think we may consider as the catatonic form of dementia praecox those cases in which the co-occurrence of characteristic agitation with catatonic stupor dominates the clinical picture."[49]

Kraepelin considered patients with the catatonic type of dementia praecox to be psychotic from their early depressive phases. At the same time as the patients demonstrate depression, "They express highly bizarre delusional notions; 'battles' and 'premonitions' are coming . . .; they feel strange, as though someone were pursuing them; their life is no longer of value; everything has failed; no-one can help them. They are mocked by wanton sluts, belittled, spat upon, cursed; they are supposed to go to jail, to be sentenced to death, slaughtered, tied to the railway track, their house blown to bits . . . the daughter will be murdered, the children executed." Then hallucinations crept in. Catatonia, for Kraepelin, was essentially a psychotic experience.[50]

This eighth edition made a distinction between flaccid stupor and rigid stupor (*schlaffer Stupor v starrer Stupor*). In flaccid stupor, the main symptom is catalepsy, with automatic obedience and stereotypies. Echopraxia, or imitating the movement of others, is included, and the patients talk so much that the actual stupor must be rather abbreviated. Kraepelin does not say that their eyes are wide open and follow movements in the environment, but others do. Set against this is "rigid stupor," the main characteristic of which, aside from stupor itself, is negativism. The patients are entirely unresponsive, and their eyes are either tightly shut or "wide open, staring with widened pupils into the distance, not fixating."[51]

Kraepelin's interest in the psychology of dementia praecox, in the "will," was by this last edition stronger than ever. "All disorders that influence psychic life find their ultimate and most important expression in the will and the actions of the patients," he wrote in 1909,[52] and proceeded to divagate on factors that increased and decreased the action of the will. It is interesting that in other medical specialties by this time the medical model was in full sway, permitting the delineation of distinctive diseases, with tests and verifications, as in cardiology and infectious diseases. Yet Kraepelin never evidenced interest in medical-model thinking—isolating distinctive diseases on the basis of biochemical, histological, and anatomical parameters—even though rapid progress was being made in these years in finding the organic bases of such diseases as pellagra and myxedema that had once belonged to psychiatry. Kraepelin's influence ensured that the field would remain true to psychology and Freudian psychoanalysis, of course, completed this divergence of psychiatry from the rest of medicine.

This eighth edition greatly widened the scope of dementia praecox. In a *mania classificatoria*, Kraepelin increased the subtypes from three to nine, one of which remained catatonia. The "simple demented form" of dementia praecox, for example, was Hecker's hebephrenia. It was perhaps a sign that Kraepelin was losing confidence in the unity of his concept, and, a few years later, in 1920, he conceded that it was not always possible to differentiate between dementia praecox and manic-depressive insanity on the basis of symptoms.[53] The nine different subtypes in this edition represented a large expansion of the concept of dementia praecox, slicing off big chunks of mood disorder, for example, and attaching them to "dementia praecox."

Gone were all the former "degeneration" diagnoses. This expansion left a toxic legacy to psychiatry, making everything that could not be considered a "psychoneurosis" into "dementia praecox" or "schizophrenia."

In this edition, Kraepelin raised a question that has bedeviled catatonia researchers ever since: How many catatonias are there? In the seventh edition in 1904, he had adumbrated a "late catatonia," identical to those surfacing earlier in life and characterized by a remote prehistory of depression. In the eighth edition, he retracted this thought and suggested that catatonia beginning late in life might be a different illness entirely: "After much experience, this [earlier] concept now seems to me increasingly untenable. It seems particularly striking that the anatomical investigation of many of these late-catatonias reveals a completely different disease process than we encounter in similar forms during youth. And at the clinical level it seems more and more the case, that at least the majority of the late catatonias show only superficial resemblance to the corresponding illnesses of the earlier periods. . . . At present, the assumption having the most to be said for it seems to be that at least a considerable part of the late catatonias are an expression of very different disease processes."[54]

The idea is an intriguing one, yet Kraepelin himself doomed it to marginality by making catatonia a subtype of schizophrenia.

Indeed, Kraepelin was so convinced of catatonia as a subtype of dementia praecox that he misdiagnosed it when he encountered it in other contexts, for example, in the context of manic-depressive illness. In manic-depression, Kraepelin identified a kind of special stage between mania and depression of "manic stupor." Alternation was among its symptoms: "Quite suddenly [the stuporous patient] becomes lively, curses loudly, and amidst boisterous laughter makes animated observations. They leap out of bed, throw their food around the room, suddenly undress, storm about through several of the wards, tear up their clothing, or mishandle without obvious reason other patients, and then immediately sink back into their earlier stupor. . . . Some patients wander in measured steps about the ward, speak almost not at all except for the occasional joke." Later, said Kraepelin, the patients remember quite precisely these episodes, but are not able to account for their strange behavior. "I didn't want to have any will, one patient told me. He refused food but . . . felt obliged by hunger to take in large quantities of milk through his nose." Kraepelin appended a photo of a patient with "manic stupor," "with her rigid facial expression staring always at the same spot; she shows clearly the inhibition that dominated her for months and made her mute."[55] In retrospect, "manic stupor" was probably the alternation of agitation and stupor of garden-variety catatonia.

Yet these nuances and reservations were quickly forgotten. For the next hundred years, catatonia would be a type of schizophrenia.

5

EUGEN BLEULER

We knew [as Bleuler went to work on schizophrenia] that the diagnostic utility of catatonic symptoms had been impermissibly overextended. But we didn't have a new, unitary classification to which all the clinical pictures of "dementia praecox" could be assigned. So it was great progress that now emphasis could be placed on the diagnosis of a schizophrenic personality and on the analysis of schizophrenic thinking.[1]
—Oswald Bumke, professor of psychiatry in Leipzig, 1924

Eugen Bleuler, professor of psychiatry in Zurich, made schizophrenia into a common disease, and catatonia, part of the schizophrenia package, increased greatly in frequency as well. If Kraepelin had assigned dementia praecox and catatonia to a specific age group, Bleuler democratized things. Everybody at any age was at risk.

Eugen Bleuler (pronounced BLOY-ler) is venerated by the Swiss in the same manner as Freud is venerated by the Viennese: both figures put provincial capitals on the psychiatric map. Bleuler's most notable achievement was plunging the diagnosis of chronic psychosis into chaos as catatonia became something called an "accessory symptom."

Bleuler was born in 1857, one year after Freud, into a farming family in the village of Zollikon near Zurich. He graduated with an MD in 1883 from Zurich, after also studying in Berne and Munich. He trained in psychiatry with Bernhard von Gudden in Munich and at the large Zurich cantonal psychiatric hospital, called the Burghölzli. In 1886, he became, at age 29, director of the huge Rheinau asylum, a chronic care facility for patients transferred from the Burghölzli and other institutions, where he encountered numerous young men with chronic psychosis that he diagnosed as catatonia. Twelve years later, in 1898, he was called to the professorship of psychiatry in Zurich as Oscar Forel's successor. Bleuler's main publications were written in Zurich, yet with the influence of the Rheinau as the wind behind him. In contrast to Kraepelin, who at the Heidelberg *Klinik* emphasized rapid turnover and saw mainly recent acute cases, Bleuler worked with end-stages. And his intimate knowledge of these patients, some of whom had been ill for decades, sensitized him to such issues as "autism" that are less apparent in the recently ill.

Bleuler is understandable only in the context of his times, and the color of the day was Freud's psychoanalysis. Bleuler corresponded with Freud, visited him, and plunged into psychoanalysis fully. By 1906, Bleuler's colleague Carl Jung could report to Freud that Bleuler was "now completely converted."[2] In all of Bleuler's writings, his belief in the unconscious mind and its influencing of the ego came through clearly.

If Bleuler did not buy the whole intellectual apparatus of psychoanalysis, he did absorb much. Bleuler's theorizing about unconscious "splits" in the mind did not come out of nowhere. Later, he became so sensitive to the charge that he had sold out to psychoanalysis that he said, "I have only taken those parts of Freud's theories that subsequent research has verified."[3] Critical observers might well have wondered what parts those were. In any event, Bleuler brought Freud to mainline psychiatry, and his own work swims in psychological speculations that acquired a reputation among Bleulerians as fact.

BLEULER DESIGNS SCHIZOPHRENIA

Two years after arriving at the "Bli," Bleuler steered his student August Müller toward a doctoral dissertation on "the periodic catatonias," a term that Müller and his advisor Bleuler seem to have coined.[4] The cases took place in the context of "dementia praecox," and Bleuler and his students seem not yet to have started using the term "schizophrenia." (In a lecture Bleuler gave to the Medical Society of Zurich Canton in May 1900, Bleuler used the term "dementia praecox" and said that he "essentially follow[s] the views of Kraepelin."[5])

By 1902, Bleuler began laying out the design of his "schizophrenia." He noted the patients' strangely changed "emotions" (he would later call this "affectivity"). "At times [as the illness progresses], one single emotion remains, but may be inadequate and not in conformity with the ideas of the patient's mind. They may speak of the persecutions, to which they imagine themselves to be subject, not only with indifference, but even laughingly and with an air of boasting. They are apt to cry over cheerful events. Such alteration of the emotions in patients with an unimpaired consciousness and orientation is found in no other psychic affection."

He also began to dilate on "splitting": "The association of ideas in dementia praecox is disturbed in such a way that on the one hand, the mental connections are interrupted here and there in an irregular manner; on the other hand, there appear thoughts, the linear connection of which, either in part or as a whole, is not traceable." "The ideas," he continued, "appear as if they had all been mixed up in a bag and that the patient took them out as chance presented them."

A third new theme was the distinction between core symptoms and accessory symptoms that would play a large role in his 1911 book: "The clinician can always separate . . . the fundamental characteristics of the disease from the accidental symptomatic accompaniments."

Nor did Bleuler, in 1902, have much use for the Kraepelinian subtypes, though they do appear in his 1911 book: "The hebephrenia of today may become a catatonia tomorrow, and the latter form may figure as a typical paranoia a few days later. In a word, there does not exist any definite line of demarcation between the different varieties of the disease."[6]

BLEULER DIFFERED FROM KRAEPELIN: 1908

In April 1908, at a meeting in Berlin of the German Psychiatric Society, Bleuler announced that dementia praecox was a member of the "group of schizophrenias." Bleuler later disclaimed that his schizophrenia differed much from Kraepelin's dementia praecox.[7] Yet there were differences. Bleuler was outlining a much milder disease, in contrast to Kraepelin's relentless dementia-mongering.

Bleuler proposed "schizophrenia" not only because it lent itself better than dementia praecox as an adjective ("schizophrenic"), but because "I believe, notably, that the tearing in half or splitting of the psychic functions is a cardinal symptom of the entire group." "Intrapsychic splitting?"[8] What did that mean? Bleuler said it represented a disruption in the supposed mental "associations" and in "affectivity." Kraepelin, though psychologically minded, thought dementia praecox was an organic brain disease. Bleuler, entwined in the coils of Freud's psychoanalysis, gave preponderance to the psyche. Bleuler dismissed heredity and "degeneration," the latter term having stood Kraepelin in good stead.

Available for study were 475 patients seen at the Burghölzli and the Rheinau. A huge difference from Kraepelin lay in the prognosis. While Kraepelin thought the cases went irreversibly downhill, Bleuler said that, of the cases with acute onset, 73 percent could be discharged as capable of work while not necessarily being fully recovered. But Bleuler set the bar rather low, saying, "There are patients completely capable of work who during months of gibberish have not been able to utter a sensible sentence."

Bleuler retained the three Kraepelinian subtypes and added one. He found that 30 percent of the catatonics ended in "severe" dementia (in contrast to only 19 percent of the paranoids and 20 percent of the hebephrenics). Particularly ominous were the patients of the "paranoid" subtype who developed catatonic symptoms as their downhill slide began.

Bleuler was not as attached to the subforms as was Kraepelin. He found them useless in predicting prognosis (catatonia excepted) and said that they transitioned so easily into one another that "We should probably give up . . . trying to find distinctive disease pictures within dementia praecox."

In an article published with Carl Jung in 1908, Bleuler said: "In every case we could examine, we found the content of the psychic symptoms linked to an affect-laden symptom complex and understandable in those terms. The complex must therefore be the relevant psychic cause, which determines the content of the symptoms."[9] This was not language dear—or even comprehensible—to Kraepelin.

What made for a good prognosis? For one thing, the patients should demonstrate no catatonic features, nor encapsulate themselves in their own little universes. Here, Bleuler anticipated the "autism" concept that he would shortly launch: "The patients must [not] lose contact with their surroundings, not dwell in a fairy tale that cannot be brought into connection with their reality, not close themselves off . . ." For Bleuler, catatonia was the great bugbear: the appearance of these symptoms meant chronicity and ultimate dementia.

Perhaps the greatest difference from Kraepelin was Bleuler's view that schizophrenia was a relatively mild disease, with many "latent" patients in the community. "Latent schizophrenias are very frequent, if one might conclude from the patients with episodes of temporary, externally caused excitement who come into the asylum for short stays, or whom one sees in the office hour. One is also mindful of the large number of schizophrenics who, after a stay in the asylum, get married and are considered healthy."

Kraepelin would have said that these patients are not recovered but in remission and that, sooner or later, a new episode will tip them onto the downhill slope. Bleuler recognized some truth in this: "I myself have seen no patient, who, at the time of discharge or at a later careful interview, was entirely free of the symptoms of the disease."

In contrast to Kraepelin, Bleuler said that many of these patients, though not fully symptom-free, did well in life: "I know patients who have achieved quite spectacular things, although I shouldn't have called them recovered—merchants who develop a large business, government officials, pastors, one novelist of worldwide reputation who has already had two episodes of catatonia."

"Dementia" leapt off virtually every page of Kraepelin's work. Yet Bleuler's sensitive assessment of what this actually meant should give heart even to those who struggle today with these issues: "The schizophrenic is not at all demented across the board, but rather is demented in connection with certain questions, at certain times, in certain illness patterns [Komplexe]." "Bleulerian schizophrenia" became a forgiving diagnosis simply because it did not foretell catastrophe, did not end invariably with shredding one's clothing and smearing feces on the sanitarium back wards.

Finally, Bleuler distinguished between the "primary" symptoms of schizophrenia, "which belong to the illness process," and the "secondary" symptoms, which "arise through a reaction of the sick psyche to the influences of the environment or to the patient's own thoughts." He would shortly pin down exactly what he meant, yet the very existence of Bleulerian schizophrenia would always depend on the hypothesized presence of these vague, intangible, "primary" symptoms.

This primary–secondary distinction was of the utmost importance in differentiating Bleuler from Kraepelin. While Kraepelin had proposed a series of unweighted phenomena, such as withdrawal, psychosis, and so forth[10], Bleuler was saying there is a hierarchy of symptoms. First came the primary, such as disturbances of affect, association, and volition; then came secondarily what were, as Heinz Lehmann pointed out, Kraepelin's "entire clinical picture" of hallucinations, delusions, negativism, and stupor.[11]

Bleuler concluded the 1908 article by asking his readers' pardon for "complicating rather than simplifying the discussion of the end-stages of dementia praecox."[12] But was it true? Was it really just fiddling at the edges of Kraepelin's dementia praecox?

BLEULER AND PSYCHOLOGY

Despite his enthusiasm for Wundt's psychometrics, Kraepelin was not interested in the psychology of individual patients, in their "minds." Bleuler was. And, in this 1908 paper, he touched very briefly on an underlying mechanism of schizophrenia, namely the patients' "affectivity," or "affective complexes" or "affect-laden complexes."[13] This was a radical displacement of attention from metabolism (Kraepelin) to psychology (Bleuler) that would fundamentally separate the Zurich school from the Heidelberger.

In terms of psychology, the 1908 article's invocation of "splitting" as the basic mechanism also meant dragging Freudian psychology onto the stage, front and center.[14] Karl Wilmanns, who in 1918 had succeeded Nissl (and before him Kraepelin) as chair of psychiatry at Heidelberg, said in 1922: "Bleuler was the first, basing on Jung's views, to dare to attribute the panoply of the schizophrenic mind to certain basic symptoms."[15]

Ideas about divided consciousness, one half of the mind losing track of the other half, were current coin in European psychology and psychiatry in those years. In

1900, Carl Wernicke, still at Breslau, codified for a general psychiatric public ideas he had been brewing about "sejunction" as the basic mechanism of psychosis—the supposed association pathways becoming separated. "We shall designate this process of the loosening of associations with the name sejunction," he told the students.[16] (In his 1908 paper, Bleuler accepted Wernicke's sejunction theory as "very related" to his own.[17]) French psychiatry in these years was filled with speculation about "double personalities" and the like.[18] Bleuler's "splitting" theories landed on fertile ground.

How revolutionary was this, really? Two Swiss historians of medicine say of the 1908 contribution, "Bleuler's 'schizophrenia' is indeed a genuinely new disease concept and . . . he can thus be described as a revisionary nosologist." In our view, this overclaims. Very little of Bleuler's semi-psychoanalytic musings about "splitting" has survived. The four subtypes are now dead as subtypes. As with catatonia, they continue to exist as independent diseases. As for the Swiss authors' accompanying boast that Bleuler "can also be called a pioneer of evidence-based psychiatry," there were in fact numerous predecessors.[19] True, German psychiatric articles often went on for endless pages with few if any numbers. But other workers, Kraepelin included, had analyzed "data," as we understand the term, and Bleuler seems less innovative here.

When Bleuler gave his schizophrenia paper at the 1908 meeting, there were murmurs of approval among the audience. Kraepelin had pioneered the primacy of clinical course. Here was a second brave attempt. Yet there was one loud dissent, and it came from Clemens Neisser, who two decades previously had rescued Kahlbaum's catatonia from a premature burial. "I want to warn urgently against adopting the name 'schizophrenia.' Certainly, the name dementia praecox is not entirely satisfactory. But we know exactly what is meant by it and are able well to work with it clinically. What I have against the name schizophrenia is that . . . it does not relate immediately to any clinical observation of apparent phenomena, but rather makes assumptions about the theoretical nature of the disease process."[20] Schizophrenia, Neisser implied, was a construct in the clouds, not a clinical entity.

In July 1910, Bleuler added ambivalence and autism to the list of primary symptoms. Of "schizophrenic negativism": "All these patients are extremely autistic, that means, detached from reality. They have withdrawn into their dream world, or the essential part of their bifurcated ego ("*Ich*") that lives in a world of subjective notions and wishes, so that reality can only bring disorder for them. Many patients are fully aware of assigning to this [world] the reason for their behavior. They want to be left undisturbed and it can anger them in the extreme if the attendant comes merely into their room with a meal."[21] The term "autism," since Bleuler coined it in 1910, has undergone such migrations that today's autism is no longer recognizable in this account. Yet "other world" is what Bleuler originally meant.

In "ambitendency," patients wanted to do something and, at the same time, not to do it. This related to a postulated "splitting" of the mind. "With every drive [*Antriebe*], there comes from within or without a certain inclination to do the opposite . . . I should like to call this entire concept '*Ambitendenz*.'" So, ambitendency concerned the will. "Ambivalence," by contrast, was the notion that every *idea* had two opposing affects attaching to it, a positive one and a negative one. Bleuler called this "affective ambivalence."[22] "Ambivalence" went on to have a stellar career in psychoanalysis; "ambitendency," by contrast, became one of the postulated symptoms of catatonia and, indeed, gave rise to a clinical test: the patient gives you his hand, then hesitates and withdraws it.[23] (Bleuler may have the priority with the term "ambitendency," but as early as 1902 Wilhelm Weygandt, a staffer at Würzburg, had described the behavior as "active negativism": "The performance of a task that is directly contrary [to the requested one] may be termed 'active negativism.'" Further, "When it comes to shaking hands, this person extends only one finger, that person gives the left hand, a third reaches out the hand stretched out like a chicken [*Gigerl*]; many draw back the extended hand or touch only with their fingertips."[24])

BLEULER'S BIG BOOK (1911)

In 1911, Bleuler published his big book on schizophrenia, which placed the diagnosis definitively on the psychiatric map. Prompted by the article favorable to dementia praecox that Bleuler had published in 1902, Kraepelin's ally Gustav Aschaffenburg asked Bleuler to write a full-scale treatment of the subject for a series that Aschaffenburg was editing.[25] From this emerged the 1911 book. (Vienna psychiatrist Erwin Stransky was thereafter forever bitter that Aschaffenburg had asked Bleuler rather than himself. Stransky believed that his own concept of "intrapsychic ataxia" had preceded Bleuler's notions of "splitting" and that Bleuler had, in effect, stolen his ideas. It also irked Stransky, who was Jewish, that Bleuler had become Freud's "Showcase Aryan" [*Renommierarier*].[26])

Bleuler said that he had no interest in "refuting" Kraepelin, and he seems sooner to have revered him for his already huge reputation.[27] In several important points, the 1911 book did differ from Kraepelin. For one thing, Bleuler detached the onset from youth. For him, schizophrenia was a disease that could strike at any time in life, and he attached no particular causal importance to the period of late adolescence and early adulthood. Kraepelin, of course, had named dementia praecox on the basis of its youthful onset. Among Bleuler's patients, only 44 percent had fallen ill before age 25; among Kraepelin's, 62 percent.[28]

Another difference was the much broader scope of Bleuler's schizophrenia. Among accessory symptoms were "bursts of anger," mood disorders of any color, heavy drinking, and a "lowered state of consciousness." Kraepelin's dementia praecox seemed frequent indeed, but Bleuler's schizophrenia threatened to become an illness that would gobble up all of psychiatry. This was already visible at the Burghölzli before Bleuler's retirement in 1927. Said Max Müller, a prominent Swiss psychiatrist who had trained at the Bli, "With Bleuler it was sometimes a real addiction, seeing schizoids and schizophrenias everywhere. . . . His whole comportment, the way he behaved with a patient, consisted of suggestive questioning to demonstrate that the patient really had hallucinated, which would seal the diagnosis of schizophrenia and finish off the case."[29]

The point that differentiated Bleuler's schizophrenia from Kraepelin's dementia praecox is that schizophrenia was a very common affliction. "It is very important to realize, that there are many transitions to normal, and that the mild cases, the latent schizophrenias with symptoms that are little pronounced, are far more numerous than the manifest forms."[30]

The book traced in detail many points that Bleuler had adumbrated in the two articles in 1908. "Schizophrenia" was the preferred term "because I wish to demonstrate that the splitting [*Spaltung*] of the various psychic functions is one of the most important qualities."[31] The discussion distinguished notably between the "basic symptoms" of schizophrenia such as disturbances in the mental associations, affectivity, and ambivalence, and the "accessory symptoms," which were largely equivalent to Kraepelin's own symptom list: delusions, hallucinations, and the group of catatonic symptoms.

Thus began Bleuler's elaborate psychological analysis that would link the clinical symptoms to hypothesized intrapsychic processes; this culminated in an almost hundred-page analysis of "the theory of the symptoms" at the end of the book that laid bare the presumed psychic roots of such disorders as "autism," "catatonic symptoms," and "distortions of reality" that had now all become "secondary symptoms." "Ambitendency of the will" figured among the symptoms of schizophrenia but was not yet linked to catatonia.[32] Of autism, Bleuler wrote, "The autistic thought content [of the fantasy world] remains incapable of being changed and represents for the patient the full reality, while the subjective reality of the real world may drop to zero."[33] Bleuler found such speculation of greatest importance, and, in 1912, as co-editor (with Freud) of the *Psychoanalytic Yearbook*, he penned a lengthy article on "autistic thinking" that dilated upon the "dream world" theme and invoked sexual motives: "Autistic thinking, at least in pathological cases, serves predominantly erotic complexes."[34] Subsequent generations of more critical observers dismissed the primary–secondary distinction as clinically useless. Paul Hoch at the New York State Psychiatric Institute said later, "Most of the diagnoses [of schizophrenia] are based on secondary symptoms and not on primary symptoms ... because the diagnostician has no clear conceptualization of any of the basic standards."[35]

For all the handwaving about the "schizophrenias" plural, in Bleuler's view, there was the core illness of one schizophrenia. Discerning different schizophrenias within the main type remained aspirational. Bleuler said, "The reduction [*Zerlegung*] of the schizophrenia group into its component parts is a task for the future. . . . Within this group we recognize no natural boundaries; what people have proposed for boundaries up to now are current clinical pictures, not diseases."[36]

BLEULER'S CATATONIA

"Under the catatonic symptoms are grouped phenomena that Kahlbaum found in his catatonia," Bleuler said. Bleuler's package of catatonic motor disorders was the same as Kahlbaum's: "motility issues, stupor, mutism, stereotypies, mannerisms, negativism, automatic obedience, spontaneous automatism, impulsivity." He added, "More than half of the schizophrenics in our asylums demonstrate chronic or transitory catatonic symptoms." All symptoms were attributive to "the psyche."[37]

Bleuler added "impulsivity" to the growing list of symptoms that could be considered catatonic.[38] For Bleuler, one subgroup of impulsives often acted violently to release growing inner tension. In another subgroup of "impulsive affective actions. . . . The patients become mildly agitated; the splitting of associations means that inhibiting factors are often not activated; thus all kinds of ill-considered actions occur, physical attacks, immoderate cursing, and pranks, the sudden leaving of the workplace, bouts of drinking, etc." Bleuler added a "buffoon-psychosis" to the list of accessory symptoms of agitated catatonia (*Faxenpsychose*, from "*Faxe*," or prank). In the same manner that Bleuler enlarged Kraepelin's dementia praecox, he also expanded catatonia, which now included a hyperkinetic form of clowning around, taking off from work, and going drinking.[39]

Yet the core of what Bleuler described was the full-blown disease of "Kahlbaum's catatonia," as Kraepelin had first designated it. The patients had the full panoply of delusions and hallucinations, and, though recovery or remission could eventuate at any stage, it was quite normal for the patients to remain in a negativistic stupor for years as they passed into the end-state.[40]

By the time of Bleuler's 1916 psychiatry textbook, one sees how very wide his definition of catatonia had become. "In catatonia there are disorders of the will. . . . What we call 'will' appears of its own accord to have run along false pathways. The patients cannot do what the conscious part of their ego wants; they cannot will [*wollen*] what they would like; these behaviors are not automatic but conscious. In particular, the following disorders may be included: hyperkinesis, akinesis, impulsive actions, automatic behavior, negativism, obsessive-compulsive behavior."[41]

"Schizophrenia" became wider still: "To schizophrenia," Bleuler said, "belong many of the mixed melancholias and manias of other schools; . . . most of the hallucinatory confusions; much of what is termed elsewhere 'amentia'; part of the disorders that have been assigned to acute delirium; Wernicke's motility psychoses; primary and secondary dementias of no definite type; most of the paranoias of the other schools; namely all of the hysterical insanities; almost all of the incurable 'hypochondrias'; many 'nervous' and obsessive-compulsive patients, and the impulsive." And therewith the list was not complete; Bleuler went on to include in schizophrenia the "juvenile and masturbatory forms . . . . "[42] All this embraced quite a large chunk of psychiatry. Wilmanns said in 1922, "Bleuler's schizophrenic basic symptoms include all transitions to normal psychic life, and his schizophrenia reaches much farther than Kraepelin's dementia praecox into the non-psychotic life of the mind—into psychopathy, into abnormal character qualities, and into the normal." As for Bleuler's "latent schizophrenia," Wilmanns mocked, "Yeah, you can't really exclude a latent schizophrenia in anyone, just as little as a latent tuberculosis."[43]

So now, Bleuler and Kraepelin were saying there is a real disease called schizophrenia and its symptoms are mental "splitting" and the autistic construction of a fantasy world. How could this possibly be invalidated? It troubled few at the time that there was little evidence for any of these assertions about things "splitting" in the mind, and "ambivalence," otherwise, was a normal human quality. Later, there were eyebrows raised. Said Joseph Zubin, who founded the biometric study of psychiatric disease in the United States in 1959, at the New York State Psychiatric Institute, "We took the old dementia praecox concept and broadened it through Bleuler's efforts . . . to the kind of spectrum that makes it impossible to try to do anything specific with it as a disease entity. I can't understand why that happened."[44] By Zubin's time, "schizophrenia" had become a diagnosis of rock-solid certainty, and catatonia was buried even further within this granite tomb.

DID BLEULER ADD OR SUBTRACT?

How much did Bleuler add, or subtract, from the concepts of catatonia of Kahlbaum and Kraepelin? In retrospect, Bleuler's imagination was great, but his science was poor. He brought in psychoanalysis, a concept that Kraepelin despised. He democratized the diagnosis of catatonia, which Kahlbaum and Kraepelin both considered a severe psychosis. And he enlarged "schizophrenia" to the point that it became the final resting diagnosis for almost all chronically ill patients. When the patients with bipolar and unipolar depression failed to remit, they ended up in the schizophrenia box.

Thus, Kraepelin's and Bleuler's efforts gave rise to an immense "schizophrenia" literature, an industry that continues even today. It is an outpouring that can be compared only to the enormous "hysteria" industry that existed before DSM-III abolished the diagnosis in 1980. The effect is striking: one moment the profession believes implicitly in a disease so huge as to dominate the literature; the next moment the disease no longer exists. We have not quite reached that point with schizophrenia. In 2013, DSM-5 abolished the subtypes, and, as the component parts of "schizophrenia" such as catatonia and paranoia are peeled away, little more will remain than the concept of chronic psychosis of youth that Hecker described as "hebephrenia." And even that may vanish as we discover that the long-term prognosis of youthful-onset psychosis is actually quite favorable.

6

KIDNAPPED!

People are talking about dementia praecox in all the university psychiatric hospitals and asylums; it is being passionately discussed in the German, American, French psychiatric press—and in our own [Italian]. It has been in recent years the favorite theme in national and regional neurology and psychiatric meetings in England, Germany and France.[1]
—Sante de Sanctis, professor of psychiatry in Rome, 1906

Catatonia was kidnapped by dementia praecox and schizophrenia, the Bonnie and Clyde of the diagnosis world. For the next century, the two diagnoses would be the face of catatonia. Kraepelin and Bleuler were the master builders of psychiatry, and their work lasted, unusual in medicine, for a hundred years.

But schizophrenia and dementia praecox were so vague and unspecific as to be little more than signposts of something going seriously wrong in psychic life. Catatonia, by contrast, was a specific combination of motor and mental symptoms. Making catatonia a "subtype" of schizophrenia relegated it to the same incoherence. Accordingly, in the century following the publication in 1911 of Bleuler's big book, catatonia hovered on the margin of visibility. Most authors blithely accepted the catatonic subtype while according it little importance; a few thought it independent, and it was these few who made a difference after catatonia started to become treatable in the 1930s. "Schizophrenia," of course, has never been very treatable because it doesn't exist. It is a wastebasket for the unclassifiable and untreatable psychiatric ill.[2] And it was a disaster of historic proportions that catatonia was thrown into this wastebasket.

THE PRAETORIAN GUARD

How could this intellectual error have happened? One reason was the immense personal authority of Kraepelin and of the "Heidelberg School" that he figuratively founded. There was never a physical Heidelberg School apart from the University Psychiatric Hospital in Heidelberg in the Voss-strasse (which still stands today). But, conceptually, Kraepelin's students in turn became authoritative figures and argued for the solidity of the master's work.

We have already met some of these disciples. Gustav Aschaffenburg and Kraepelin were close personal friends. Aschaffenburg, 29, had won his Habilitation at Heidelberg under Kraepelin's supervision in 1895, proceeding then to Halle. Aschaffenburg was Jewish; Kraepelin was somewhat anti-Semitic, yet Aschaffenburg trusted Kraepelin to help him find a job.[3] So when, in 1898, Aschaffenburg was among the earliest to weigh in on behalf of Kraepelin's new dementia praecox, it may have been from a sense of obligation. Kraepelin made catatonia a subtype of dementia praecox in 1899, but Aschaffenburg encouraged him a year earlier to do so. As we have seen, in 1898, Kraepelin said that catatonia and hebephrenia were very similar and possibly represented the same subtype of dementia praecox. But the psychosis of catatonia was special. It was not a mania, not a paranoia, "but rather just a specifically colored catatonic excitement, delusional ideas on a catatonic basis." "Dementia" could include various outcomes, including "deepest *Verblödung*" (the German term for severe dementia): "patients who never again awaken from their loss of contact. Mute, dirty, and negativistic, they sit dully in the corners of chronic care facilities, in forced postures, repeating monotonously for hours the same movements, cutting the same grimaces." On the other hand, we might find them living in the community, "someone who earlier was a merchant reduced to a factory worker, the teacher to a laborer, the student to a clerk, the worker to a vagabond."[4] Kraepelin's own views were more catastrophic, and others reproached him for having stamped "madness" across the entire face of psychiatric illness. Aschaffenburg was a faithful lieutenant, with different opinions about some matters, but a forceful and influential advocate of Kraepelin's dementia praecox.

Georg Ilberg, whom we met previously, had trained with Kraepelin at Heidelberg in the mid-1890s, then went on to serve as an assistant physician at the Sonnenstein asylum (ultimately becoming its director in 1910). In 1898, he endorsed the subtypes and noted that they all ended in dementia. One new note, however, was Ilberg's comment that hebephrenia and catatonia might also exist in very mild forms and that these patients went on to become vagrants, beggars, or emigrants to America.[5] This becomes a major theme: apparently recovered patients who were not really restored and harbored traces of their illness for years (in 1898 as well, Ilberg privately told Kraepelin that he agreed that stereotypies had an invariably downhill course: "All previous remissions . . . sooner or later turn out to be of a transitory nature."[6]) (Later in the book we see that successfully *treated* patients often become entirely symptom free between episodes.)

Karl Wilmanns, 29, came to Heidelberg in 1902, as an assistant physician at the very end of Kraepelin's tenure, becoming a ward chief under Nissl in 1904 after Kraepelin had left for Munich. In 1906, Wilmanns wrote his Habilitation under Nissl, and, in 1907, he suggested that catatonic symptoms appeared in manic-depressive insanity in addition to dementia praecox.[7] Wilmanns succeeded Nissl as professor of psychiatry in Heidelberg in 1918, and, under Wilmanns' regimen, much more manic-depression was diagnosed than previously. Yet Wilmanns approved of the split between dementia praecox and manic-depressive insanity, and even later, in 1922, as he turned his pen again to "schizophrenia," he said that dementia praecox, as a "disease of its own," lay at the core even though the subtypes were a handful of smoke: "Let's admit that Kraepelin's dementia praecox is a group of diseases that is held together only through external similarities; nonetheless its core is a unitary disease [*eine Krankheitseinheit*]."[8] He was a loyal trooper.

Wilmanns did not accept the subtypes. He argued in private to Kraepelin in 1907: "A sample of [dementia praecox] patients turns up a large number who have misdiagnoses. Many of the catatonics who were considered incurable and demented have recovered sufficiently, often after years, that even with the best will it is impossible to detect a defect."[9] In that same year, Wilmanns stated that many catatonics did respond to treatment and that all were not "burned out craters." "Even apparently advanced catatonic dementias may still experience substantial recoveries."[10]

Finally, Robert Gaupp belonged to the Heidelberg core group under Kraepelin. Gaupp had been trained in Tübingen, yet, in 1900, Kraepelin brought him to Heidelberg, where he wrote his Habilitation; in 1904, Gaupp followed Kraepelin to Munich, becoming then in 1906, at age 36, professor of psychiatry in Tübingen. In 1903, Gaupp said the Heidelberg data showed that even apparent "recoveries" of catatonic patients sooner or later ended in dementia, which was exactly what Kraepelin preached. Yet, Gaupp added, all psychomotor disorders were not necessarily catatonia.[11]

Aschaffenburg, Ilberg, Gaupp, and Wilmanns, trained or worked directly under Kraepelin and became powerful figures in their own right. And even under Nissl and Wilmanns, the "Heidelberg School" continued to be loyal to Kraepelin's dementia praecox.

Outside of Germany today, such names as Ilberg and Wilmanns have been forgotten. The member of the Heidelberg School who has not been forgotten is Karl Jaspers, who published in 1913 the foundational volume of modern psychopathology and went on to become a world-famous philosopher. Jaspers graduated in medicine from Heidelberg in 1908, then trained in psychiatry under Nissl. His "General Psychopathology" (*Allgemeine Psychopathologie*), written at age 30, was his Habilitation and marked a new departure in psychiatric theory: making patients' phenomenology the focus of study rather than Kraepelin's objectivizing approach to symptoms and diseases. Jaspers situated catatonic agitation somewhere between psychiatry and neurology. "[The patients] appear to be aimless, without any euphoric or anxious affect or any other mental condition. These motionless patients have sometimes the appearance of Egyptian statues, or of lifeless machines. Their movements are situated between motor inhibitions on the one side, which may be investigated neurologically; and on the other side we have meaningful emotional expression that one might approach empathically [*verständliche Ausdrucksbewegungen*]."[12] Thus, for Jaspers, catatonia was a mixture of neurological activity at the physiological level and behavior that one could understand and sympathize with psychologically. There is no good English translation for Jaspers's concept of patient actions that are "*verständlich*," but it means that, in an empathic leap, the investigator can interpret the current symptom picture in the patient's past personal events.

It would be tedious to review each of the Heidelberg graduates under Nissl who endorsed the dementia praecox concept, with or without subtypes. One, Willi Mayer-Gross, we encounter later after his flight to England in 1933. (In 1932, Mayer-Gross produced an authoritative account of schizophrenia, together with its catatonic form, in the massive Bumke series of handbooks; it was a contribution that would have stamped the field for decades had the Nazis not seized power the following year.[13]) We are aware of no Heidelberg clinician, except perhaps Wilmanns, who rejected the Kraepelinian concept of catatonia as a dementia-praecox subtype. And some of the defenders had more than a bit of the Old German Dogmatism. Martin Pappenheim, a Heidelberg junior clinician, argued in 1908 that if the patient recovered, it would constitute ipso facto evidence that the original diagnosis of dementia praecox was "in error."[14] More hubristic than this it doesn't get. The point is that this group around Kraepelin constituted a powerful disease lobby on behalf of dementia praecox-schizophrenia.

And the almost universal adoption of catatonia as a subtype owes much to the relentless flacking of these workers.

BACKLASH: SUPPORT FOR CATATONIA AS A SEPARATE DISEASE

Kahlbaum, who died in 1899 without stating his views, would never have consented to the subtype argument, and neither did many other influential clinicians. They were, in the end, overwhelmed by the "subtype" vogue, but the very presence of these insubordinates shows that catatonia *sui generis* had some advocates.

Theodor Ziehen, one of the founders of child psychiatry, told the International Congress of Medicine in 1900 that a catatonic variety of adolescent psychosis, "characterized by stereotypic movements and postures" had been proposed by various authorities as a form of dementia praecox. "This strikes me as impermissible," he said, "because catatonia also occurs in later years and dementia praecox often occurs without catatonic symptoms."[15] (Yet by the time of his textbook, in 1915, when Ziehen had temporarily abandoned academic medicine and was a practicing psychiatrist in Wiesbaden, he had ceded to the vogue for "schizophrenia" and agreed that a "catatonic variety" existed.[16])

In 1904, Otto Binswanger, professor of psychiatry in Jena (a member of the Binswanger dynasty and brother of Robert Binswanger, founder of the private nervous clinic in Kreuzlingen, Switzerland, where "Anna O"—of psychoanalytic fame—and Russian ballet dancer Vaslav Nijinsky were interned), dissertated upon "disturbances of action," which included Kahlbaum's catatonia, with no reference to Kraepelin's schizophrenia.[17] In later editions of this textbook (of which Binswanger wrote about a quarter), other authors did discuss schizophrenia, yet Binswanger remained an influential disbeliever.[18]

The principal scoffer about dementia praecox—and upholder of catatonia as an independent disease—was Vienna psychiatry professor Richard von Krafft-Ebing, at the time of his death in 1902 one of the world's most distinguished psychiatrists. He did not even deign to recognize the term "dementia praecox" (Bleuler had not yet coined "schizophrenia"), but was a complete enthusiast about Kahlbaum's catatonia, which he believed to be a "degenerative psychoneurosis."[19] Krafft-Ebing did accept Hecker's hebephrenia, but of Kraepelin's dementia praecox, not a word. Had he lived beyond 1902, would he have endorsed Kraepelin's creation as virtually everyone else did?

An early advocate in the years 1909–12 of the view that schizophrenia and catatonia were different was Polish psychiatrist Maurycy Urstein. He trained in Germany at Heidelberg and Munich, practiced in Berlin at the Schweizerhof private asylum, then had an office in Warsaw—until his disappearance in 1940 in the Holocaust. An undeservedly ignored figure, Urstein subsequently became briefly known for the "Urstein psychoses,"[20] psychoses with a cyclical course developing into a defect state.[21] In two big books on dementia praecox (1909) and catatonia (1912), Urstein set out to demolish the Kraepelinian system, claiming that manic-depressive insanity often turned into catatonia and might end in dementia.[22] Catatonia thus became for Urstein the master diagnosis and dementia praecox an epiphenomenon. One of Urstein's critics, Georges Dreyfus, an attack dog of the Heidelberg school, said mockingly that Urstein had set out to show "the complete fiasco of the psychiatric vision of Kraepelin and his acolytes."[23] (The idea being, well, of course, Urstein failed.) Urstein didn't like the term "dementia praecox," but distinguished between catatonia, which was often recoverable, and dementia praecox-hebephrenia, which ended catastrophically. Urstein observed that, "For someone who recognizes the Kraepelinian doctrine and makes diagnoses on that basis, a catatonic, demented manic-depressive should be an impossible thing." But for Urstein, it was reasonable that depressives became demented and that depression turned into catatonia. Urstein thus used catatonia to dismantle the Kraepelinian firewall between mood and psychosis. He concluded, "Now it is time for catatonia to come into its own."[24]

One last doubting voice was that of Oswald Bumke, who in 1924 succeeded Kraepelin in the psychiatry chair in Munich. There was little love lost between the two men. And while Bumke gave plenty of space to "schizophrenia" in his textbook, in collegial communications he was less forthcoming. In 1924, on the verge of going to Munich, he said: "Our view of syndromes, which, it seems to us after years of clinical experience might at least be conceivable, has long been blocked by the dogma that in psychiatry only unitary diseases exist, and that the 'unity' of these diseases is always determined on the basis of course and outcome." This clearly was a dig at Kraepelin. Bumke continued, "I simply want to show today that it would be good to place the schizophrenic processes in close vicinity to the organic brain diseases. That 'dementia praecox' would thus give up even more of its unity is, it seems to me, the likely result. I merely think that schizophrenia should be dissolved in the exogenous kinds of mental reactions [cause coming from outside] and not belong to the psychopathic constitutions."[25] By contrast, Bumke was a firm advocate of catatonia.[26]

Kraepelin died in 1926, leaving to Johannes Lange, 35—a staffer at the Schwabinger Krankenhaus, the clinical arm of the German Research Institute that Kraepelin had recently founded—the task of completing the ninth edition of Kraepelin's textbook. Lange might have made sense as a collaborator because, in 1922, in his Habilitation thesis directed by Kraepelin, he had written about catatonia in manic disorders; Lange acknowledged, however, that not many catatonia cases had a schizophrenic "coloration."[27] As Kraepelin and Lange went to work on the ninth edition, Kraepelin himself managed to get through the section on neurological psychiatry—head wounds and brain diseases—before expiring. Kraepelin did not complete any of the clinical psychiatry sections that had made earlier editions of the textbook such compelling reading.[28] Lange finished drafting Kraepelin's neurology sections and took over responsibility for the "general psychiatry" volume that laid out basic principles of psychopathology without getting into disease classification. In any event, Lange had a poor opinion of the idea of specific diseases and produced something that would have been not at all to Kraepelin's liking. The ninth edition appeared in 1927, safely a year after Kraepelin's death. It is of interest that Lange in his chapters had virtually nothing to say about either manic-depressive insanity or dementia praecox; he did, however, concede that a "catatonic syndrome" seemed to exist independent of dementia praecox.[29] Thus, as far as Lange was concerned, the subtypes were uninteresting. Five years later, the Nazi seizure of power closed down this entire discussion. Lange, who had long previously acquired a racist interest in genetics, went on to become the professor of psychiatry in Breslau and died prematurely in 1938.

Here ends the list of contemporary opponents of dementia praecox-schizophrenia who simultaneously accepted catatonia. The story reached a provisional end with

Budapest psychiatrist Ladislaus von Meduna, the originator of chemical convulsive therapy in the 1930s, who remained a doubter. For Meduna, schizophrenia and catatonia were separate diseases. Writing in 1950, from the safety of Chicago, where he had sought refuge, Meduna said in a book on "confusional states" that "[t]he existence of Kahlbaum's catatonia as a separate disease, though repudiated by the Kraepelin-Bleulerian school, can hardly be denied."[30]

HOW MANY CATATONIA PATIENTS WERE PSYCHOTIC?

What distinguishes Kahlbaum's catatonia from the catatonic syndrome is the presence of stupor plus psychosis. And it was psychosis that led so many to accept the classification of catatonia under "schizophrenia" despite the large motor component in catatonia—which otherwise made no sense at all in the context of the hypothetical "splitting" of schizophrenia.

In 1898, Georg Ilberg, whom we met previously, said, "The diagnosis [of catatonia] is complicated in a number of cases because in the initiation of the disease and later on, the patients develop hallucinations and delusions.... The delusive ideas of the catatonics usually appear in the stage of stupor and have a depressive content.... If the patients had experienced a complex, systematic delusion—being thus deluded, or paranoid, in a psychiatric sense—they would not really be catatonics."[31] This points to a central issue: catatonics who developed psychoses often had their diagnoses changed.

At the Bicêtre Hospice, patient P had catatonia plus psychosis. P, 30, was admitted for a second time to Bicêtre in 1899. He had developed ideas of persecution, thought that his brother was about to poison him, and advanced on the brother with a knife. On the ward, he became mute, held postures for days at a time, and alternated stupor and agitation. His delusional system developed further, thinking that two families were out to rob him. He started refusing food completely and had to be fed with a nasogastric tube.

A note from P's chart: "Ordinarily, P stands upright, immobile and stiff, his arms held alongside his body, fists closed, the head forward, his eyes lowered, almost closed, his brow creased, his lips projecting outwards (*Schnauzkrampf*). He remains fixed in this attitude for hours."

P displayed negativism. "Another time, the patient spontaneously draws his handkerchief and raises his hand to blow his nose. It suffices to say to him, 'Hey, you need to blow your nose', to cause his oppositional tendency to make him stop the movement and immobilize his arm in the air with the handkerchief."

P also demonstrated hoarding (*collectionisme*): "P always has his pockets filled with old bits of paper, old newspapers that he keeps meticulously. He always carries a folded newspaper; sometimes he holds it up to his eyes, in the position of someone reading; but his eyes remain stubbornly closed and often the newspaper is held upside down."[32] P evidently had Kahlbaum's catatonia: the full raft of catatonic symptoms plus psychosis.

In 1905, Paul Albrecht, a staff psychiatrist at the Treptow/Rega asylum in Germany, identified among their dementia praecox patients 64 with catatonia. (An apparently downhill course rather than the presence of psychosis was the basis of the dementia praecox diagnosis.) Of these 64, 51 had delusive thinking and hallucinations.

"Usually [the psychosis] was only transitorily expressed, often changed, and in later disease phases was often difficult to ascertain on account of the incoherence of all expressions."[33] The point is that psychosis in catatonic patients was quite common.

TWO CATATONIAS: A DISEASE AND A SYNDROME

Fritz Freyhan, later an investigator at the US National Institute of Mental Health (NIMH), had trained with Eugen Bleuler in Zurich before the Second World War. Bleuler insisted that all the residents establish "contact" with the catatonic patients in conversation, an often arduous task. But then, after the war, the sodium Amytal interview came in and this painful contact-seeking was no longer necessary. The patients began speaking spontaneously. Freyhan recalls, "In some instances this method has a 'normalizing' effect, meaning that the patient verbalizes in a seemingly rational manner. In the case of catatonics, however, the verbalizations, not surprisingly, mostly consist of bizarre delusions."[34] This was the psychotic penumbra of Kahlbaum's catatonia.

Like a red thread, there ran from Kraepelin onward the distinction between *catatonic schizophrenia*, a psychomotor disease entity involving psychosis, stupor, and negativism and a *catatonic syndrome*, a mixture of catatonic motor symptoms that might well appear in any psychiatric or medical illness. We're thus dealing with two traditions here. In one, catatonia itself was the disease *sui generis* (but still part of "schizophrenia"); we join others in calling this Kahlbaum's catatonia. But catatonia as a truly independent disease entity virtually vanishes after the turn of the century, and, for the next hundred years, it would piggyback on the disease schizophrenia. Whether one considers the independent disease to be catatonia *sui generis* or catatonic schizophrenia, we are dealing with the one-disease tradition of Kahlbaum's catatonia.

The other tradition is the *catatonic syndrome*, found widely in medicine as well as psychiatry. An example: August Bostroem, who had been a protégé of Oswald Bumke in Munich, captured the difference between catatonia as a disease and as a syndrome clearly in 1928, in an article on "catatonic disorders" in Bumke's massive *Handbook*. He said that, after Kraepelin, "the term 'catatonic' was used either as a designation for a motor symptom complex, or more or less served as a synonym for the disease dementia praecox; and catatonic phenomena included in this sense all the symptoms that occur in dementia praecox."[35] So here, catatonia was not just a subtype but a synonym for schizophrenia, unlike the catatonic syndrome seen elsewhere. This is interesting because Bostroem, who owed nothing to Kraepelin, seems ready to make catatonia as described by Kraepelin, with its motor symptoms and psychosis, a "unitary psychosis" (*Einheitspsychose*), *the* major psychiatric illness.

Kraepelin's great inheritor was Kurt Schneider, not a graduate of the Heidelberg School but professor of psychiatry in Heidelberg after the Second World War. In 1914, Schneider, then at Cologne, separated "catatonic pictures," which can occur "in every form of mental illness," from catatonic "schizophrenia." For Schneider, "catatonia" had become almost a synonym for schizophrenia, noting that it had very little in common with Kahlbaum's original catatonia.[36] Schneider said much later that they called all patients with schizophrenic defects "Old Catatonics." It was unclear, he continued, whether they had ever been "Young Catatonics."[37] He said, "It is precisely the catatonic element that runs through all forms of dementia praecox and characterizes the clinical picture, sometimes in coarser, sometimes in finer form." This would be what we and others have been calling "Kahlbaum's catatonia." But Schneider noted that Kahlbaum's original catatonia had been "completely submerged" by Kraepelin's catatonia of dementia praecox.[38]

THE INTERNATIONAL VIEW

In no country did catatonia survive as a disease entity separate from schizophrenia. The international reception of Kraepelin's dementia praecox and Bleuler's schizophrenia was enthusiastic. All previous terms for acute psychosis gave way to dementia praecox and schizophrenia. In 1895, Philippe Chaslin at the Bicêtre in Paris surveyed the international literature, identifying 36 different terms for acute psychosis, ranging from Louis Delasiauve's *confusion hallucinatoire*, through Carl Westphal's "acute primary insanity" (*acute primäre Verrücktheit*,) to American psychiatrist Edward Spitzka's "acute hallucinatory confusion."[39] *All 36 were forgotten as dementia praecox triumphed!* (Chaslin, quite misjudging the future, failed to include "dementia praecox" on the list.) By the 1930s, madness had become dementia praecox and schizophrenia. But what of catatonia?

France

In France, the general trend was to accept "dementia praecox" and "schizophrenia" but to carve out large exclusions for the chronic psychoses that did not deteriorate. Such diagnoses as the "chronic systematized delusional disorders" that Valentin Magnan proposed in the late 1880s became current in France but were not adopted internationally.[40]

As for dementia praecox, it was, after all, the French who coined the term. Bénédict-Augustin Morel introduced "*la démence précoce*" in 1852. Why would the French have opposed the concept, or, at least, the narrow concept of deteriorating psychosis with onset in adolescence?

In 1888, Jules Séglas, a psychiatrist in training at the Salpêtrière Hospice, and Philippe Chaslin, his friend and counterpart at Bicêtre Hospice, discounted Kahlbaum's catatonia as a specific disease. They rejected Kahlbaum's view that *Attonität* was found only in catatonia and said, "The great majority of published observations of melancholia with stupor show no traces of catatonic phenomena."[41] Following this unpromising beginning, in 1895, in a book on *Clinical Varieties of Madness*, Jacques Roubinovitch, an attending psychiatrist in the Paris system, devoted an entire chapter to catatonia, delivering the solemn verdict that it had no status as a disease. "As you see, none of the symptoms taken one by one has anything pathognomonic and when we nonetheless find a number of these symptoms in the same patient, their coincidence is purely accidental and constitutes in no manner a syndrome on a clinical, physiological or anatomical basis."[42] (In his doctoral dissertation in 1899 on pediatric psychiatry, Marcel Manheimer had a slightly more positive appreciation, silent on Kraepelin's dementia praecox but mentioning catatonia as a real disease in children.[43])

It was *la démence précoce*, meaning the original Morelian version, that dominated the early discussions.[44] The Germans played no role. At a congress in 1890, Eugène Charpentier at Bicêtre dilated upon "*les démences précoces*" beginning in adolescence and including epilepsy and neurosyphilis. Mixed in among these adolescent diseases were patients who "continually rub their hands together or against a part of their bodies or even better alongside the cranium to the point that the hair stops growing . . . partial muscular rigidity. . . . They avoid looking at the person they are speaking to; questioned, they turn their head and eyes away." Some, he said, were "absolutely mute, contenting themselves with repetitive gestures." Charpentier made no reference to catatonia, and the concept clearly had not penetrated to the Bicêtre.[45]

The first breakthrough of Kraepelinian dementia praecox in France, together with the subtypes, was the review in 1900 by Paul Sérieux, a staff psychiatrist at the Ville-Evrard asylum in Paris, of the fifth edition (1899) of Kraepelin's textbook. The big advantage, said Sérieux, of Kraepelin's attention to course and outcome was giving "the prognosis of psychoses the certainty that had been previously lacking." Sérieux reviewed the entire Kraepelinian nosology, summarizing without commentary the chapter on dementia praecox and its subtypes.[46] Then, two years later, in 1902, Sérieux ventured an assessment of Kraepelin's dementia praecox that made Sérieux the sherpa of German-style dementia praecox in France. Rather curiously, Sérieux incorporated a stage-type progression that echoed more of Kahlbaum than Kraepelin. But Sérieux gave French clinicians an exact account of what they would encounter when they looked for catatonia. This first such description in France took catatonia seriously as a disease of its own—as a form of another disease, but nonetheless a real disease—not just a misplaced expropriation of the symptoms of other diseases that had been assembled as something new (as dementia praecox had previously often been pooh-poohed). Sérieux praised "the value of this recent conquest of contemporary mental pathology. More and more, one tries to substitute, in the place of purely symptomatic groupings, clinical types with a well-described course. . . . It is thus appropriate to stop denying to dementia praecox the legitimate place that it deserves in the nosological schema."[47]

In 1902, Jules Séglas at Bicêtre articulated some of the refinements of Kraepelin's diagnosis. For Kraepelin's doctrine of the "will," Séglas added a French touch: the common denominator behind the symptoms, he said, was aboulia (*l'aboulie*), or weakness of will, a term that Pierre Janet was in the process of popularizing in France. Séglas distinguished between the "catatonic syndrome," as seen in a number of diseases, and "*la catatonie de Kahlbaum*," which Séglas saw, not as an independent disease itself, but as a part of dementia praecox.[48] Later, it would require little to detach catatonia from dementia praecox and make it free-standing.

Now that Sérieux and Séglas had stamped approval on the German dementia praecox, it won wider acceptance among French psychiatrists, quite surprisingly in a country hostile to things German. When Raoul Leroy, chief psychiatrist at Ville-Evrard, presented his patient Yvonne, 20, to the Clinical Society of Mental Medicine in 1908, his diagnosis was catatonia. Because of her mutism, the clinicians at Ville-Evrard couldn't really investigate her mental state. Over the next seven years, her symptoms remained the same: not psychotic but "a true automaton, a true articulated doll, maintaining the most improbable positions," and mute. Then, in the fall of 1915, she developed tuberculosis. But three weeks before her death, a change happened: "Yvonne was transformed: speaking readily, interested in everything . . . the catatonia had disappeared" and "she gave the impression of having a normal mentality." Interesting in the case, however, is not the transformation in Yvonne, but in Leroy's diagnostic assessment. He said she was "inhibited, dulled, stuporous and apathetic," and her final diagnosis was dementia praecox.[49] Clearly, among these French clinicians, catatonia was being pushed aside by dementia praecox.

One large exception to the disappearance of the diagnosis of catatonia in France is the work of Henri Baruk, chief psychiatrist of the French state asylum at Charenton, which he and his students conducted in the 1930s. With electromyography they established that the mind was implicated in the "psychomotor" aspects of movement in catatonia. Baruk determined in catatonic stupor that "Their will is not free and the patient finds himself compelled to act as if under the influence of some force that commands him and that he cannot resist. This force sometimes takes the form of a command hallucination." One female patient later reported voices ordering her to remain immobile. "That's why I contracted my muscles with all my power."[50] Baruk and Henri Claude, the professor of psychiatry at the Ste. Anne Hospital (where the professorship of clinical psychiatry was located), collaborated in 1928 on the use of the barbiturate combination drug Somnifen in catatonia (which had no therapeutic effect).[51] From 1928 on, Baruk and the Dutch physiologist and psychiatrist Herman De Jong undertook experimental research on catatonia with the alkaloid bulbocapnine, duplicating in animals many of the symptoms of humans, together with emotional expressions.[52] Baruk accepted the diagnosis of "catatonic dementia praecox," but he was highly dubious about "schizophrenia" as an entity[53] and dedicated a lifetime of research to catatonia *sui generis*.

After the Second World War, Jean Delay, now in the psychiatry chair at Ste. Anne, investigated the treatment of catatonia with various agents including the amphetamines.[54] So it is not the case that interest in catatonia in France expired. Yet it was almost always seen in the context of dementia praecox or schizophrenia.

United Kingdom

Catalepsy had long been recognized in Britain, as elsewhere. The 1888 article by Séglas and Chaslin was translated into English and published in *Brain* the following year.[55] In 1892, Daniel Hack Tuke's *Dictionary of Psychological Medicine* gave a definition of catalepsy that would have been recognizable anywhere: "An intermittent neurosis, characterized by the patient's inability to change the position of a limb, while another person can place the muscles in a state of flexion or contraction as he will (*flexibilitas cerea*). The patient is unable to speak. Insensibility is common. . . . The mental functions are to a great extent or altogether suspended in relation to the external world." The entry, written by Tuke himself, went on to dilate upon the condition in some detail.[56]

Catatonia, by contrast, got a rather mixed reception in the *Dictionary*, in an entry written by Clemens Neisser. Neisser had been an initial enthusiast—or perhaps he merely wished to demonstrate his learning to this English audience, as he mentioned Kahlbaum's *Gruppirung* of 1863 and in general praised Kahlbaum as "the first to give us an objective and clinical symptomatology." As for "Katatonia," Neisser said, "Kahlbaum's scheme has been rejected by many renowned authors." And perhaps it was not even "a special disorder."[57]

Lewis C. Bruce, an Australian psychiatrist presenting to a London meeting in July 1903, provided an early touchdown for catatonia. He considered it "an acute toxic disease with a definite onset and course," then listed the standard symptoms.

The reception was enthusiastic. Robert Jones, who managed a private asylum, said, "I am astonished to see the number of stuporous cases which have come under my care recently. . . . My experience goes back nearly a quarter of a century, and it was quite uncommon to have cases of katatonia and dementia praecox many years ago, but now they have become comparatively common." William Lloyd Andriezen, pathologist and medical officer at the prestigious West Riding Asylum in Wakefield, found it "worthy of inclusion in our system of classification." And Frederick Walker Mott, pathologist and clinician who helped establish the Maudsley Hospital as a psychiatric institute after the First World War, said that Bruce, who had done experimental research as well, "is to be heartily congratulated on a move in the right direction."[58] These were not inconsiderable figures.

Historians R. M. Ion and M. D. Beer have given us an account of the rather slow reception of dementia praecox in textbooks and journals before the First World War, without touching on catatonia. Bleuler's schizophrenia, it appears, was ignored, as no English translation was available.[59]

David K. Henderson, later professor of psychiatry in Edinburgh, whom one authority judged "the most eminent psychiatrist in this country, and probably in Europe, between the two world wars," had studied with Kraepelin in Munich and Adolf Meyer in Baltimore and, during the First World War, was an assistant psychiatrist at the Royal Mental Hospital in Glasgow. In 1916, he wrote a powerful endorsement of catatonia. The article planted the disorder right onto the middle of the British map, without claiming that it was a subtype of dementia praecox. (Unsurprisingly as a Meyer student, he endorsed Meyer's vague and antiscientific views about every case being special).[60]

Not being great systematizers, the British did not dissertate on whether catatonia was a subset of dementia praecox and schizophrenia, but they certainly used the clinical diagnosis of catatonia. Yet schizophrenia did begin to march in, and, in 1928, Hubert J. Norman, superintendent of the private asylum Camberwell House in London, said that among the symptoms of "schizophrenia" was waxy rigidity of the "catatonic state."[61]

Catatonia became much more firmly a subtype of schizophrenia in the UK when Willy Mayer-Gross—who fled Heidelberg in 1933 for England (he ended in Scotland)—published in 1954 with two English collaborators what became the main English textbook of psychiatry after the Second World War. The huge schizophrenia chapter contained a long section on "catatonic schizophrenia," with various supposedly schizophrenic patients displaying the diagnostic features of catatonia[62]. Therewith, Mayer-Gross brought British psychiatry right in line with German.

United States

Psychiatrists in the United States, especially under the influence of Adolf Meyer at Johns Hopkins University, warmed quickly to dementia praecox. By contrast, writes Richard Noll, a foremost historian of the subject, "Americans were slow to welcome schizophrenia."[63] Indeed, Noll sees a social function of the dementia-praecox diagnosis that may have been absent in other lands where psychiatry breathed more the spirit of science than of desperation, "Dementia praecox was the vehicle through which American psychiatry reentered general medicine," said Noll.[64] Not until 1950 was Bleuler's 1911 schizophrenia book even translated into English.[65]

Early accounts of "dementia" in young people tended to bow to Kraepelin's dementia praecox while remaining silent on catatonia. In 1901, George P. Sprague, superintendent of the High Oaks Sanatorium in Lexington, Kentucky, described "primary dementia" as "a grouping based upon the teachings of Kraepelin." The clinician might see symptoms as the patient "rapidly becomes confused, refuses food, becomes mute, or at least ignores questions, neglects his person, removes his clothing, resists every attention and may even pass into . . . a stuporous condition with catalepsy." Sprague added that verbigeration, negativism, "and peculiar attitudes and movements" might also enter the picture. Could this be catatonia? Sprague was silent on the subject.[66]

There were two big exceptions to the American refusal to countenance catatonia as a separate diagnosis; they were comparable to Baruk in France. In 1913, George H. Kirby, an attending psychiatrist at the Manhattan State Hospital on Wards Island in New York City, argued that catatonic symptoms, especially stupor, were more common in manic-depressive illness than in "deteriorating psychosis." "Marked catatonic syndromes may appear in otherwise typical manic-depressive cases. In some cases a catatonic attack apparently replaces the depression in a circular psychosis. . . . There can be little doubt that Kraepelin over-valued catatonic manifestations as evidence of a deteriorating psychosis, and that many of these cases have served to unduly swell the dementia praecox group."[67]

Eight years later, in 1921, August Hoch, who followed Kirby at Wards Island, built on Kirby's work in a book on *Benign Stupors*. On the basis of 40 cases, he said there were two kinds of stupor: *deep stupor*, meaning the cessation of activity as seen in the catatonic depression of manic-depressive insanity, and *stupor reaction*, a lesser version. He compared the two to the difference between mania and hypomania. Both kinds of stupor, he said, had a good prognosis and were part of manic-depressive insanity, as Kirby had argued.[68] Hoch died before his book was completed, but, unfortunately for his historical reputation, in 1935 Hyman Rachlin, an attending psychiatrist at Wards Island (later at Hillside Hospital on Long Island) went back and looked at the subsequent course of 13 of Hoch's supposedly benign-stupor patients (from Hoch's description, he was unable to identify the others). "The study reveals that the greater number of these cases have suffered from psychoses which have had unfavorable outcomes," he found. "There seems little reason to believe that the stupor described by Hoch is fundamentally different from catatonic stupors [in schizophrenia]."[69]

With the exception of these admittedly dim points of light, the rest of American psychiatry was overwhelmingly committed to the theory that catatonia was a subtype of schizophrenia. One example among many: Daniel C. Main, the clinical director of St. Elizabeths Hospital in Washington DC, a government psychiatric hospital, commented in 1923 on "the bizarre delusional ideas, the negativism, the muscular tensions, the untidiness, the refusal to cooperate, the wild excitement and the deep stupors" of patients with "catatonic schizophrenia. . . . The routine treatment in the past has been to shut them in a room when they were excited, feed them when they were stuporous and thank God and discharge them when they recovered, which some of them did for no assignable reason."[70]

The many émigré psychiatrists who, after 1933, found shelter in the United States were composed of two contingents. The psychoanalysts had little interest in catatonia and, led by Silvano Arieti, himself an émigré from Mussolini's Italy, steered the American discussion in the direction of the theory of schizophrenia and of the neuroses.[71]

A considerable number of non-psychoanalytic émigrés had been very much under the influence of the Heidelberg School of phenomenology yet found the American audience almost entirely unfamiliar with these views. Ulrich H. Peters, who has studied the post-1933 situation, writes, "The émigrés who adhered to the [Heidelberger] camp, found a more complex situation, one little comprehensible to them, than was the case in other areas of knowledge."[72]

Yet, given the inadequacy of hospital statistics, differentiating among pure catatonic cases, catatonic depression, and catatonic deteriorating psychosis is a difficult proposition. Hospital statistics on the frequency of the catatonic "subtype" are virtually worthless. Whereas in the mid-1930s in Massachusetts, 30 percent of the new admissions for schizophrenia were classed as catatonics, in Illinois, only 2.7 percent were. Commented one student, in Massachusetts it was the agitated patients who received the diagnosis "catatonia"; in Illinois clinicians would look for catalepsy.[73]

Nor was there a separate place for catatonia in the classification systems used in American psychiatric hospitals. In the *Statistical Manual for the Use of Institutions for the Insane*, published in 1918, there was a place for "dementia praecox" and its four subtypes (the "catatonic type" meant negativism plus stupor and excitement)[74]. A successive edition, published in 1936, changed nothing, save to add "schizophrenia" in parentheses to "dementia praecox."[75] Another big compilation in these years said the exact same thing.[76]

By the mid-1950s, the American concept of "schizophrenia" diverged profoundly from the British and the Continental. Schizophrenia and its subtypes had ceased to be defined by the symptoms, as Charles Peters puts it, but rather by the "severity of functional impairment."[77] This was perfect for the psychoanalysts—those who were less impaired were candidates for "the couch," the more impaired for the asylum. Any scientific content the term might have formerly possessed had evaporated.

Yet the blackout of catatonia was not complete. At places such as the University of Wisconsin, new treatments were being discovered, such as sodium Amytal to relieve stupor (see Chapter 13). And at the government-run Veterans Administration Hospital in Lexington, Kentucky, Erwin Straus, an émigré from Hitler's Germany, was thinking anew about what happens in stupor and posturing. He wrote in 1955, "These patients are not immobilized in the panzer of their musculature but hold themselves immobile. There is no irreducible increase of tone as in patients with paralysis agitans [Parkinsonism] or in a pallidum syndrome [some dystonias]. If this were so, the patient could not change his attitude from one moment to the next, from a stuporous negativistic posture to well-coordinated movements and back to frozen attitudes with mannerisms."[78] Straus did not manage to puzzle out what was going on in catatonia, but neither has psychiatric science 50 years later.

CLASSIFICATION AT THE INTERNATIONAL LEVEL

There can be no more dramatic testimony of the extent to which dementia praecox and schizophrenia had abducted catatonia than, in the 38 classifications of disease that were produced by official and semiofficial bodies and prominent investigators from the 1930s to the 1950s, *not a single one* mentions catatonia as an independent disease entity. Virtually all incorporate "schizophrenia." Some shell out catatonia, together with hebephrenia and paranoia, as subtypes of schizophrenia. But none recognizes Kahlbaum's epochal diagnosis.[79]

The standard international guide to disease classification was the *International Classification of Disease* series of the World Health Organization, which began incorporating psychiatric diagnoses in the sixth revision, adopted in 1948. It contained separate entries for "catatonic schizophrenia" and for "catalepsy."[80]

This situation did not change by the time of the seventh revision in 1955, when "catatonia" became a "type" of "schizophrenic disorders (dementia praecox)."[81]

In the ninth edition in 1975, things did, however, change. To be sure, the "schizophrenic psychoses" were the master classification. But one of these psychoses was "the catatonic type," and under this type were listed some of the main symptoms of catatonia: agitation, stupor, and waxy flexibility. A little monograph even told clinicians what features to look for.[82] Technically, catatonia remained a subtype, but a stroke of the pen was all that would be required to cut catatonia loose. (There was in 1978 a ninth edition—called "CM" for "clinical modification"—specifically tailored for American audiences that did not contain even this refinement. It was rich in the kind of jargon favored by psychoanalysts—for example "acute hysterical psychosis"—but maintained the standard catatonic subtype of schizophrenic disorders.[83])

In the tenth revision in 1992, the disease designers at the World Health Organization did in fact liberate catatonia. Technically, it was still listed as a subtype. Yet they added the portentous sentence: "It is vital to appreciate that catatonic symptoms are not diagnostic of schizophrenia. A catatonic symptom or symptoms may also be provoked by brain disease, metabolic disturbances, or alcohol and drugs, and may also occur in mood disorders."[84] Could catatonia also occur on its own? That would be going, in 1992, a bridge too far.

By the end of the Second World War, the term "schizophrenia" had lost whatever specificity it might once have possessed, and catatonia in schizophrenia had shed its distinctiveness as a treatable motor syndrome. As Meduna wrote in April 1946 to a correspondent in India of the American situation, "The psychiatrists of today have forgotten any other diagnosis and if the patient is not epileptic or paretic [neurosyphilitic], or does not belong to the manic-depressive group, he is classified as schizophrenic, which word today doesn't mean anything more than 'crazy' or 'cracked.'"[85]

7

PSYCHOLOGY

During an attack [of stupor] the mind is almost entirely unconscious; it seems, so to speak, separated from the body.[1]
—Leon Elias Hirschel, *Gedanken von der Starrsucht* (1769)

There have always been two views about the psychology of catatonia, especially stupor: one, that there is no psychology of the disorder, it is a purely neurological phenomenon; two, that the mind is active during stupor but unable to communicate.

Until the First World War, the psychological interpretation of schizophrenia and catatonia carried the day. Kraepelin was given over to "disturbances of will," and, with Bleuler, Freud had a foot in the door. The notion prevailed that catatonia had a psychology of its own, that the personality influenced the course, and that the symptoms could be understood in terms of their symbolic value for the patient.[2] For example, in 1910, Karl Jaspers said that catatonia patients did indeed have a psychology: "The catatonic syndrome (*Symptomkomplex*) is the final, external expression of complex mental phenomena: mannered positions, repeating words, stereotypic movements, grimacing, and so forth—all are so widespread in different psychoses that these symptoms must be viewed as a constellation of objective but atypical signs. . . . If one tries to understand psychologically the catatonic syndrome in 'classic' cases, one comes to very remarkable observations, but never to a definitive conclusion. In these puzzling conditions we are dealing with the most baffling mental states. They are just as baffling to the psychiatrist as to the laity. We have no idea what is in the patient's mind."[3]

But after 1914, three events challenged the psychological paradigm and put a neurological paradigm to the fore. The head wounds of the First World War founded the cerebral localization version of modern neurology. The wounds were associated with specific deficits. Or, even without localization, it was apparent that catatonic symptoms could be generated by head wounds, by the experience of being "blown up" in the trenches.

The appearance of encephalitis lethargica, first diagnosed by Vienna neurologist Constantin von Economo in 1917,[4] turned in the early 1920s into a worldwide epidemic.[5] Encephalitis patients developed catatonic symptoms, and, in tardive postencephalitic parkinsonism, catatonia was also prominent.[6] Neither the catatonia seen in rear-echelon war hospitals nor that seen in the encephalitis patients was associated with psychology.

And then there was "Jaspers fatigue." In 1910, Jaspers distinguished between *erklären* (explaining) and *verstehen* (empathic understanding) in grasping the roots of illness. The concept of empathic understanding was based on a knowledge of the patient's previous history and the history of the present illness, and it had given psychological approaches a huge boost. But psychiatry grew weary of this distinction. For illnesses of acute onset, such as melancholia or acute psychosis, empathic understanding did not explain much. Psychiatry returned to seeing "schizophrenia"—and with it catatonia—as organic diseases caused by outside forces. In 1929, Hans Gruhle, a member of the Heidelberg School and major schizophrenia expert, voiced this impatience: "I consider schizophrenia to be an organic disease. . . . I find myself therefore in sharp opposition . . . to those authors who try to make schizophrenia 'verständlich' [empathic] as a conflict psychosis, which is to say a flight of the personality from a conflict underway in the unconscious." He spoke of the "bankruptcy of empathic psychology" in dealing with "the schizophrenic process." "We can't do anything more with deriving things, tracing back, feeling our way, or empathy." [7] Gruhle was not hostile to psychology but found Jaspers's version useless in psychotic illnesses, and Jaspers's theories, enunciated in 1910, began to lose their stranglehold of almost 20 years. (Four years later, with the Nazi seizure of power in 1933, they would vanish from Germany completely.)

GERMAN NEUROLOGY AND KLEIST

For all his talk about psychic stages, Kahlbaum had an intensely neurological approach. He felt his patients' muscles and reported "tension." In these years, German psychiatry was moving toward motor symptoms, and Kahlbaum had struck a chord. In 1886, Christian Roller, who had been medical director of a private nervous clinic in Kaiserswerth, reported on "motor disorders in uncomplicated insanity."[8] And Friedrich Lehmann, who also had come up in the asylum world, described the neuropathology of catatonia in 1898.[9]

Yet it was the work of Breslau psychiatry professor Carl Wernicke that put neurological interpretations front and center in psychiatry. Wernicke proposed his own concept of "motor psychoses" (Motilitätspsychosen) in 1892.[10] For Wernicke, there was nothing psychological about it. The term meant "abnormalities of motion and of speech which were independent of thought or will."[11] Mental disorders were caused by the "sejunction" of associations in the brain, meaning that the continuity of associations laid down by experience was interrupted by mental disease.[12]

Karl Kleist was a resident of Wernicke's in Halle for the brief span of Wernicke's tenure there, and Kleist was impressed by Wernicke's intensely neurological approach to psychiatric illness. Born in 1879, Kleist graduated in medicine in Munich, in 1903. After five years in Halle, he worked first with Ludwig Edinger, a well-known name in neurology at the Neurological Institute in Frankfurt am Main, then habilitated on "psychomotor disorders" in 1908, at Erlangen. Between 1914 and 1916, Kleist led the neurology division of a rear-echelon military hospital on the western front. In 1920, he became the professor of psychiatry at the newly founded University of Frankfurt and director of the psychiatric Klinik, where he opened several neurology wards.

Kleist's involvement with catatonia began with his Habilitation in 1908, although, following Wernicke, he did not call it catatonia but "motor disorders," and among the motor disorders were mutism, hyperkinesis (agitation being part), and akinesis. The psychological theories of previous authorities had for him no general validity, and Kleist felt it was the neurological disorders that gave rise to psychological phenomena.[13]

Out of Kleist's experiences with war casualties came a study, in 1918, of "fright psychoses" and movement disorders, which he refused to call catatonia because many lacked an organic cause. Nonetheless, the case histories involved men with agitation, ticcing, grimacing, strange movements, mutism, stupor, and negativism. Kleist's studies were among the earliest of the relationship between catatonia and what would later be called "posttraumatic stress disorder."[14]

Kleist accepted the Kraepelin-Bleuler diagnosis of dementia-praecox-schizophrenia, and was at pains to insert it in the psychoses ending in dementia ("the endogenous dementias"), one of which was catatonia. In 1919, Kleist addressed catatonia for the first time directly, which he called one of the "defect psychoses." "Psychomotor dementia ('Catatonia')" was more a diagnostic basin than a specific disease "because individual cases are highly diverse in their symptoms and course." He distinguished various forms: the stuporous, agitated, and manneristic.[15] Identifying these distinctive "forms" became Kleist's hallmark. In the years 1921–25, he saw 179 catatonia patients, of whom 80 percent did not recover (as for those who did recover, Kleist said they had been given the wrong diagnosis.)[16]

Schizophrenia, Kleist said in 1923, was a group of disorders, one of which was "psychomotor dementia (catatonia)." He called schizophrenia a "neurological system disease," a form of "heredodegeneration."[17] Some of the catatonias were typically rigid, others were primarily negativistic.[18] By 1943, he had individuated eight different subforms of catatonia, distinguishing between catatonia and "motor psychosis." In catatonia, hyperkinetic forms tended to predominate (such as agitation); in the degenerative motor psychoses, drive (*Antrieb*) was lacking and there was an impairment of active thought.[19]

The junior clinicians who gathered about Kleist became part of "the Frankfurt School" of neuropsychiatry. Kleist added several diagnostic signs of catatonia, specifically "*Gegenhalten,*" in 1927, which he called "motor negativism". (The article also described a finger-reflex that has survived as "Kleist's sign.") In now-anglicized gegenhalten, the patient resists the clinician's effort to reposition the limb. The sign was, he said, not specific for catatonia but was found in a wide variety of psychiatric and neurological illnesses.[20] By 1943, he was using "*Mitmachen*" to denote automatic muscle obedience.[21]

Few of the psychiatrists who remained in office during the Third Reich emerged with their reputations intact. A pro forma kind of de-Nazification "cleared" many, including Kleist. Yet there is no doubt that he participated willingly in the regime's sterilization program, arguing in 1936 for an *expansion* of the sterilization agenda "so that the bearers of degenerative psychoses may be made infertile."[22]

Kleist's complex and impenetrable system of classifying catatonia in the larger context of schizophrenia—and filled with eugenic blather about "heredodegeneration," some of which continued to be repeated in German psychiatry into the 1960s[23]—had little impact abroad, save for "Kleist's sign." He explained his psychiatric system in 1960 to what must have been a puzzled British audience[24]; otherwise his publications were largely in German. Kleist figures in the catatonia story with the impact of one of his students, Karl Leonhard.

LEONHARD

Kleist actually had two important students. One, the first academic German female psychiatrist, Edda Neele, has been forgotten. The other, Karl Leonhard, has given us a classification of endogenous psychiatric disorders that even today challenge the Diagnostic and Statistical Manual of Mental Disorders (DSM) system. In 1947, in her Habilitation, Neele, 37, introduced the distinction between "unipolar disorders" and "bipolar disorders," above all in connection with mood diseases, a distinction that has had far-reaching consequences for psychiatry.[25] Catatonia was not an immediate interest of hers, but Neele's work demonstrates the historic impact of the Frankfurt School.

Leonhard had doubtless become familiar with this distinction at the same time as Neele, given that both were Kleist's students, but it was Leonhard who incorporated it into a larger system. Karl Leonhard, Bavarian by origin, was born in 1904 and finished his medical studies in 1929 at Erlangen. After training there in psychiatry, he took a junior post at the asylum in Gabersee, filled with chronic patients, and it was here that Leonhard conceived the idea of studying the course of psychiatric illness starting with the end stage and going backward, rather than, as Kraepelin had done, starting with the patients at admission and then going forward. In 1936, Kleist brought Leonhard, then 32, to the Frankfurt *Klinik*. In that same year, Leonhard completed his Habilitation on end-stage schizophrenia[26] and began a fruitful collaboration with Kleist.

In Gabersee, Leonhard had conceived the distinction between the "systematic" and the "unsystematic" schizophrenias (as he later called them), the former with grim prognoses, the latter, often periodic ("cyclic") in nature, occurring intermittently and frequently having a benign course.[27]

Leonhard's involvement with catatonia started in 1935, in a population of end-stage catatonics in Gabersee. He identified two subtypes in the end stage: patients with rigidity and those who were hyperanimated (*"faxenhaft"*). He likened both to certain neurological disorders of the subcortical corpus striatum in the brain.[28]

A year later, in his Habilitation in 1936, Leonhard advanced the classification of the "end-stage" (defect) catatonias to six: slow-speech defect catatonia (*sprachträge*), speech-prompt defect catatonia (*sprachbereit*, a verbal form of automatic obedience), negativistic, socially accessible, rigid, and hyperkinetic (*faxenhaft*). Several of these he took over from Kleist; the two relating to speech and the rigid subform were of his own devising.[29] It may seem to some readers that these are distinctions without a difference and that all of the catatonias respond alike to therapy, so what would be the point of making such fine differentiations? Kleist and Leonhard both argued that these various subtypes were clinically well-defined and represented genetically distinct phenotypes as well. Yet the investigators produced little in the way of what we would recognize as data.

In the years ahead, Leonhard occupied himself more with other pieces of the Kleistian agenda, such as the cyclical psychoses (illnesses that flipped into their opposites, then back again), and he did not return to catatonia until 1957, after he had left Frankfurt for the East German "Academy" of Erfurt, then two years later becoming professor of psychiatry at the famed Charité Hospital in East Berlin. His "Classification of the Endogenous Psychoses" that appeared in 1957 even today is admired by Leonhardians around the globe.[30]

Even though Leonhard classified the catatonias under "schizophrenia," he had second thoughts. "The systematic and unsystematic schizophrenias," he said, "are not intrinsically related to one another. The common name is justified solely on the basis of tradition, because ever since Kraepelin and Bleuler, people have been accustomed to seeing all the endogenous psychoses that lead to a defect as schizophrenia."[31]

His final synthesis on catatonia in his 1957 book went considerably beyond that of the Gabersee discussion. Under the influence of Kleist, there were now three kinds of psychotic psychomotor disturbances: motility psychosis (nonschizophrenic), unsystematic catatonia (schizophrenic), and systematic catatonia (also schizophrenic, though of a different kind). Periodic catatonia was the only unsystematic catatonia, occurring intermittently with a range of outcomes. These patients demonstrated much alternation between stupor and agitation.[32] The six systematic catatonias were outlined in 1936, and they were characterized by an irreversible downhill course. (Periodic catatonia seems to have a much higher genetic risk than systematic catatonia.)[33]

The Leonhardian classification is important for two reasons. It tended to re-establish catatonia as a practically independent illness; the sections describing catatonia make little reference to schizophrenia, and Leonhard insisted that each form of catatonia was a separate disease *sui generis*.

And Leonhard deviates from the Kleistian tradition in his emphasis on a psychological component of catatonia. Of the systematic catatonias he said: "In the 'peripheral' [neurological-seeming] catatonias, the systemic connections run towards the top [towards the mind], the systems no longer possess solely a neurological significance but also a psychological one."[34]

PUSHBACK

Against this neurological chorus from Frankfurt, there was some pushback. Polish neurologist Maurycy Urstein said, in 1912: "I don't think an organic disease is the cause of catatonia. . . . How are we going to explain the repeated cases in which the patient has not a single pathological symptom inbetween uncommonly powerful attacks of catatonia over decades?" And between these severe episodes of catatonia, he questioned: "the cells of the cerebral cortex all function normally?"[35]

After the Second World War, the rejection of the Wernicke-Kleist-Leonhard approach was extensive. Kurt Schneider, by now the professor at Heidelberg and the doyen of German psychiatry, said, in 1956: "With great respect, I see nothing convincing in Leonhard's careful clinical efforts nor any benefit in all of that; also, not to mention the practical unmanageability of the whole thing, with its different constructs that are so hard to separate one from another."[36] Three years later, in 1959, Karl Conrad in Götttingen added, "[Leonhard] feels compelled to 'sharply' delineate his forms of disease in numberless sub-forms, as if we were dealing with genuine biological or even genetic entities. But for us . . . such a classification, as sharp as he constructs it, is impossible; at the end of the day we consider it an almost arbitrary question of judgment, whether you put the case record in this box or that one."[37]

International judgments—to the extent that Leonhard's system was known abroad—were no less shattering. Said Erwin Stengel, formerly of Vienna and now, in

1959, just retired from the Maudsley Hospital in London: "This classification has no prospects of acceptance before the observations underlying it have been confirmed."[38]

THE PSYCHOLOGICAL APPROACH

Henri Baruk had a different take on stupor than Karl Jaspers. He wrote in 1959, "We see from these concrete details that the psychological state of these [catatonia] patients is not as mysterious and impenetrable as it seemed to Jaspers.[39]"

What happens in stupor? Do the patients simply go blank, or is there an active inner life that the patient is unable to communicate? Of those who, unlike these German neurologists, made a careful study of the subjectivity of the stupor patients, opinion overwhelmingly endorsed the active inner life.

Even before Kahlbaum, numerous patients and their physicians mused about the source of symptoms of "chorea." One of Rudolf Arndt's asylum patients in Greifswald, who believed he was persecuted by the Freemasons, mumbled nonsense, bobbed his head around, and felt his muscles contract. After the fellow was partially restored, Arndt reported in 1868, "In tears, [the patient] said he could do nothing about it. Everything just suddenly came over him against his will; he himself did nothing. Before he knew what was happening, suddenly he was shaken; without any warning, his head suddenly flew to one side; without being able to stop himself, he felt a need to say crazy things. . . . Before he burst forth with them, he had no idea of them. For precisely that reason, they must have been made for him."[40]

Stupor is an interesting theme because patients are unable to communicate while it is in progress and often afterward are reluctant to do so. In 1869, Viennese neurologist Moriz Benedikt described cataleptic patients who said, "They wanted to move but couldn't."[41]

Kahlbaum, though neurologically focused, was not entirely silent on the psychology of stupor. In his 1874 book: "In some cases patients say, as they emerge from the condition of silent Attonität, they had not spoken because a voice (an 'interior' voice, a voice they heard clearly, thus hallucinated) ordered them not to speak; in other cases the patients complained about the absence of any thought and about their incapability of understanding. In still other cases, they were unable to make any statement at all." He noted the pattern of alternation: the pressure of speech and verbigeration alternating with muteness and the tonic muscle contractions. So it is not that Kahlbaum was indifferent to his patients' mental states but rather that he wanted to demonstrate the larger patterns of symptoms.[42]

Caspar Max Brosius, director of the private mental hospital in Bendorf on the Rhine, in 1877 said that he detected signs of inner psychic life in his stuporous patients whom others were inclined to write off as "lifeless lumps." "You often see these inward-turned patients slightly moving their lips, and if you look and listen very closely you will discover it's exactly the same lip movements, the same words that the patient is whispering countless times. And if you consider these mute, inwardly-turned patients, who sit there motionlessly, to be melancholic, you will be surprised, when it's the same words and sentences, that the content is not of a painful nature, and includes such words as, "Clever fellow!" or "God how wonderful!" that the patients whisper dozens of times in succession."[43]

In the 1880s and '90s in German-speaking lands, the level of consciousness in catatonia was "reduced" (but maybe not in some stupor patients, judging from the alertness of the eyes). Kraepelin's contribution to the discussion began in 1896, in the fifth edition of his textbook, with his views about "psychic inhibition" (*psychische Hemmung*, later *psychomotorische Hemmung*): "a general inhibition of the chain of thought." Common to the various stupors, "is inhibition. Sometimes it is accompanied by powerful inner tensions, sometimes by a simple slowing of the process of thought, sometimes again with a will-less dependence on exterior or interior stimuli that might surface incidentally."[44]

Carl Jung reviewed this literature in 1907 and added his own Freudian notions.[45] This subject would probably have been forgotten as unfounded speculation had it not spilled into psychoanalytic concepts of "blocking" that powerfully influenced later psychological interpretations of schizophrenia. In any event, it was with Kraepelin's "psychomotor inhibition" and Bleuler's "incapacity to move" (*Bewegungsunfähigkeit*)[46] that the psychogenic interpretation of catatonia took root. Bleuler's student Jakob Klaesi was confident in 1922 that repetitive movements and verbigerations were not pointless and meaningless. "They are expressive movements that we . . . can understand [*verstehen*] only after a period of observation and empathy [*Einfühlung*]."[47] This was Jaspersian rhetoric.

FRANCE

Just as the neurology of catatonia was dominated by the Germans, its psychology was led by the French. As early as 1833, the trainees in psychiatry were asking patients what they recalled from their stupors. Mme C, 30, had been much upset by the July Revolution in Paris of 1830, followed by problems with her mother and her sister. "Soon her reason left her. She hears the cannon, sees the wounded, the blood, the dead. She gradually becomes overwhelmed," said intern Gustave-François Étoc-Démazy at the Salpêtrière, "She stays motionless, her eyes fixed, mute, barely murmuring a few incoherent words." Then Mme C came out of her stupor. What did you remember? "She tells us that she thought she was in the galley-ships or in the desert. She saw wagons filled with coffins passing by, but she could not remember exactly. In her head, which remained heavy and painful, there was only vagueness and confusion. A lot of ideas occurred to her, but she couldn't bring herself to articulate them. Other times, she didn't speak because she didn't feel the need to speak. She let everything happen to her without offering any resistance; she felt vaguely as though she were stupefied but didn't feel a need to change."[48]

Étoc-Démazy's thesis was widely cited, and it may have inspired several senior clinicians to take a look at the psychology of stupor (*stupidité*). In 1843, Jules Baillarger at the Salpêtrière and Charenton, in the first volume of the new psychiatry journal, the *Annales Médico-Psychologiques* that he and colleagues had just founded, discussed the subjective experiences of patients in stupor. A 25-year-old man seen at Charenton compared his experiences to "a long dream." "Around him everything had been transformed, all in a general stupefaction. The ground trembled and opened under his feet. At every moment he saw himself about to be swallowed up in bottomless crevasses. When he restrained people near him, it was to keep them from falling into the precipices that resembled craters of a volcano."

A 23-year-old prostitute had arrived at the Salpêtrière in stupor, believing that she was at the Botanical Garden amidst the animals. "Her head was full of noises; she heard church bells, drums, confused voices, that caused her much suffering. She was preoccupied with ideas of suicide. One day she tried to strike herself with a knife, and on another tried to starve herself to death."[49] These typical stories came from Baillarger's wards.

The interpretation by Louis Delasiauve at the Bicêtre hospice offered a perfect counterpoint. Delasiauve, the nihilist, said in 1843 that, in *stupidité*, "Thought is not merely irregular; it is suspended, abolished; the exercise of intellectual functions is shackled . . . . [The patient] is like a machine reduced to immobility by the fouling of its gears. . . . These unfortunates have been reduced to a vegetative state."[50] Several years later, Delasiauve added that the *"stupidité"* patients in stupor reminded him of the Psalm about, "They have mouths, but they speak not; eyes have they, but they see not. They have ears, but they hear not." Thus it was with catatonic stupor: Patients "who have eyes but cannot see, ears but cannot hear. . . . They are powerless to block the impressions that strike their imagination; they preserve the memory of these, as spectators who recollect the blast of the cannon, the fusillade, the melee of the combatants. . . . In a word, stuporous patients [*les stupides*] are unwilling and passive witnesses to scenes that unfold within themselves."[51] (Between Delasiauve's two accounts in 1843 and 1851, the Revolution of 1848 in Paris intervened!)

Delasiauve notwithstanding, it slowly became a part of French mental medicine to look at the psychology of stupor. The theme is virtually omnipresent in any discussion of patients' experiences. In 1862, Monsieur "X," emerging from a catatonic stupor, described his experience for Henri Dagonet, chief psychiatrist of the Stéphansfeld asylum in Strasbourg: "I imagined," he said, "that both my parents were dead, that my native city had been flooded; and that a new deluge had submerged the land. I was always hungry, and I believed that people were going to let me die of starvation. In the garden where I was taken for walks, I was afraid of the patients around me; to my eyes they looked like brigands and assassins, and I lived in continual anxiety. In walks outside the asylum I would walk slowly, with loathing; I was convinced that people wanted to drown me, or else have me crushed on the railway tracks that passed nearby."

Dagonet added of the *"stupidité"* patients in general, "Phantom images pass ceaselessly in front of their eyes; the ground trembles under their feet; they see in front of them a yawning chasm, a precipice ready to swallow them; they hear death threats; they're buffeted by alarms, and gun shots that echo in their ears."[52]

Pierre Janet, a student of Jean-Martin Charcot, gave psychological approaches a kind of Charcotian magisterial blessing in 1889, with his book *L'Automatisme Psychologique*. At the time, Janet was still a high school teacher in Le Havre, not yet having begun the medical studies that would take him into psychiatry. But the book on automatism was his doctoral thesis in psychology, a book that today evokes the miasma of hysteria, double personality, and automatic writing that settled over French medicine in the last third of the nineteenth century. But Janet was also interested in catalepsy and saw an intimate relationship between minimal consciousness and stupor: "Acts carried out during catalepsy are under the control of psychological phenomena."[53]

Charcot died in 1893, and Janet, with all of his references to hysteria at the Salpêtrière, was soon seen as clinging to a past that Parisian psychological medicine would prefer to forget. By 1900, the leading light was Paul Sérieux at the Ville-Evrard asylum in Paris, and it was Sérieux who introduced Kraepelin's dementia praecox to France. Sérieux's students began carefully administering psychological tests and interviewing post-stupor patients to see what they had experienced. In 1902, one student, René Masselon, asked the catatonic dementia praecox patients at Ville-Evrard batteries of questions about word associations and arithmetic, but he had poor pickings on stupor: Mlle Bi, 24, could remember nothing, only that "she was afraid."[54]

Another Sérieux student, Gustave Monod, encountered Mlle YN, 30, who kept a journal of the first three months of her stay at Ville-Evrard, experiencing alternations between semi-stupor (saliva dribbling out of her mouth) and agitation. An extract: "All the feelings that I have are false. This doesn't have a name. Me neither, I don't have a name, I don't have a name. I no longer exist. My soul is used up. Nothing is nothing. Nothing is good for anything. The brook is in the field, the pretty river, clear, full of pretty fish. The baker bakes bread."[55] The ten folders of the journal are evidence of a lively, if psychotic, intellectual life in catatonia.

FEAR?

In order to get a young woman of 17 who had been mute for three months to speak, Carl Ideler, professor of psychiatry at the Charité in Berlin in the mid-nineteenth century, trickled hot wax on her hands and back. She didn't cry out at this treatment (and recovered after getting her menses). Asked later if the hot wax didn't hurt, she replied, "Certainly, and I wanted to cry out, but I couldn't. It was as if a demon had taken hold of me."[56]

What emotions trigger catatonia? Georg Northoff cites "the intensity of emotions" that provides the trigger. "One can also have very positive emotions that are extremely intense and can lead to catatonia as in mania. It is the emotional valence (negative vs positive) that makes the difference." He continues: "I had a patient who became catatonic each time she fell in love and was very happy."[57] The point is an important one and deserves further study.

But in our research there has been little happiness, and, like Carl Ideler's teenage patient, lots of fear in evidence. Fear seems almost always to have played a cardinal role in the ideation of stupor. This does not mean that stupor is caused by fear, but certainly that fear looms prominently in the stupor content.

For Kahlbaum, the psychology of catatonia was encapsulated in the traditional term "melancholia attonita," or thunderstruck melancholia: "The so-called melancholia attonita is the condition in which the patient sits silently, completely mute and unmoving, with rigid countenance, immobile body, gaze fixed upon a distant point, motionless and apparently completely without will, without a reaction to sensory impressions. . . . The overall condition of such a patient gives the impression of someone who has turned to stone [*Erstarrung*] in deepest mental pain, or in extreme fright."[58] To the extent that Kahlbaum concedes a psychology to catatonia, it is to mental pain and fright.

Kahlbaum hypothesized psychic stages through which catatonia would progress, beginning with melancholic depression, advancing to mania and to psychotic excitement and stupor, which he called *Attonität*. Then, in the event that recovery failed to eventuate, to dementia. He conceded, however, that very exceptionally the illness could begin with *Attonität*: "In very infrequent cases the entire disease progression seems to commence with the picture of *Attonität*, following a very severe mental or physical insult, or following a very great fright, such as, to take one case from the literature, after an attempted hanging."[59]

Kahlbaum traced the range of emotions that might trigger a melancholic initial phase. "Usually it's chagrin and worry and a depressive mood that is directed against oneself that give rise to catatonia. A particularly large portion comes from chagrin over love, and self-reproach on account of secret sexual sins [masturbation]. . . . There follow concerns about money and wounded honor (shame), which constitute the content of the initial symptoms." He indicted "the other melancholic symptoms: fear of being poisoned, delusions of persecution, religious delusions about sinfulness, and so forth."[60]

Was Kahlbaum right about fear? Yes, indeed.

In August 1759, Francisco Mazars de Cazelles, a physician in the Pyrenees, was called to the bedside of a shepherd boy, 17, who lived in a village near the (later) spa of Lamalou. The lad was thin, of a vigorous constitution. Six months previously, he had been "terribly frightened" by a neighboring peasant who attempted to assault him while the boy was out with his flock. With great exertion, the boy had managed to save himself. Three months later, the shepherd, "his mind still very upset from the first incident," became greatly taken as "a wolf, in a least suspected moment, suddenly appeared and carried away a lamb." The boy gave chase and ended up in a tug-of-war with the wolf, which the boy finally won. Despite this display of courage, the shepherd was terribly alarmed and, the next day, after an awful night's sleep, he "showed signs of *stupidité* [stupor]."

For the next three months, this vague feeling of "indifference and taciturnity that surprised his friends" continued. "He began speaking in monosyllables and resisted all efforts to cheer him up." Then one day, rather than arising early, the boy stayed in bed. "A few hours later, people lost patience with this sleep; dinner time had arrived; he was called but failed to respond; the family shook him, pinched him; he was unresponsive; they seated him on his bed—although he offered some resistance, and a kind of stiffness came over his body in this position. He remained motionless; people examined him: his eyes were open and stared fixedly at the same object." He managed to swallow a bit of soup that was spooned into his mouth. "Once this sad meal was over, people interrogated him very firmly, but he was unresponsive to prayers, tears and cries. . . . This automatic diner [*mangeur automate*] was put to bed again. He remained unmoving all night in the position in which he was placed." The parents, in consternation "at the sight of this new statue," summoned Dr. Mazars. After telling the story in a medical journal, Mazars concluded: "The manner in which the passions act on us may be viewed as a problem that remains to be solved." The passions, he noted, affected many areas of life: "But beyond these disorders of the spirit [*l'âme*], physicians have observed that the animal machine itself is in various ways the victim and the plaything of these furies." This was an early, powerful statement of the role of fear in what Dr. Mazars correctly diagnosed as "catalepsy." (The family diagnosed demonic possession.)[61]

But it was not merely that fearful events could give rise to stupor. Rather, the imagination could create terrible scenes during the stupor. Delasiauve captured this well in 1854: "These hallucinations [*phénomènes fantastiques*] that his imagination evokes are for the most part of a sinister nature. Most commonly, he believes he sees phantoms, assassins, robbers, obscene and repellent spectacles, which frighten him, irritate him or make him indignant; in his terror he cries out, struggles, seeks to flee, and even is given to violence against others or himself. . . . When the hallucinations subside, the patient is plunged into a sad prostration; his face is doleful, stupefied, despondent and reflects the terrifying thoughts that have arisen within him and the persistent memory of the false perceptions."[62]

At mid-nineteenth century, fearfulness surfaced often in French psychiatry. Bénédict-Augustin Morel at the Maréville asylum in eastern France said, in 1852: "Terror, fear and anger often act in the same pathological manner on general conditions of health. More than once, excessive terror has plunged people into a true state of stupor." "Our asylum," continued Morel, "offers numerous examples of the influence of fear on disorders of the mental faculties." Morel cited a merchant who saw his factory burn down. "He fell into a sad stupor. He awakened as if from a coma and his first cry was, 'I am ruined!' "[63]

It occurred to George Kirby, in 1913 an attending physician at the Wards Island asylum in New York City, that the catatonic stupors of his fearful patients were akin to "the phylogenetically old reaction seen in animals that in time of danger lie motionless as if feigning death." He said that "the most typical catatonic manifestation, the negativistic stupor, has the general characteristics of a defense reaction or of protective mechanisms whereby the individual practically shuts out the external world." A young woman of 16 had undergone a previous attack of psychosis and was brought to the hospital "where for five months she showed stuporous behavior and catatonic symptoms. She was mute, resistive, gazed vacantly, refused food, paid no attention to pin pricks. . . . She recovered with good recollection for the stupor period, during which there had been hallucinations and various dream-like ideas; e.g., that she was dead and in a cemetery, had a cross inside of her body which interfered with the beating of her heart." Her psychoanalytically oriented clinicians immediately referred this back to a previous breakup with a Christian boyfriend.[64]

Quantification begins. August Hoch, who continued Kirby's work on Wards Island, found that 35 of their 36 stupor cases had "thoughts of death or closely related conceptions."[65] Of 100 patients with "catatonic dementia praecox" admitted to the Hudson River State Hospital between 1927 and 1931, 48 had ideas "expressing fear": fear of being killed, 18; vague fears, 15; of castration, 10, of homosexuality, 6; of being buried alive, 5, and so forth.[66]

The picture sharpens with the introduction of the sodium Amytal interview in 1928 in France and in 1929–30 in the United States. With a few grains of the barbiturate drug, mute patients would begin to speak, requesting food (after they had been tube fed for weeks) and behaving amicably even after weeks of negativism. In this narrow window, which opened for an hour or two, the patients related what they had been experiencing during the stupor. In 1932, Erich Lindemann at the Psychopathic Hospital of the State University of Iowa, who helped pioneer the Amytal interview after William Bleckwenn and William Lorenz introduced it at the University of Wisconsin in 1929, reported his experiences. A woman, 38, who had been mute, refusing food and muttering to herself for four weeks: "lost the suspicious and apprehensive expression in her face," two minutes after the Amytal injection. "She appeared relieved, looked around in an interested way, and spontaneously asked the examiner,

'Where am I? Who brought me here? Where are my children? Can I go home?' She reported that something terrible was pressing down on her, that she had a tremendous fear of impending danger, that she heard God's voice talk to her, that she was in a coffin which was prepared to take her to hell, and that she had a profound feeling of guilt with reference to autoerotic habits in her adolescence." (This guilt about masturbation was well-nigh universal.) She remained alert for about two hours, then relapsed into her previous condition.[67]

THE TRANSMISSION BELT OF FEAR?

What is the meaning of this fearful ideation? How does intense fear metamorphose into the motor behaviors of catatonia?

The Australian psychiatrist Richard Perkins described four patients with systemic physical illness who exhibited catatonia in association with intense fear.[68] Two patients were paraplegic after falls, one had recurrent seizures, and one was surgically treated for a cerebral abscess. Each was under enormous psychological and physical stress. The presence of organic brain disease lowered the threshold for the release of catatonic behavior. Although the patients improved with treatments for catatonia, recovery depended, he believed, on the treatment of the psychological stressors.

In a unique experimental study of catatonia, Georg Northoff and his colleagues in Frankfurt compared the thoughts and motor signs of akinetic catatonics with the signs in Parkinson patients. Of 22 catatonic patients, 13 were relieved by lorazepam within 24 hours. On day 21 after treatment, the patients were questioned as to their recollections of their akinetic states. Compared to the Parkinson patients, the catatonic patients were not fully aware of their deficits in motor functions, were more concerned about the loss of control of their movements, and were overwhelmed by feelings of anxiety and by the blockade of their movements by emotions and feelings of isolation from their environment. The patients' greatest fears were their inability to control intense anxiety. They felt threatened and feared dying and were less concerned about their lack of control of body movement or of self-care.[69,70]

We are dealing here with two kinds of "fear" situations. In one, the fear is a realistic response to a shattering life experience or trauma, such as being bombed on the roads of France by the German Stukas in 1940. In the other, the fear is a fantasy and does not arise from trauma. In the madness of fear, reality and fantasy interlace. Experience gives rise to realistic fears, fantasy to unrealistic ones. The catatonic response, however, seems to be the same.

AN EVOLUTIONARY RESPONSE?

Recognition that clinical catatonia is present in 10 percent of acutely ill psychiatric inpatients, that it is relieved by anxiolytic drugs, and that patients give the appearance of intense anxiety, led the psychologist Andrew Moskowitz, now teaching in Berlin, to propose in 2004 that catatonia is "a relic of ancient defensive strategies, developed during an extended period of evolution in which humans had to face predators in much the same way many animals do today and designed to maximize an individual's chances of surviving a potentially lethal attack."[71] Seven years later, in 2011, Eliane Volchan and a group of Brazilian researchers asked, "Is there tonic immobility in humans," and, on the basis of evidence from victims of traumatic stress, answered in the affirmative.[72]

Such behavior is labeled "tonic immobility"—the involuntary, reflexive state of muscular rigidity, inability to move, with suppressed vocal behavior. It is a defense seen in animal behaviors when threatened by a predator. It can also be experimentally elicited by slowly and quietly stroking an animal, then gradually releasing it, with the animal now remaining immobile with limbs in the unusual postures in which they are placed. The phenomenon is demonstrated in chickens and other fowl, frogs, snakes, guinea pigs, rabbits, and other prey animals. A tradition of pretending to be dead is described as the behavior of the Virginia opossum—"playing possum"—as enshrined in childhood play.[73]

The defensive postures called forth in prey animals by a threat are described as freeze, flight-or-fight, fright, followed by flag-and-faint. Freeze and flight occur when a predator is at a distance; fight is an option when escape is not possible—these behaviors are accompanied by fright—followed by "shut-down" labeled flag and faint.[74]

Sexually assaulted women recall an overwhelming fear, feeling physically re-strained and immobile, rigid and unable to move or resist, to call out, to move away, or to fight.[75] More than a third of rape survivors experienced paralysis.[76]

After the prolonged immobilization inherent in cardiac surgery, one patient was "immobilized and almost like a statue"; another "was frozen and expressionless. She spoke barely audibly in a monotone with long pauses and made no spontaneous comments." The postoperative reaction has been described as experiencing a catas-trophe, the patients resembling "the photographed faces of survivors of civil disasters, the countenances present staring and vacant expressions of seeming frozen terror. Immobile, apathetic, and completely indifferent to their fate, they respond to inquiries in monosyllables devoid of affect."[77]

A "resignation syndrome," marked by severe stupors, is reported among refugee children coming to Sweden from the Syrian wars.[78] In the Uganda conflicts, a similar stuporous, repetitive "nodding syndrome" is observed.[79] Some patients in this Uganda study were relieved by lorazepam, the effective treatment for catatonia.

The present view focuses our interest on the psychology of catatonia rather than on pathology of the nervous system. In this image of catatonia as a response to threat and fear, the role of the autonomic nervous system is to be considered. The freeze-fight-flight defenses call for increased activation of the sympathetic autonomic pathways. The shift to flag and faint positions are activated by the parasympathetic system. In the special form of catatonia expressed in adolescents with autism, Dirk Dhossche, a child psychiatrist in Mississippi, has identified activation of vagal activity as supporting the behavior.[80]

Catatonia is a behavior that is recognized by observation and by responses to simple commands. Changes in movement, posture, and speech identify the syn-drome. It does not result from a structural defect in a body organ, nor is it associ-ated with an identifiable physiologic dysfunction, although vegetative dysfunctions are common accompaniments. It occurs in the context of systemic medical illnesses and is frequently associated with manic-depressive disease. After catatonia is relieved, we see no residuals; it is as if the blackboard had been erased with a few smudges left at the corners. Catatonia is a behavior of the whole organism, arising suddenly and vanishing without a trace. It is similar to crying, an inherited behavior that expresses a strong emotion.

Catatonia is not a disorder in thought or emotion, although such accompaniments are common. Some authors consider catatonia an "end-state" whole-body response to imminent doom, a behavior inherited from ancestral encounters with carnivores, an adaptation that remains an inherent feature of living. This would make catatonia an atavism precipitated by psychological disruptions.[81]

8

DELIRIOUS MANIA AND FEBRILE CATATONIA

The ultimate court of appeal is observation and experiment, and not authority.
—T. H. Huxley[1]

For more than two centuries, clinicians have described patients acutely excited and delirious, dangerous to themselves and to others, so severe as to result in death. Many are febrile with a story of stupor, mutism, negativism, and motor signs of catatonia. A spontaneous lethal or malignant febrile catatonia is also described, often associated with systemic illnesses. A specific variant sprang to the fore with the introduction of chlorpromazine and the successor neuroleptic drugs in eliciting an identifiable and treatable toxic response labeled the *neuroleptic malignant syndrome*. This experience is described in the next chapter.

"Mania" once meant inchoate violence, not euphoria and flight of ideas. In 1913, Emil Kraepelin described an agitation that he considered part of "dementia praecox": "Anxious patients pray, kneel, run away at night, hide in the forest, try to strangle themselves, leap out of the window... As a rule there is no probable motive to be discovered for the often extremely bizarre behavior of the patients; rather, they seem to be following blindly some drive that has surfaced within themselves. They wander aimlessly about, try to go to America, run around naked, tear the bedding apart, destroy the stove, burn up important documents, smash windows, bite into plates and glasses, suddenly grab someone about the neck and kiss them, then spit in his face or give him a tremendous swat on the head. They pull other patients out of bed, hit out wildly, throw their shoes, dance around holding the room door, gallop about in fencing style with great leaps, bite a neighbor, push around the furniture, seize some object with brute force, climb up frantically on a table or window sill in order to defecate there."[2]

Kraepelin called it "mania under conditions of delirium." It entailed a "deep, dreamlike disturbance of consciousness and violent, confused hallucinations and delusions." "The attack usually begins quite suddenly; there may be insomnia, agitation or mood anxiety for one to two days, more seldom a few weeks. Consciousness is quickly clouded; the patients are severely stuporous, confused, puzzled, and lose completely their orientation with respect to time and place. Everything seems different to them; they believe themselves in heaven, in the Palace of Herod, in the 'Clinic of the Christ Child.'"[3] They hallucinate. "Angels appear... the coffee smells like death; their hands are rotting; there's a smell of smoke in the house; the food tastes like goat or human flesh."[4]

Then Kraepelin described catatonic features: "These patients are heedless of the surroundings, don't follow orders or respond to questions, hit out." One patient yelled out spontaneously, 'I am Justice; don't touch me; I am all-knowing; get away from me!'" This would be negativism. "Frequently, waxy rigidity, echolalia and echopraxia are demonstrated." Often there is "alternation of agitation and stupor." At the end of an episode, the patients typically remember nothing.[5] Kraepelin did not emphasize violence in this account of manic delirium as a mood disorder, but perhaps merely because the presence of violence sufficed to establish the case as one of dementia praecox.

Kraepelin's descriptions of violent, senseless agitation have long been known as demonic possession, psychotic agitation, or paranoid schizophrenia. Delirious mania is synonymous with catatonic excitement or agitation.[6] Much of this agitation involves repetitive motor activity, vanishes like many catatonic symptoms without a trace, and responds to anticatatonic remedies. "Delirious mania" was a common term for it in the nineteenth century, and the passing years have not really improved on this label. It is mania in the old sense, meaning out of control behavior, not in the new sense, meaning euphoria. It is delirious because consciousness is usually clouded, and it may go as suddenly as it comes, leaving the patient with no memory of it. Many psychiatrists today are unfamiliar with delirious mania because it is the police, not the clinic, who see these patients in the midst of some maddened spree, and it is the police who shoot them down rather than delivering them to care.

Psychiatry has extraordinary difficulty coming to grips with delirious psychotic activity, preferring to leave insensate violence to the police. Yet, as a combination of motor symptoms and psychotic ideation, the behavior is clearly within the realm of psychological medicine. In 1962, Frank Fish, then at the University of Edinburgh, described "pernicious catatonia": The beginning was sudden, preceded perhaps by a brief prodrome of "dejection." "This is followed by a sudden onset of senseless excitement which is often associated with self-mutilation. The patients do not speak, beat wildly at everything around them, and bang their hands or heads on the wall or on the floor. Sometimes they tear their hair out in handfuls and bite their own arms and hands." It was, he said, quite impossible to make contact with them, and, if not given electroconvulsive therapy (ECT), they would be dead in 14 days. He considered it a form of schizophrenia.

Fevers develop. Much is uncertain in psychiatry, but nothing is less certain than the relationship among fever, motor symptoms, and death. There is probably a basin in the brain where fever, catatonic symptoms, and death sit, but exactly how they are related is obscure. Historically, we know that, in their agonal moments, patients with "catatonic schizophrenia" sometimes experienced a remission of their catatonia and psychosis before dying of tuberculosis.[7]

We are in the Allenberg asylum in East Prussia. It is 1881. Kahlbaum left it some time ago to found his own private clinic in Görlitz, but his colleague Julius Jensen remained and became director. Jensen describes a catatonic patient who lay "stiff and staring in bed," but who, "with his fingernails, ripped open his scrotum and retrieved one of his testicles, all this concealed beneath the covers." An attendant, suspecting masturbation, came running, but the deed was done. "A few months later, the same patient, after his attack of stupor had lost its force, sat mute and rigid with his fellow patients at table, and while the attendant ladled out the soup, no-one noticed that the patient had removed his right boot and sock underneath the table. People probably did notice that he had his dull and undangerous table-knife in hand as he leaned down, as if he wanted to get something off the floor. And in fact he had, as he raised his hand again atop the table, a rather bloody object between his fingers, which he laid beside his plate. It was the small toe of his right foot that he had severed with a quick cut through the joint. The whole thing happened in a moment, and, as the patient started to eat his freshly served soup, his companions recognized the nature of the bloody object. Later, the patient was unable to give a reason for this self-mutilation as he began again to speak. The whole thing gives the impression of a simple, driven automatic action."[8]

In Jensen's view, the patient had given us an example of automatism in catatonia, yet the whole affair, in its incoherent violence, could have as easily been ascribed to delirious mania.

The delirious mania story resembles the catatonia story. It begins with a dozen different diagnostic rivulets that then converge on catatonia as clinicians identify an underlying theme.

Vienna's Joseph Leopold Auenbrugger, who is remembered for describing in 1761 the diagnostic value of percussion, gave an account 20 years later of "the silent fury." An officer, 52, healthy during a lifetime in the military, developed a "spasmodic" disorder of the abdomen. In August 1771, he was invited to a friend's for lunch and underwent a psychological attack (*Tiefsinn*). He didn't eat. "Suddenly he sprang up and cried, 'With me it's over! I'm past saving!'" He thereupon went into a stupor, and Auenbrugger was called. Scarcely had Auenbrugger left the bedside, however, than a messenger hurried after him: "The patient has suddenly sprung from bed and attempted to plunge out the window." Baulked at this, the patient began ramming his head against the wall. (Catatonic alternation and self-injurious behavior.) He became mute, then, supremely agitated, began yelling, "I am eternally damned" and started cursing and blaspheming. Several episodes of agitation followed before the patient finally responded to the laxatives that seem to have been Auenbrugger's therapeutic mainstay. Asked about his mental status at the end of the illness, the officer said that: "His internal anxiety and torment had become unbearable, and had brought him so much out of himself that he could no longer even remember what he had actually done."[9]

FRANCE

In 1809, Philippe Pinel stamped the next century of French psychiatry with the concept of "mania without incoherence" (*la manie sans délire*). Mania, for Pinel, meant not euphoria but violent eruptions of insanity, and "*délire*" meant incoherence: the total loss of reasoning capacity. Thus, mania without madness meant insanity but not the abolition of mental function. The disorder began with a burning sensation in the stomach that spread to the neck and the brain. "It is then that the patient is dominated by an irresistible drive for bloodshed; he may grab a suitable weapon, sacrificing the first person he sees in a kind of rage. Otherwise, he enjoys the complete exercise of reason, even during the attack. He responds directly to questions, lets slip no incoherence of thought, no sign of *délire*; he even feels profoundly the entire horror of his situation; he is stricken with remorse, as if he were to reproach himself for this violent penchant."[10]

Pinel laid down the doctrine. Recognizing "maniacal fury," "acute delirium," and the like began to flourish in France. In 1817, François Fodéré, professor of psychiatry in Strasbourg, proposed "maniacal fury, or mania without incoherence" (*manie sans délire*) as a diagnosis. "The blind impulse to rob, insult, provoke, and even to spill blood, without the ability to assign to this fatal drive any idea other than doing harm; it is a true periodic rage . . . of which a violent fit of anger is an exact description." Fodéré described a perfectly composed society lady subject to periodic fits. "Everything changes as soon as her attack begins, which happens every six months. Her eyes bulge from her head; she curses and hits everyone; she exaggerates the wrongs supposedly done her, and is no longer able to write a single consecutive sentence; now, this patient can foresee very well the arrival of these attacks, of which she is ashamed."[11]

In 1819, Pinel's pupil Étienne Esquirol narrowed Pinel's concept, making it a kind of delusional disorder. He said of "instinctive monomania": "Troubled by hallucinations, driven by violent and even ferocious passions, there are patients who give themselves over to extreme behavior, who commit acts of the most atrocious ferocity, driven by a fury of which they are well aware. . . . They believe they are obeying the voice of heaven, which orders up for them the most painful sacrifices. Immersed in hallucinations, they cede to an interior voice that cries to them kill, kill; although they may not understand the motives that drive them, they are compelled to commit acts of fury the consequences of which afterwards they can only deplore."

And now came the violent part: As early as 1833, Louis Calmeil at Charenton alluded to the insensate violence of the "furious" patients (*les furieux*) who had sought "to batter their servants or friends, to wound or mutilate them; these episodes did not upset the patients greatly and were soon forgotten."[12]

Several years later, in a volume in the same dictionary series published in 1839, Calmeil developed this point more fully: "Fury" was a type of "manic delirium" (*délire maniaque*), often induced by intolerable conditions of confinement, common in the provinces where manic patients are still chained. "Some furious patients take out their rage on trees, on walls, they bite the ground, emit terrible cries, crush everything that comes under their hand. I saw a patient with manic fury throw himself twenty times against the ceiling of his cell, grab and tear to pieces a cat, which put up strong resistance. One unfortunate woman, in a behavioral excess, bit off a part of her tongue, her lips, and several shards of skin that she spat in the face of other patients; to prevent a resumption of such incidents, we were obliged to proceed to the extraction of all of her incisor teeth."[13]

In a discussion of monomania, Calmeil said, "The fury of monomaniacs is the more to be feared when it manifests itself impulsively. . . . There are monomaniacs, as if driven by a suicidal fury, by an imperious needed to exact a cruel vengeance on those who irritate them, who writhe until they fall over from fatigue; they exhaust themselves against the personnel who try to restrain them. Others tear their straight-jackets to pieces or the ropes which were thought sufficient to head off a terrible event . . . I might cite as an example of homicidal fury . . . the cruelty of a hallucinated soldier, who, before his ghastly aims were known, ground under his feet on the pavement the chest and the limbs of a sweet and inoffensive idiot, and who every day threatened to create yet more victims."[14]

Delirious mania also sailed under the flag of "acute delirium" (*délire aigu*), which originally was a catch-all for brain inflammation, then came to mean stupor, agitation, and the other signs of catatonia.

"MENTAL EPILEPSY"

The concealment of manic delirium under the label "epilepsy" is suggested in the French literature. Epilepsy is common in catatonia; as Fink and Taylor have reported, "about 15 percent of adult patients with catatonia not due to a mood disorder have epilepsy," as verified by electroencephalography (EEG).[15] The reverse is true, too. Posturing occurs in partial complex seizures; in other epileptic states not marked by grand mal seizures, such catatonic symptoms as negativism (tightly clamping jaws or eyelids), grimacing, mutism, and immobility are not unusual.[16] Yet before the introduction of the EEG in the 1930s, the diagnosis of partial complex seizures, petit mal seizures, and petit mal status epilepticus was difficult (if not unknown—these differentiations are ascertainable only with EEG). Historically, the diagnosis of "epilepsy" was much broader and covered a multitude of sins, including delirious mania.

In 1853, Morel distinguished between "instinctive fury"—a dangerous instinctive monomania—and fury "motivated" by hallucinations." In epilepsy, both were equally perilous, either before or after the seizure. Thus, in "epileptic fury," agitated behavior and deep stupor were the norm. In one of their male patients at the Maréville asylum, as the attack approached, "his eyes became brilliant; the convulsions of the muscles of his face intensified, and he was unrecognizable under a grimacing mask. When the rage of this epileptic patient reached its maximum, it was necessary to put him in a straight-jacket, and for eight to ten days we had before us the most horrifying spectacle that one could imagine." He was finally restored only after, as people said, "using up all his epileptic fluid."[17] Thus began Morel's doctrine of "atypical epilepsy" (*épilepsie larvée*), in which convulsions were replaced by psychosis.

In 1854, Louis Delasiauve, an epilepsy expert, summarized the literature: "All the authors correctly remark that epileptic mania has a very distinctive tendency to take on the furious form. Its manifestations are clamorous and wild. The face is animated, the pulse strong, the skin burning, the eyes haggard, frequently ferocious." He described patient G: "We are much less secure with him, as the explosion of delirium is often instantaneous, and his violent acts strike with the promptitude of lightening. With one kick, he almost broke the leg of one of the orderlies, who was laid up for a month. He would certainly have killed a patient with a bowl that he threw at his head if by misfortune he had hit him. When, at its height, the agitation is transformed into incoherence, nothing equals the fierce expression of his features . . . the vehemence of his words. Finally, when in his rage he is restrained and can no longer cause harm, G spits in the face of those who come near and tries to bite them."[18] For Delasiauve, this was "epileptic" rage.

BELL'S MANIA

One American contribution to the delirious mania story loomed overprominently: It was "Bell's mania." Luther Bell was 31 in 1837, when he became superintendent of the McLean Asylum, a private nervous clinic in Belmont, Massachusetts. In 1849, he described "a class of cases, not unfrequently [sic] presented, and of the gravest moment, but of which I had had no previous experience, and the authorities offered no distinct recognition."[19]

In the McLean records for 1836–49, he found 40 cases, three-quarters ending fatally, among 1,700 admissions. The patient is brought in. "He sinks into a chair, with his shoulders bent forward as if very feeble. When informed where he is, his mind appears to comprehend the fact dimly. His hands and tongue are tremulous. . . . The face is pinched up, yet florid and greasy. The expression is anxious. . . . There is loathing of food, with suspicions of it's being filthy or poisoned." Nor does he drink. Thus far we have grimacing, motor twitchings, and the negativism of food refusal. Moreover, the patient "makes constant attempts to get out of bed, and if permitted to do so, will stand until exhausted."

A "sensation of danger will exhibit itself in the patient's attacking any one who approaches him, with a blind fury." On the ward, he exhibits "constant restlessness and anxiety," an agitation of a catatonic nature. In a few weeks, this food-refusing patient has sunk into inanition and dies. If, however, the patient recovers, he becomes quite well again with no signs of the previous illness. "The cure is permanent as well as complete."

Bell reported stupor, mutism, violent outbreaks of glass-shattering and attacking staff and other patients, verbigeration, "howl[ing] and stamp[ing] which continued all night." One patient "yells because he is just about to be crushed." There is self-injurious behavior—"beats his head most furiously"—and "paroxysms of fury." Another patient, a woman of 49, "has continued highly excited; screaming most of the time and perfectly incoherent." In another female patient, the family had hoped, "from the suddenness of the attack that it might prove merely hysteria." Alas, no. "Her violence was extremely great, attacking wildly and indiscriminately all who approached her, until it became necessary to remove her here." Leeches failed to remediate her, and she died with symptoms of dysentery.

It required two attendants to keep a 30-year-old male patient in bed. "Strikes and kicks; attempts to smash his head against the walls of his room; vociferates; eyes wild; expression of countenance wild and fierce."

Of another male patient of 30, Bell said, "Hands in constant motion. Refuses food; fixes eyes on one object; takes no notice. Pays no attention to calls of nature."

In the differential diagnosis, Bell ruled out delirium tremens, brain inflammation, and typhoid fever. Mania? Bell saw the disorder as delirium, as it was rare for mania to terminate in death. Bell concluded "that [the case] must be regarded as one of the nervous derangements which has hitherto been overlooked and undescribed."

While Delasiauve and the other delirious-mania authorities sank into oblivion, the memory of Luther Bell and his eponymously named "disease" or "mania" have survived almost to this day. The 1975 edition of the World Health Organization's *International Classification of Disease* included "Bell's disease" and "Bell's mania" (code 296.0). They recognized "maniacal delirium" as well; it had the same code.[20]

UNITED KINGDOM

How to deal with "the angry and irascible excitement of maniacs"? asked Edinburgh physician and nosologist William Cullen in 1798. "Inspiring them with the awe and dread of some particular persons," seemed to him a capital remedy. "Sometimes it may be necessary to acquire it even by stripes and blows," he added. But there was one exception: "That is, when the maniacal rage is either not susceptible of fear, or incapable of remembering the objects of it; in such instances, stripes and blows would be wanton barbarity."[21] Later generations might have quarreled with Cullen's therapeutics. But it is clear that, in Cullen's Edinburgh, some kind of maniacal rage was familiar.

It was likewise familiar at Bethlem Hospital in London (the storied "Bedlam" of history). In 1798, John Haslam, the apothecary of the hospital, described a young man, 25, admitted in September 1795, "in a very furious state, in consequence of which he was constantly confined. He got little or no sleep—during the greater part of the night he was singing, or swearing, or holding conversations with persons he imagined about him. Sometime he would rattle the chain with which he was confined for several hours together, and tear everything within his reach." "Completely exhausted by his exertions," he died early in November.[22] Haslam later described "the gusts of violence from the furious maniac."[23] He pointed out to the Governors of Bethlem Hospital what might happen if patients of "irritable temper" are not confined in an institution such as the hospital: "Then the unhappy victim of this calamity is to be abandoned to his own guidance, floating through society without the compass of discretion, or the rudder of reason, in order that in due time he may add to the wreck of incurables, if he should fail to terminate his miseries by suicide, or discover the irritation of his temper by the commission of murder."[24]

In 1823, some insider, possibly Haslam himself, wrote an account of the patients at Bethlem. William Gammage, for example, 40, admitted in 1818, had murdered two people and arrived at the hospital "under strict vigilance to prevent mischief from any sudden paroxysm of that dreadful mania." Thomas Dowle, 28, admitted in 1822, had lost his reason after a practical joke. He had fainted away. "He was taken up and conveyed home, delirium ensued; and confirmed madness followed, which has ever since continued without abatement, to a degree not only pitiable, but dangerous to all who approach him. His propensities are fierce and vicious; he tries to kick at all who come near him, and even to bite at them, with all the rabid fury of an enraged dog. . . . He seizes and tears rugs, blankets, his own clothes, and anything within his reach." Tearing things into fragments is typical of the psychotic excitement of catatonia. But as yet the English had no specific diagnosis for such "manic" behavior, aside from "frantic derangement."[25]

The first effort in England to assign precise diagnoses to violent unreasoning behavior comes with a German physician, Hermann Weber (MD Bonn, 1848), who in the early 1850s migrated to England, settled in London, and soon had a large society practice. In 1865, he described "the delirium of collapse," a kind of postinfectious delirious mania. "I couple the term 'acute insanity' with that of 'delirium' because the nature of the mental aberrations . . . [is] not the same as in the common febrile delirium, but resembles much more those which accompany the aberrations usually comprised under the term 'insanity,' and especially those described under the head of mania." He continued: "The suddenness of the outbreak of the mental derangement is mentioned in all the cases; and the form approached, more or less, what may be termed maniacal delirium, with delusions of an anxious nature and hallucinations of the senses."[26]

The English were not caught up in the diagnostic complexities of the Continent, such as differentiating fatalities in "acute delirium" from those in "catatonic schizophrenia."

In 1867, Henry Maudsley pooh-poohed some of the fashionable maladies arriving from Europe yet granted that "A *furor transitorius* lasting for a few hours or days, and accompanied by vivid hallucinations and destructive tendencies has been attested by so many trustworthy observers that it is impossible to doubt its occasional occurrence; the outbreak is comparable, indeed, with an attack of epilepsy."[27]

By 1874, Thomas Clouston, physician to the West London Hospital and among the founders of biological thinking in English psychiatry, was discussing manic delirium in disease terms, calling it "homicidal insanity." "Homicidal insanity," he said, was a "form of homicidal mania or monomania in which the patient is possessed with an impulse to kill somebody . . . yet exhibits no other mental derangement." Pinel had called it *"manie sans délire,"* and Esquirol had labeled it "instinctive monomania," distinguishing it from "intellectual monomania" with its delusions.

"Affective monomania" meant "moral insanity," said Maudsley. The homicidal urge, he said, was merely symptomatic of a larger form of insanity: "In all forms of the disease, paroxysms of impulsive violence are common features; without assignable motive, insane patients suddenly tear their clothes, break windows or crockery, attack other patients, and do great injury to themselves; they exhibit unaccountable impulses to walk, to run, to set fire to buildings, to steal, to utter blasphemous or obscene words."[28] With Maudsley, delirious mania crystallizes in England into a regular diagnosis.

In 1889, W. Bevan Lewis, medical director of the West Riding Asylum in Wakefield, found the exact diagnosis as "acute delirious mania." It was the acute delirium of the French. "The disease is often most sudden in its onset, and frequently appears to follow upon some moral [psychological] cause—shock or fright." Lewis differentiated it from "ordinary acute mania" in its "intensity" and in "the absolute oblivion in most cases and in the rapid course and frequency of a fatal termination." Ordinary acute mania was almost never fatal and usually eventuated in "a certain and rapid recovery. Not so, however, in acute delirious mania; here the outlook from the first is ominous, and the gravest prognosis must be given." He described the lips covered with sordes, food refusal, and negativism. The patient becomes incomprehensible, psychotic, and shows verbigeration The utterances are a broken strain of completely unintelligible jargon. The fever is now 102°F, urine and stool pass involuntarily, and a rapid and fatal termination ensues.[29] The description is harrowing.

Daniel Hack Tuke's *Dictionary of Psychological Medicine* in 1892 was fairly awash with delirious mania–style diagnoses. The section on "acute delirious mania" went on for four pages and gave as synonyms Bell's disease, *délire aigu*, delirious mania, acute delirium, mania gravis, and so forth. The entry for "mania, moral" said "see moral insanity." *"Manie sin delirio,"* "maniacal delirium," and "maniacal fury" were all cited.[30] The rivulets were now swelling into a great stream. Interestingly, the section on "katatonia" dwelt entirely on Kahlbaum and mentioned none of these cases. But that may be because it was only Kraepelin who, in 1904, dragged delirious mania into the catatonia spotlight.

In this manner, "acute delirious mania" became a standard diagnosis in England. In 1928, Hubert J. Norman, superintendent of Camberwell House, a pricey private nervous clinic in London, was describing "delirium," with its confusion, psychosis, and restlessness. "A specially acute variety," he said, "is that known as acute delirium, acute delirious mania, or Bell's mania. It usually comes on rapidly and the patient passes into a grave condition. The mental confusion is complete; there is entire incoherence with a tendency to repeat certain words or acts." He then painted a picture of "severe physical disorder," with temperatures of 102° to 103°F, sordes, and negativism. "The outlook is always bad, and death takes place in the majority of these cases."[31]

GERMANY

Delirious mania was as well-known in German-speaking Europe as elsewhere, and it is unnecessary to dwell on the disparate diagnoses flowing together into a single disease entity. By way of illustration, in 1829, Johann Baptiste Friedreich, at 33 an associate professor of psychiatry in Würzburg and an early biological thinker, said of "mania" (*Tobsucht*): "You will find with him everything smashed up, his clothing torn to shreds, he himself often naked."[32]

With time, the diagnoses begin to sharpen. In 1878, Heinrich Schüle, superintendent of the Illenau asylum who in 1867 had launched in Germany the French "acute delirium"—anticipating Kahlbaum's catatonia—asserted that *delirium acutum* had a specific maniacal form, with numerous motor symptoms, clouding of consciousness, fever, and might end fatally.[33]

The following year, 1879, Richard von Krafft-Ebing, professor of psychiatry in Graz, produced a more elaborate differentiation. He distinguished between nondegenerative and degenerative kinds of delirium and *stupor*. Among the nondegenerative, he listed *"mania transitoria"* (caused by *epilepsia larvata*), hallmarked by "furious excitement" or "maniacal confusion"; there was also "stupidity or primary curable dementia," where mental activity was largely suspended. Among the degenerative forms, he listed the stupor and psychosis of "epileptic insanity."[34] In these years, Morel's concept of degeneration was coming into play, and Krafft-Ebing was among the main German apostles of the doctrine.

But it was Kraepelin who built a bridge between manic delirium and catatonia, and he did it via Hermann Weber's "delirium of collapse." From the very first edition of his textbook in 1883, Kraepelin incorporated Weber's postinfectious "acute condition of collapse," with its confusion, flight of ideas, agitation, and hallucinations.[35] In a second edition in 1887, he extended the concept of collapse delirium to the (presumably febrile) puerperium—in an epoch when postpartum infection was so common as to be routinely called "milk fever." He said of collapse delirium: "The patients leap from bed, run about the room with grimacing countenance, blather much nonsense, do not answer questions directly, fail to recognize the surroundings, and are not to be calmed. The mood is highly changeable but is usually predominantly anxious."[36]

By the fourth edition in 1893, Kraepelin had changed the delirium of collapse to being a consequence of "exhaustion," not just fever. "The first thorough description of collapse-delirium came from Hermann Weber, who observed it in falling temperature after acute illnesses. Further observation has revealed, as I believe, that the same syndrome may arise, where any kind of severe external pathology produces a sudden exhaustion."[37]

In 1903, in the seventh edition, Kraepelin linked agitated delirium to catatonia. In the section on "infectious diseases," he wrote, "In a large number of cases of mental disorders following somatic diseases, we are dealing with forms of insanity that in reality arise from quite different causes. The acute lesion provides here only the trigger for the eruption of a disease that was already more or less long underway. That is the case in the various forms of manic-depressive insanity and of catatonia, also in melancholia and senile dementia." Apparently postinfectious delirium could be catatonia.[38]

In the eighth edition, in 1910, Kraepelin abandoned entirely the postinfectious collapse-delirium explanation: "Most of the cases that I earlier considered collapse-delirium have, as a result of more careful observation of the clinical pictures, turned out to be other diseases, namely circular or catatonic excitement."[39] This was the bridge between manic delirium and catatonia.

DELIRIOUS MANIA IS ESTABLISHED
AS A FORM OF CATATONIA

The middle third of the twentieth century was a time of confusion. Was catatonia really a subtype of schizophrenia? What did fatal catatonia (or fatal delirious mania) have in common with the other catatonic pictures, or was it a disease of its own?[40] And the catatonias caused by other diseases—did they offer the same picture as Kahlbaum's catatonia? Even today, these questions have not been clarified. But the now-forgotten clinicians of the past century made a start.

As we saw earlier, Kraepelin adumbrated the link in 1910. Yet he was rarely cited on this. In 1919, Paul Ladame, a staff psychiatrist at the Bel-Air nervous clinic in Geneva and associate professor of psychiatry, proposed "acute idiopathic fulminating psychosis" as a distinct variety of acute delirium. Its distinguishing characteristic was that it ended fatally. (This is in contrast to patients with "acute delirium," most of whom survive, he said.) He reported eight female patients in mid-life between 1901 and 1912 who had died of "acute psychosis." Their common clinical features: "intense motor agitation," precipitous cachexia (their flesh "literally melted" from their bodies), mental confusion and psychosis, and apparent brain inflammation. Some exhibited negativism as well; others, food refusal and stereotypies.[41]

Linking catatonia to fatal outcomes was Werner Scheidegger's retrospective study of 43 deaths from catatonia between 1900 and 1928 in the Zurich University Psychiatric Hospital. The main symptoms were "conspicuous physical deterioration, intense motor agitation, anxious affect, fever, self-injury or suicide attempts, food refusal, severe clouding of consciousness, alternation of catatonic rigidity with pronounced motor agitation, pressing at the door, racing around, ideas of sinfulness, and loud screaming and aggressivity." Four of the deaths were owing to encephalitis lethargica, the others to "schizophrenia."[42]

Interest in fatal outcomes in "schizophrenia" was rising. In October 1934, Hermann Stefan reported four deaths from "agitation" and "exhaustion" in a private nervous clinic in Westphalia. Case number one, a woman of 22, had manic delirium. She maintained that she had a mission "to protect Hitler." After 10 days of agitation, she suddenly died. Case number 2, a woman of 28, kept crying "Hitler is my brother." She kept up the monotonous repetition of this and other nonsense phrases, "raged and cried the entire night and was not to be calmed." She died suddenly nine days later.[43]

The argument that fatal delirious mania was a form of catatonia was presented in 1934 by Karl-Heinz Stauder, who had just finished training at the Munich University Psychiatric Hospital, with 37 cases of "lethal catatonia" (die tödliche Katatonie).[44] The

37 cases had an age at onset of 18 to 26; the illness, in previously healthy individuals, came suddenly; the catatonic feature was extreme agitation and violence, and, as the patients lay dying, they gave the appearance of "animals hunted to death"—the author acknowledged Schüle's phrase (see below). They were also negativistic, refusing food, and striking out when approached.

The violence of Stauder's patients was extraordinary. A farmer, 23, had just finished writing a warm note to a friend. "He put the pen aside, spoke the mealtime prayer, took knife and fork in hand. Suddenly he sprang up and attacked his family members with the knife. His speech was incomprehensible, except for the phrase that 'he must soon die.'"

A 25-year-old shoemaker had raved for a week before admission. On the ward, he was in stupor. "Suddenly he screams wildly, hits out around himself, and fast as lightening before an attendant can reach him he falls out of bed onto his face." Blood is now running from his nose. He's put into the hydrotherapy bath, where a whole team of orderlies can scarcely restrain him. Out of the bath, "He drums with his arms and legs ceaselessly against walls and floor, tries to spring head first onto the floor. Is extremely dangerous to himself."

Patient number 3, a 19-year-old woman, was admitted for catatonic excitement. On the ward, "She suddenly springs up and leaps upon other patients. Hammers ceaselessly with both fists on herself."

Muscular rigidity was striking. As the end approaches, "The patients lie mostly in bed in cramped positions or throw themselves back and forth with clamped jaws. Every muscle is tensed to the extreme." (None of the patients responded to barbiturates.) The only antemortem physical findings were extensive petechial hemorrhages into the tissue and cyanosis of the extremities. At autopsy, no recognizable pathology was found.

Stauder is among the earliest authors to offer evidence that fatal catatonia was not a subtype of schizophrenia but possibly a disease with its own pathological anatomy. "It is justified to assert the unity of this catatonia group; because in the last analysis it is this differentiation that opens the way to the first pathological-anatomical findings [in catatonia]."

Stauder's article touched off a wave of research on "fatal catatonia" and secured for him an acronymic place in medical history.

In the years 1935–47 there were 142 cases of "acute fatal catatonia" at the Steinhof asylum, Vienna's large public psychiatry hospital. Otto Arnold achieved a therapeutic landmark when he reported in 1949 on the remarkable efficacy of ECT for these patients. (See Chapter 13; he actually confirmed previous findings.) He described the patients' state of fear. "Frequently they expressed thoughts of death in very specific forms." Thoughts of suicide were rare. "But it rather seems to me as if the patients were surrendering themselves without resistance to an awaiting fate, indeed formally fleeing into death."

The life-threatening catatonia ran its course beginning with extreme agitation, then fading into stupor. "Such true manic delirium [*Tobsucht*] with its ruthless and pointless violence presents the most memorable images in psychiatry. When we consider the frequently high temperatures in this stage, the cyanoses, the hemorrhages . . . which I found in every patient, sometimes in mild, sometimes in the most severe form, it is the case that these symptoms constitute a picture that I should like to call the syndrome of threatening fatal catatonia." Given its treatability, the correct diagnosis was of capital importance.[45]

But freeing catatonia entirely from schizophrenia was a different story. Fatal catatonia was probably the first chunk to come off the schizophrenia mass. Two workers at the Szeged University in Hungary said, in 1953, of the ECT treatment of fatal catatonia, "Of the different forms of schizophrenia, the so-called acute fatal catatonia is the most unitary clinical syndrome. . . . The pathological changes evident in all forms of schizophrenia demonstrate most clearly here, that with this psychosis we are dealing with an illness of the whole body."[46] Indeed, this would be an illness different from "schizophrenia."

FATAL NOSTALGIA

There is one more rivulet to run into the great stream that becomes delirious mania, and that is "nostalgia."

Nostalgia had cousins. Understandably, the first clinicians to grapple with the biological consequences of fear and regret were not able to hone their concepts finely. Samuel Tissot in Lausanne was fully aware of the biology of these emotions but expressed it as "remorse." "I have seen remorse kill a very strong man in five weeks," he wrote in 1779, "sleep abandoning him totally." "He could take only a bit of milk and water mixed together. . . . He passed sometimes a full twenty-four hours in continuous agitation in his room; when he was no longer strong enough to walk, he would roll; other times, he would spend an equally long time without changing position; but in the last ten days he lost completely his strength and could not get out of bed; he no longer had the strength to see, to understand and to speak. . . . He was given over to very strong spasmodic movements in the last five days and frequently to delirium. The idea of trying any medications was odious to him."[47] The catatonic elements of alternation, food refusal, negativism, and "convulsive" muscle twitching are familiar.

Yet the principal rivulet leading to this stream of fatal delirium was "nostalgia."[48] The term entered medicine in 1688, with Johannes Hofer's Basel dissertation on "Heimwehe," the German for nostalgia.[49] The term was rooted in the Swiss experience of sending young men and women to distant places for military or domestic service and then seeing them fall ill with homesickness, often a sickness unto death. Clinically, it was quite striking to witness an otherwise healthy young man become ill with stupor, lie abed psychotic, his circulation failing, then develop a fever and die. Fever seems to be highly present in fatal cases of nostalgia (though not universal, and we are loathe to loan it the scientific status of a sentinel symptom).

In 1745, Ernst Anton Nicolai, who had just completed a dissertation at Halle on "The Connection of Music with the Practice of Medicine," noted "the disease which arises from a heartfelt longing to see the Fatherland again and that is called Heimweh [homesickness]. Those notably plagued with it are the Swiss. . . . When these good people have to leave the Fatherland, one can well imagine how difficult it is for them to come together with strangers and change their lifestyle. The most curious aspect, however, is that Heimweh arises in them through a certain song, that they call 'Kühe-Reyhen' [literally, "cow-series," but meaning calling for the cows] that they have often heard at home." This was such a problem among Swiss mercenaries in France that the government had to forbid the playing of the song.[50]

Fatal Nostalgia in France

The wars of the Napoleonic Years saw much fatal nostalgia among young troops, not in advance, but in retreat, who would fall by the wayside and die. There were numerous causes of death in Napoleon's terrible retreat from Moscow in 1812, but one certainly was nostalgia, as the expeditionary force was whittled from the 400,000 men who went out to the 3,000 who returned.[51]

In France after the Napoleonic Wars, references to fatal nostalgia begin appearing in the literature. Two workers said in 1819 that, in the years of war, it was especially "peasants from the west of France who failed to thrive in the inaction of an army camp and soon began to long for the home hearth. The nostalgia to which they were prey, rendered fatal the slightest wounds, even simple scrapes, while the young people of the cities felt no threat from this malady." The authors continued, "We have seen soldiers die the day that home leave was refused. But these cases are rare." They said that ordinarily a fever seized the patient, followed by marasmus "that finally puts an end to the suffering." At autopsy, little is found. This chain of events may be reversed, however, if the physician can assure the patient that soon he will go home.[52] In 1821, Philippe Pinel said of "simple nostalgia" (not complicated with another disease): "He is vulnerable to it to the extent that he has been separated from all that he holds dear in the world. The state of solitude, which becomes daily more terrifying for him, plunges him into the blackest of reveries; the memory of the past worsens his lamentations; he fears to look into the future; he suffers, languishes, and dies."[53]

In 1852, Bénédict-Augustin Morel said "Nostalgia represents the most serious of the physiological and psychological perturbations that sadness can bring to the spirit. . . . It can sometimes cause death when the return to the cherished places of birth does not occur quickly enough."[54] But, not quite a decade later, in his large psychiatry textbook, Morel gave nostalgia little attention and said it was acute delirium, in any context, that produced psychosis and death.[55]

Thus, nostalgia was on its way out, and acute delirium, as a means of linking fear and death, on its way in. In 1912, Philippe Chaslin was able to write of "*nostalgie*": "This sad emotion is scarcely found anymore save among the Bretons and is disappearing with the new ways. It has no importance in pathology."[56]

Yet the twentieth century had not yet finished subjecting the French to trauma. Two terrible world wars lay still in store. In the "Great Fear" of May and June 1940, as the Germans dive-bombed terrified refugees on the roads of France, psychiatric hospitals received cases of "acute delirium" with fatal outcomes such as had not been seen in France for decades. In 1940, the psychiatric hospital at Auxerre admitted 17 such cases, many of which ended fatally: "On May 20 arrived a female refugee from the Department of the Meuse, in 'agitated confusion' with a temperature of 38°5 C. She died May 25. She was 55."

"On May 23 a female refugee, 45, arrives from the Aisne Department. She is confused; she doesn't know where she is or where she has come from; she has multiple bruises; she mutters incomprehensible words; she is frightened as if she were looking at menacing forms . . . The 6th of June: she is very agitated, screams without cease, her temperature is 40°; her lips are dry, covered with sordes . . . her tongue is dry. Despite efforts to rehydrate her with sodium bicarbonate, her temperature remains high. She dies the 8th of June."[57]

Nostalgia, Acute Delirium, and Death in Germany

In Germany, homesickness (*Heimweh*) battled with acute delirium as explanations of fatal cases. In 1803, Johann Christian Reil, professor of medicine in Halle with an interest in psychiatry (to whom students of neuroanatomy owe the "Island of Reil"), theorized that "Homesickness is a true emotional disorder [*Gemüthskrankheit*]. . . . The Catholics of Appenzell Canton are simple shepherds, but are extremely attached, as are their cows, to the Alps of their Fatherland." And so, observed Reil, a melody such as the "*Kuhreihen*" suffices to abolish all their nervous power, a kind of "nervous consumption," or tuberculosis.[58] There are cases on record of nannies who tried to murder their charges out of homesickness, in the psychotic belief that once the children were dead they could depart.[59]

Acute delirium, on the other hand, had a big following in Germany, as in France. Viennese psychiatry professor Ernst von Feuchtersleben described, in 1845, a kind of furious mania that could end fatally ("*ira furor brevis*"). He didn't use the term "acute delirium," but the Viennese version corresponded to the Parisian: "The heat climbs from the breast, to the throat and head, which hurts; the ears ring or buzz; the countenance becomes anxious; the patients say 'they've got the heat in the front of their eyes'; they often warn the people around them, and even themselves ask to be rendered harmless." Finally, the process reaches the brain: "and in this instant arises the blind irresistible urge to murder, to commit suicide, robbery, arson . . . . "[60]

In 1861, Wilhelm Griesinger, about to go from Zurich to Berlin as professor of psychiatry, laid it out clearly. The attacks that the French call acute delirium "are characterized by the sudden onset, a furious delirium with continuous incoherent, meaningless babble, by repetitive expressions of great anxiety—namely frequent paranoid ideas about being poisoned—by dizziness, by clumsy, tremulous movements as though half-intoxicated, often by light muscle contractions, insomnia, a pale countenance, dry tongue, and rapid exhaustion. . . . These are often febrile, may last 6–8 weeks, and often end fatally, after the patients suddenly collapse."[61]

This clear statement set the stage for reports in the German literature about acute delirium ending fatally. Heinrich Schüle at the Illenau asylum apparently encountered it often: "In [the maniacal form of acute delirium], death may eventuate in as quickly as a few days: It is the exhaustion death of a hunted deer."[62]

In 1880, at a psychiatry meeting at the Crown Prince Hotel in Karlsruhe, Carl Fürstner, who preceded Kraepelin as head of psychiatry in Heidelberg, told colleagues about three recent cases of "acute delirium": Two had ended fatally. Details of one case: "excessively increased and quite purposeless muscular activity, which continued to the lethal termination, also conspicuous tension and rigidity of the muscles . . . stubborn food refusal, a severe . . . increase in temperature, early collapse, decubitus ulcers [bedsores]."[63]

These cases establish that delirious mania and its fatal variants were a rock-solid part of traditional psychiatric diagnosis. By the 1960s, almost everywhere in the UK and Europe, fatal delirious mania, pernicious catatonia, or whatever label one chooses, was an accepted part of psychiatric diagnostics that a clinician would ignore at the patient's peril. How this sturdy European concept was replaced by the much more anodyne American notion of "intermittent explosive disorder" is told elsewhere.[64] In 1982, Heinz Häfner, a Mannheim psychiatrist, scoffed at views that lethal catatonia had somehow gone away. Not at all, he said. It was merely treated in internal medicine services in the absence of psychiatric emergency care.[65]

9

THE NEUROLEPTIC MALIGNANT SYNDROME

The history of science is one long series of tournaments, of champions and challengers, of pledges and surrenders and rewards beyond compare in chivalry. The conquests and captures of the knights errant of natural history, the feats of backroom squires and laboratory heroes, are also legendary. . . . The Round Table of Science has room for all who can find their way to it—the rim of it is a snowflake curve.
—W. Grey Walter, 1956[1]

THE AMERICAN CENTURY

In the second half of the twentieth century, America became the new epicenter for psychiatry. Yet, after the 1950s, previous European scholarship, together with the diagnoses and treatments that flowed from it, was largely ignored by an American psychiatry focused on psychoanalysis, then on psychopharmacology. For the psychoanalysts, delirious mania and lethal catatonia were abstractions as remote as "moon madness." And for the budding psychopharmacologists, catatonia was a form of schizophrenia that, like all others, would respond to the new antipsychotics. Three threads emerged: one, the recognition that Kraepelin's and Bleuler's marriage of catatonia with schizophrenia was inadequate, as catatonia was clearly recognized in other psychiatric illnesses; two, a febrile neurotoxicity was noted, caused by the new neuroleptic agents, which became known as the *neuroleptic malignant syndrome* (NMS); and, three, the recognition took hold that NMS and delirious mania were the more lethal forms of catatonia, identified by catatonia signs, verified and validated by the response to catatonia treatments of sedatives and electroconvulsive therapy (ECT). The impetus to these recognitions came from the post-1950s flood of psychoactive drugs.

THE INFLUENCE OF PSYCHOPHARMACOLOGY

The active interest in psychopathology and identifying disorders among clinicians in the nineteenth century—the Karl Kahlbaums, Ewald Heckers, and Emil Kraepelins— waned with the Freudian belief that psychoanalysis was the treatment for psychiatric illnesses regardless of the symptoms, signs, or history of the illness. Faced with many new psychoactive substances with different effects on behavior, clinicians sought guides to prescribe each medication. Syndromes were labeled by symptoms defined by rating scales and clustered by statistical factor analyses. By default, Kraepelinian labels became the lingua franca of clinical psychopharmacologists who recognized schizophrenia, manic-depressive illness, and anxiety states as broad labels for which different new drugs could be prescribed. Randomized controlled trials (RCTs) compared medications, and soon populations were identified that were more responsive to one agent than to another. An RCT trial of chlorpromazine, imipramine, and placebo in a broad sample of psychiatric ill at New York's Hillside Hospital in the 1950s by Max Fink and Donald Klein identified useful predictors for the two active compounds.[2,3] The trials confirmed that chlorpromazine reduced the aggression and disordered thought of psychotics and that imipramine lessened the inanition and suicide drive of melancholics and relieved the neuroses of adolescent girls. Chlorpromazine also relieved patients with psychotic depression, showing a broader influence of chlorpromazine and raising doubt as to the significance of labels such as "antipsychotic" for the primary psychiatric disorders.[4] These studies were accompanied by detailed electroencephalograph (EEG) recordings that characterized the effects of each agent on the brain.[5]

More specific diagnostic labels were welcomed to pinpoint therapeutic effects in clinical practice. These treatment differences were particularly important in catatonia. Treatments with barbiturates and ECT had been effective for catatonia but were ineffective in schizophrenia. Physicians had to identify catatonia and prescribe either the effective anticatatonic treatments or the new "antischizophrenic" neuroleptic drugs that soon became associated with a neurotoxic syndrome.

Viewing catatonia singularly as a type of schizophrenia was challenged early in the psychopharmacology era. Applying Sydenham criteria for diagnostic validity, Earl D. Hearst and colleagues at Washington University in St. Louis, in 1971 argued that the label of catatonic schizophrenia did not specify an identifiable syndrome nor offer a guide to treatment. Catatonia was heterogeneous with many causes; it was often associated with affective features not characteristic of schizophrenia. It warranted attention outside schizophrenia.[6] We return to this subject in the following section.

THE NEUROLEPTIC MALIGNANT SYNDROME CHALLENGES THE CONNECTION OF CATATONIA AND SCHIZOPHRENIA

By 1960, Jean Delay, the Parisian doyen of chlorpromazine and a member of the *Académie française,* and his associates at the Centre hospitalier Sainte-Anne had described a *syndrom malin* when they first administered haloperidol.[7] The patients suddenly became febrile, rigid, posturing, mute, and either stuporous or excited. Discontinuing neuroleptic treatment led to a slow recovery.

Similar reports increasingly appeared. Mutism, rigidity, incontinence, fever, and coma followed the injection of the depot antipsychotic fluphenazine enanthate in a college student. She improved slowly with discontinuing the medication and persistent nursing care.[8] A similar syndrome following treatment with haloperidol was next reported.[9] Anticholinergic treatments that at the time were prescribed to relieve the dyskinesias and motor signs associated with neuroleptic drug use offered no benefit.

In 1980, Stanley Caroff at the VA Hospital in Philadelphia summarized 60 case reports of neurotoxic responses to neuroleptic drugs. He offered the label of "neuroleptic malignant syndrome" (NMS), a name that has been widely accepted, to describe the lethal syndrome of acute onset of fever, autonomic instability, altered consciousness, stupor, rigidity, and posturing.[10] The role of potent neuroleptics, particularly haloperidol as the most toxic, was quickly identified.[11] As the syndrome became increasingly recognized and neuroleptics withdrawn, the mortality rate reduced from 25 percent before 1984 to 12 percent by 1989.[12]

Sudden deaths in psychotic patients treated with potent neuroleptic drugs raised little interest until the Caroff report. After reading Caroff's description, Fink at the University Hospital at Stony Brook recognized the neurotoxic syndrome in three patients treated with neuroleptics.[13] Each story was marked by repetitive motor movements, mutism, posturing, rigidity, negativism, fever, and autonomic instability. Neuroleptic medications were discontinued and bromocriptine prescribed, following Caroff's guide. The syndrome persisted. One patient slowly recovered with nursing and medical care. Intravenous diazepam and lorazepam transiently relieved the motor signs of two subjects, but both required ECT for complete remission.

At the height of the summer of 1976, a 23-year-old agitated and aggressive psychotic man under Fink's care at the Central Islip Psychiatric Center in Long Island refused food and fluids and required restraint and sedation. Intramuscular haloperidol was administered. The ward was incredibly hot; the patient became stuporous, dehydrated, hyponatremic (low sodium), febrile, suffered a seizure, and died within 12 hours. Neither physical nor psychological postmortem reviews offered understanding, as the NMS syndrome had not yet been defined and the toxic response to haloperidol was waiting to be discovered.

Another retrospective example of NMS was the death of Ms. Libby Zion, an 18-year-old Bennington College student being treated for depressed mood with phenelzine. In the summer of 1984, she was visiting New York City and developed an acute febrile, agitated, and disoriented state with abnormal motor movements. Admitted to New York Hospital, meperidine was administered; her agitation worsened and parenteral haloperidol added. Now in stupor, her temperature quickly rose to 107°F and she died. Her family sued the hospital for malpractice, and, in 1993, Fink was asked to review the records as an expert witness in the hospital's defense. Her many initial diagnoses did not consider NMS, but, by the time of the legal case, her experience was recognized as a tragic example of neuroleptic-induced malignant catatonia.[14]

Neurotoxic syndromes were increasingly recognized, usually appearing within the first two weeks of exposure to antipsychotic drugs in about 1 percent of patients treated.[15–20] One patient had similar toxic responses to three different antipsychotic drugs.[21] More men than women were affected (3:2), but male patients typically received higher drug doses, possibly explaining their increased risk.[22] Persons under age 20 and over age 65 were underrepresented in the reported cases, probably as a result of practitioners limiting their use of antipsychotic drugs in these age groups.[23]

The pathophysiology and effective treatment of NMS became widespread clinical concerns. Stanley Caroff and his colleagues Stephan Mann and Arthur Lazarus ascribed the syndrome to excessive dopamine blockade and recommended the prescription of dopamine agonists, such as bromocriptine and amantadine. [24] As some patients exhibited fever and muscle weakness reminiscent of malignant hyperthermia (MH), the toxic genetic-based response to inhalational anesthetic agents that was popularized at the time, these authors encouraged simultaneous treatment with the muscle relaxant dantrolene. The discontinuation of neuroleptic administration and prescription of bromocriptine and dantrolene became the recommended treatment for NMS.

Discontinuing the offending neuroleptic was essential to relief, but the prescription of the other medications added little. These ministrations were often ineffective, and patients languished in mutism, stupors, and abnormal motor movements. As more case records were described, the signs of mutism, rigidity, stupor, posturing, and negativism were increasingly seen as catatonia; the connection to malignant catatonia became more apparent—what clinched it was that the administration of ECT resolved the fevers, stupor, and catatonia within the first few seizures.[25] Once the response to ECT was acknowledged, assuring clinicians that NMS was a form of catatonia, clinicians began successful treatment with lorazepam or diazepam after trials with bromocriptine and dantrolene had failed.

NMS REMINDS CLINICIANS OF MALIGNANT CATATONIA (AND THE ROLE FOR ECT)

As we have seen, excited states of delirious mania of acute onset and malignant outcome were historically well described, often with the diverse labels of malignant, lethal, or fatal catatonia, or Bell's or Stauder's mania. Similar acutely ill, delirious, and overactive patients were described in the popular literature as having frenzy, furor, and catatonic excitement.[26]

Malignant catatonia was increasingly recognized among hospitalized psychotic patients.[27-32] In each instance, neuroleptic drug administration elicited acute excitement or stupor, delirium, and fever, accompanied by systemic autonomic crises that led to death. Systemic infections with the signs of encephalitis were avidly sought in the investigation, often to no avail. Some patients were deliriously manic and uncontrollable, dying in fever, dehydration, and vegetative collapse.

Effective relief for malignant catatonia by intensive daily ECT had been described in 1947 by Borreguero and in 1952 by Arnold and Stepan, as cited below.[33] Daily induced seizures, even multiple seizures in a day, were required to save lives. Fink often treated delirious manic patients by daily, even twice daily stimuli, and cites the following story of his awakening to the usefulness of ECT in malignant catatonia.[34]

On a morning in the Fall of 1987, Fink was teaching an expert class of five practicing physicians at the University Hospital in Stony Brook. A patient from the medical service had been referred for evaluation for ECT. A restless, delirious, and febrile 25-year-old woman in four-limb restraints, with nasal and urinary catheters and intravenous fluids running was seen by the class. When alert, she was negativistic, posturing, rhythmically thrashing, alternatingly mute and screaming. She was suffering an acute episode of systemic lupus erythematosus, a chronic autoimmune illness being treated with intravenous methylprednisone and sedated with haloperidol and lorazepam. An EEG had shown seizure-like activity, and phenytoin was prescribed as anticonvulsant. She was in delirious mania.

Was she a candidate for ECT? The physicians, influenced by the severity of her systemic illness, the restraints, parenteral feeding, and manifest weight loss, thought not, that the treatment was likely to do her more harm. They demurred even after Fink described the rapid relief with ECT in three patients with the same psychiatric complications of lupus that had been reported earlier by Samuel Guze at Washington University.[35] Contrary to the class opinion, the severity of her illness supported treatment with ECT since the treatment was remarkably safe even in the most extremely ill patients.[36]

With consent of her family and her physicians, a course of ECT was begun on hospital day 28. Within 10 days and 7 treatments the delirium was relieved, restraints were lifted, and she became cooperative and pleasant. But family and physician prejudices against continuing ECT forced cessation of treatment.

She rapidly regressed, again required restraints, and a second ECT series from days 68 to 90 resolved her illness.[37] By day 100, she was discharged with some relief of lupus by her medicines and relief of catatonia by the induced seizures, to remain well and care for her family at one-year examination.[38]

Additional case reports followed quickly, each affirming the connection and citing relief with cessation of neuroleptics and treatment with benzodiazepines and ECT.[39–44] The significant connection between NMS and catatonia was made by Denise White, in Cape Town, South Africa. She described five patients in whom the signs of catatonia preceded the administration of a neuroleptic.[45] In a second report a year later, catatonia was presented as a precursor to the malignant state, raising the question whether NMS, malignant catatonia, and the nonmalignant forms of catatonia were a single pathology.[46]

Treatment of NMS by ECT became the effective alternative when medications failed.[47–51] A review in 1991 of 734 published cases of NMS reported 48 (6 percent) that had been successfully treated with ECT with no greater mortality rate (10 percent) than those treated with medications alone.[52]

In a report of a patient with malignant catatonia, Mann et al. described ECT in 27 patients with NMS.[53] Of these, 20 patients recovered, 3 had a partial response, and 4 did poorly. The four patients with poor responses developed cardiac irregularities limiting their course of treatments. Numerous reviews find similar treatment efficacy rates.[54–57]

RELIEF OF NMS BY BENZODIAZEPINES STRENGTHENS ITS RECOGNITION AS MALIGNANT CATATONIA

As various medication protocols were tested for patients with malignant catatonia, none was recognized as immediately effective until 1983, when Gregory Fricchione in Boston presented four catatonic patients who responded rapidly to intravenous lorazepam.[58] Each patient had become agitated in the hospital and was treated with haloperidol, quickly precipitating a febrile toxic state with posturing, negativism, and mutism. Diphenhydramine and amantadine were ineffective, but 2 mg intravenous lorazepam relieved all signs of catatonia.

Rosebush and her colleagues at McMaster University in Hamilton, Ontario, next described 24 cases of NMS, almost all responsive to lorazepam.[59] In their survey of psychiatry admissions, they found an incidence of 9 percent with catatonia admitted in one year, with 80 percent responsive to lorazepam.[60] The authors were satisfied that proper dosing with lorazepam relieved catatonia and that resort to ECT was rarely necessary. Similar reports came from Teresa Rummans at the Mayo Clinic.[61,62] These authors recognized NMS as a form of malignant catatonia.

Similar reports by Fink at University Hospital at Stony Brook increasingly identified and treated catatonia in febrile neurotoxic patients. A 6-month survey on the psychiatry, neurology, and emergency room services using a newly devised catatonia rating scale found 7 percent met criteria for catatonia.[63] Of 28 inpatients treated with lorazepam for up to five days, 76 percent were relieved of catatonia. For the four accepting ECT, each responded well.[64]

In 2010, Rosebush and Mazurek reviewed their 20-year experience with 180 episodes of catatonia in 148 patients, again finding an 80 percent response rate to lorazepam among those ill with mood disorders, lesser success for those with psychotic signs.[65] The patients responded to lorazepam regardless of the duration of catatonia. Treatment with neuroleptic drugs was the precipitating factor in half the cases, making cases of NMS the largest part of their experience. The authors also made the interesting note that fear was a prominent feature in 60 percent among those with mood disorders.[66]

RESOLUTION: NMS IS A CATATONIA VARIANT, AND CATATONIA IS INDEPENDENT OF SCHIZOPHRENIA

Some authors sought to distinguish NMS and malignant catatonia. They argued that the degree of rigidity, the time of onset or the presence of fever, and the abnormality of laboratory tests differentiate the two conditions.[67] Yet in a review of University of Iowa hospital records of 9 patients with NMS and 17 with malignant catatonia admitted over an eight-year period, Brendan Carroll and Robert E. Taylor could find no differences in clinical features and concluded that the distinction was not useful.[68] Other studies seeking to differentiate NMS and malignant catatonia were also unsuccessful.[69-71]

Acceptance of NMS as a form of catatonia was slow, inhibited by the different treatments offered and different explanations of mechanism. As stated, Stanley Caroff and his colleagues believed that NMS resulted from the neuroleptic inhibition of dopamine activity and focused on treatment with the dopamine agonists bromocriptine and amantadine.[72] And, because the fever, muscle rigidity, and weakness simulated malignant hyperthermia, they augmented treatment with the muscle relaxant dantrolene. Despite poor responses and continuing deaths, many authors favored this prescription.

A national debate ensued, carried on for more than two decades, whether NMS was best considered an abnormality of dopamine metabolism and treated with dopamine agonists or an example of malignant catatonia and treated with ECT.[73] The debate turned around Fink's argument that NMS was best seen and treated as a form of malignant catatonia, with benzodiazepines as the primary treatment and ECT as the effective backup.[74]

An NMS internet hotline was created with catatonia scholars responding to queries.[75] For more than a decade, the responders advised discontinuing neuroleptic treatment and ending the prescription of dopamine agonists (bromocriptine, apomorphine) and dantrolene for the relief of muscle rigidity.[76] As the experience with benzodiazepines and ECT showed greater success, the guidelines increasingly preferred these treatments.

Essential to the different views was the failure to recognize the signs of catatonia. For many observers, the essence of NMS was the fever, autonomic instability, and muscle rigidity, encouraging belief in the overlap with malignant hyperthermia. Interest in catatonia was minimal, blocked by the prevailing belief that catatonia was schizophrenia, despite the reality that few of their patients met the criteria for the thought disorder, impaired speech, delusions, and hallucinations that characterized what people were calling "schizophrenia." Furthermore, treatments with barbiturates and benzodiazepines were considered still more risky, as it was believed that their use caused the development of tolerance and dependence; these beliefs were reinforced by the restricted prescribing rules set by the US Food and Drug Administration for the benzodiazepines. Dosing was limited to a few milligrams of lorazepam, often inadequate for the relief of malignant catatonia.

The debate was ongoing at meetings of psychiatric societies and in the literature, with the two camps soon distinguished by the ready availability of ECT for Max Fink, Gregory Fricchione, Teresa Rummans, Michael Taylor, and Denise White, compared to the necessity to refer their patients to other services for Stanley Caroff, Stephan Mann, Patricia Rosebush, and Gabor Ungvari. Also, many hospitals lacked ECT treatment units, so the clinicians could not prescribe this treatment, but all could prescribe dopamine agonists and dantrolene.

The awareness that catatonia was independent of schizophrenia and best considered a free-standing category in the psychiatric disease classification system developed slowly; these questions soon became issues in the American Psychiatric Association's revisions of the *Diagnostic and Statistical Manual* in 1994 and 2013.

10

SYMPTOMS AND DIAGNOSES

We are far from knowing why some are struck down overnight in a pandemonium of catatonic excitement while others exhibit an insidious and subtle departure from the tenets of reason.[1]
—Reg Ellery, 1941

Buffeted by psychoanalysis and blinded by the prestige of German learning, clinicians let catatonia languish in the quagmire of schizophrenia. Meanwhile the science of catatonia was under way. Some investigators thought they could use catatonia as a lance to pierce to the heart of schizophrenia, others took it as a disease *sui generis*. Useful leads were discovered, but almost none was followed up as psychiatry contorted itself in issues of early toilet training, guilt of the mothers, and patients who felt "empty."

Then the spirit of science began to reinfuse psychiatry. The profession began searching for its place as a specialty of medicine, not as an obscure offshoot of speculative philosophy. In the post-psychoanalytic era, psychiatry began to rediscover, as one wag put it, "that the plural of anecdote is not data; It is anecdotes."

WHAT ARE THE MAIN SYMPTOMS OF CATATONIA?

How to diagnose catatonia? Gabor Gazdag in Budapest, a leading catatonia specialist, says that all patients "with severe mood disorders or psychotic patients" should be assessed for catatonia because catatonia may not be immediately evident. Posturing is among the most striking symptoms, he argues, but it is present only in a minority of patients. The clinician should look for negativism, waxy flexibility, and automatic obedience.[2] What else to watch for today?

ALTERNATION

Around 1815, a woman of 40 was admitted to the psychiatry service of the Julius-Hospitale in Würzburg. "Initially she lay in bed for the entire day, spoke nothing more than yes and no, and that quite hurriedly, stared straight ahead with an unnatural gaze. Because she was not relieved mentally with either external or internal remedies," said chief psychiatrist Anton Müller, "I ordered her to be treated with electricity. After this operation had been applied for several days, she became so lively and exalted that she rushed continually about the room, so that I deemed it necessary to bring her down with other remedies. She lapsed back into her apathetic, inactive condition, did not leave the bed, and was mute. I took refuge again in the electricity machine. The same result followed. She danced for the entire day, as if she were stricken with tarantism [dance mania]. This dance mania then changed into erotomania, so that no male person could approach without being grabbed and being so tightly held that we had difficulty getting her off."[3] Thus, an early illustration of the alternation of stupor and agitation in catatonia, which we touched on in Chapter 2 but revisit here because of its importance as a candidate for addition to the symptom list.

No single symptom is pathognomonic of catatonia—absolutely characteristic of it—because they occur in many other illnesses as well. (It would be their *accumulation* and their response to sedation tests that makes the diagnosis of catatonia.[4]) But one temporal pattern of symptoms, that of *alternation*, is highly characteristic of catatonia. This is especially true for stupor and agitation since in no other psychiatric illness do stupor and agitation alternate.

In 1886, Heinrich Schüle, superintendent of the Illenau asylum in southwest Germany, described the alternation of agitation and stupor. "The patient lies for hours motionless on the floor, lets his limbs be moved, does not react, or only very little, to sensory stimuli, salivates freely, and stops speaking. . . . But then the tension breaks." The patient erupts in "fantasy positions and body postures, alternating with motor attacks, and then again a dreamlike quiet; later, verbigeration or echolalia. Then relapses into transitory motor rigidity and muteness. And so kaleidoscope-like, his condition alternates back and forth."[5] For Schüle, this "hysteric/constitutional" alternation was of sufficient importance as to make it one of his three main subtypes of catatonia (after "religious-expansive" and "depressive/demoniac").

Kraepelin added alternation to the signs of Kahlbaum's catatonia. In earlier editions of his textbook, Kraepelin had mentioned this alternation in passing. But in the fifth edition, in 1896, he made it a frequent feature of the course of catatonia. "Commoner than immediate dementia is the periodic appearance of singular states of agitation. Sometimes these insert themselves quite temporarily in the stupor. The patients suddenly become boisterous, gay, garrulous; they start to sing, to dance, to laugh stupidly, to destroy, to smear, to become violent, and then after a short period, just as quickly they sink back into their earlier immobility. . . . In many cases there is a frequent and irregular alternation between rigidity and agitation."[6]

By the eighth edition, in 1913, alternation had become the defining characteristic of catatonia: "I think we might characterize the catatonic forms of dementia praecox as the domination of the clinical picture by the linking of this singular agitation with catatonic stupor." He said, "Often enough we see in the stuporous patients some of the driven kinds of behavior that otherwise characterize agitated conditions. Suddenly the patients throw a cup into the room, run around the table, then fling themselves headfirst into bed and lie there still, or they may emit animalistic noises, or cry hurrah."[7] These descriptions are so graphic that it is quite surprising that this pattern of alternation did not survive in subsequent lists of individual catatonic symptoms.

Alternation was recognized as a fundamental characteristic of catatonia in the entry for "Katatonia" in Daniel Hack Tuke's 1892 *Dictionary of Psychological Medicine*: "Just as the immobility is frequently interrupted by stereotypical movements, so the mutism may be interrupted by the monotonous utterance of incessantly repeated words—verbigeration."[8] The entry, to be sure, was written by a German psychiatrist, Clemens Neisser, but it provided for the British readership a take on alternation. In

1914, Henry Devine, an attending at the West Riding Asylum in Wakefield, Yorkshire, began an article on "katatonia" with, "Under the heading of 'katatonia' are included certain peculiar states of stupor and excitement, which tend to alternate irregularly with one another."[9]

In France, Bénédict-Augustin Morel, at the Maréville asylum, described in 1853 this alternation in his patients without giving it a name. "They remain for weeks, or months, glum and silent, taking no initiative, and evidently deprived of all intellectual activity. Then at periodic intervals, they suddenly emerge from this state to precipitate themselves upon those around them, to hit, tear and bite. Some are moved to commit these acts by external circumstances. Others find in their pathological constitution the elements of an agitation so powerful as to move them to accomplish acts of great danger."[10]

"Acute delirium" was the French equivalent of catatonia, and Paul Guiraud, by 1938 at Ste. Anne, listed "inchoate motor agitation" and "somnolence" as principal symptoms. Motor agitation involved the violence we have been reviewing. "Somnolence is the inverse of the preceding syndrome. It frequently alternates with agitation. It is not coma, because the patient emerges brusquely from the somnolence in agitation."[11]

Karl Leonhard, among Kleist's most faithful students, elevated alternation to a principal feature of one of the two main types of catatonia that he proposed. There was *systematic catatonia*, a form of schizophrenia, and *unsystematic catatonia*, which Leonhard also called "periodic catatonia." Alternation was commonly found in periodic catatonia. In 1943, he reported that 9.8 percent of the systematic catatonias had agitation and 43.5 percent of the periodic (unsystematic) group did so.[12] Later, he again emphasized alternation as a part of periodic catatonia, the episodes of which "are characterized by agitated or inhibited symptoms, which frequently alternate."[13]

Leonhard described several of these "cycloid," or "bipolar," psychoses, the symptoms alternating from one behavioral pole to another. In 1962, Frank Fish at Edinburgh, a Leonhard student, said, "Excitements may alternate with stupor and, sometimes, before the introduction of tranquilizers [e.g., chlorpromazine, 1955], the patient often passed into stupor, then back into excitement, and so on, many times." Fish charted a mild and a severe version of Leonhard's catatonic alternation: There was the mild "motility psychosis," in either "hyperkinesia" or "akinesia." Fish said that "periodic catatonia" was a more severe version of this alternation.[14]

Although Leonhard's ideas have had little impact on US psychiatry (aside from "bipolar disorder"), his international influence has been diffuse but extensive, and today these concepts are widely credited.[15]

Even among non-Leonhardians, the conviction grew that alternation corresponded to a single underlying process. Said Bernhard Pauleikhoff, head of psychiatry in Münster, in 1969: "The symptom picture can alternate between stupor and agitation, because basically these spring from the same root and are an expression of the same inner tension."[16]

Has alternation vanished today as a symptom? Not at all. A pediatric psychiatrist writes the authors, "I've seen [alternation] a lot, and I think it is really common in these autistic and otherwise disabled kids, but I've seen it in typically-developing patients, too. One of the first alternators I saw was a girl who had some unclear recreational drug vs. illness etiology to her catatonia, and would alternate between crouching like a toad in the corner and staring, repetitively running her hands through her hair (like an echopraxia of combing), and then these wild leaping and jumping episodes where she had to be put into a net bed zipped closed, and she would literally hang upside down from the top. It was really wild."[17]

It is of interest that, in 2015, two workers at Baylor University criticized the catatonia symptom-list in the just-released *Diagnostic and Statistical Manual of Mental Disorders, 5th edition* (DSM-5) as "not capturing the true clinical picture of catatonia. Very opposing (eg immobility or excessive motor activity, mutism vs echolalia) . . . are listed in parallel and are given equal diagnostic weight."[18]

An overwhelming body of historical (and current) opinion thus endorses the concept of a specific pattern of symptoms—the alternation of stupor and agitation—as a clinical hallmark of catatonia. In retrospect, this issue of alternation sounds a warning in diagnosing the supposed mania of "bipolar disorder" in patients with catatonia.[19] What looks like mania might well be the agitation phase of catatonia. This is a differential diagnosis into which a good deal of thought once went,[20] now, alas, largely forgotten.

IS "CATATONIC SCHIZOPHRENIA" DIFFERENT FROM CATATONIA?

We addressed the separation of catatonia and "schizophrenia." But one question in the study of symptoms is: Are the symptoms of "catatonic schizophrenia" different from those of nonschizophrenic catatonia? The question strikes us as outdated, as it reflects the belief that there is a single entity called "schizophrenia," the symptoms of which can be well delineated. Nonetheless, if we assume for the sake of argument that "schizophrenia" exists as a defined entity, do its "catatonic" symptoms differ from the catatonia of other illnesses? Gabor Ungvari and collaborators write, "Preliminary evidence suggests that the symptom profile of catatonia in schizophrenia is different from that of other catatonic disorders. . . . Catatonia in the chronic phrase of schizophrenia is phenomenologically different from what is usually observed in an acute episode." Yet the evidence is weak that these apparent differences reflect anything other than duration-of-illness effects and inadequate catatonia treatments.[21] We join other scholars in the growing disbelief about "schizophrenia."

VANISHING CATATONIA?

For many years, catatonia was thought to be vanishing. Clear minds were troubled. In 1974, James Morrison, who, while at the University of Iowa, had done much to revive the diagnosis of catatonia, noted that the frequency of catatonic schizophrenia seen in acute settings had declined greatly since 1920.[22] "This disorder has," he said, "fallen on hard times."[23] It seemed at the end of its days. Banerjee Mahendra at St. Bartholomew's Hospital in London stated in 1981 that catatonia "has virtually disappeared from the modern psychiatric unit."[24] Medical historian German E. Berrios at the University of Cambridge agreed, declaring in 1996 catatonia to be "rare."[25] And, in 2010, Gabor Ungvari and colleagues noted "a dramatic decline in the diagnosis of catatonic symptoms among patients with schizophrenia over the last century."[26]

Really? How could such testimony be so at odds with statistics (cited in Chapter 1), based on systematic screening, showing that a seventh to a tenth of admissions to psychiatric emergency settings involve catatonic symptoms?

Several circumstances are in play here. For many years, catatonia was tied to schizophrenia. But the concept of schizophrenia was so vague and unstable that little importance could be attached to variation in its supposed subtypes. A graph of the incidence of "catatonic schizophrenia" in Missouri as a percent of all schizophrenia shows large fluctuations from 1900 to 1979, not a straight-line decline.[27] Changes in the real incidence? In all likelihood, no. It shows the lack of consistency in making these diagnoses, with catatonia shuttling back and forth between mood disorders and "schizophrenia" at the observers' whim.

What of ascertainment? As Patricia Rosebush and Michael F. Mazurek of McMaster University point out, catatonia "vanished" only because clinicians didn't see it "on the couch" in these years, the heyday of psychoanalysis. "There was a marked decline in interest on the part of psychiatrists in the 'somatic' or motor aspects of mental illness, except to the extent that they might contribute to the psychological interpretation of a particular patient's condition." Nonverbal patients were of less interest and often hospitalized. "In this climate, catatonia was lost from view." The apparent "revival" of catatonia is explained by the decline of psychoanalysis.[28]

Once DSM-IV in 1994 began accepting catatonia as a "specifier" in mood disorders, the rout of "catatonic schizophrenia" became complete (The schizophrenia subtypes were abolished in DSM-5 in 2013). At the Vincent van Gogh Institute for Psychiatry in the Netherlands, catatonic schizophrenia as a share of all schizophrenia admissions fell from 7.8 percent under DSM-III to 1.3 percent under DSM-IV.[29] Thus, little remained of catatonic schizophrenia, either because it wasn't being ascertained in private practice or because hospital psychiatrists were putting it in other diagnostic categories.

CATATONIA RE-EMERGES AS AN INDEPENDENT DIAGNOSIS

Does it matter if catatonia is an independent defined diagnosis? Around 1987, a girl, 14, was admitted to a British psychiatric facility with a nine-day history of bizarre behavior, gathering mutism, "and an increasing tendency to rocking and other self-stimulating behavior."

On admission, she continued the rocking, was negativistic, and now "mainly mute, but once echoed the two last words of a question. She stared vacantly, occasionally looking frightened or perplexed." She became incontinent of urine and "banged her legs or head hard enough to produce extensive bruising. She remained mute, but with occasional echoing or bouts of screaming."

Her clinicians made the diagnosis of "catatonic schizophrenia" and prescribed chlorpromazine. The symptom picture continued for four weeks, but she also developed "the facial grimacing described as *Schnauzkrampf*" and displayed "other mannerisms such as pointing her index finger at others." Her clinicians ordered a computed tomography (CT) scan and, to produce a good image, they administered a dose of the benzodiazepine diazepam. Miraculously, she awakened after the injection and "for 15 minutes appeared normally orientated and rational, before reverting to her former mute state."

Given her response to a benzodiazepine, but not to an antipsychotic, at this point the case should have shouted "catatonia" rather than "catatonic schizophrenia." A benzodiazepine, of course, is not a treatment for schizophrenia but is the first-line treatment for catatonia.

Alas, the case screamed the wrong message, and she was dead several days later of inhaled vomitus caused, they thought, by "intracranial haematoma produced by repeated acts of self-injury."[30]

The case shows how completely unknown catatonia was to these clinicians, even in 1987. Equally unknown to them were its therapeutics. Today, by contrast, catatonia is edging its way back to center stage as an independent disorder. How did this happen?

Ever since Kraepelin, there had been isolated reports of catatonia occurring in other disorders than schizophrenia: in medical disorders, for example, such as encephalitis lethargica, or in psychiatric disorders, such as depression. Yet the mere reporting of such phenomena had not sufficed to break the stranglehold of "schizophrenia." What gave schizophrenia's grasp a real jolt was the work from 1928 onward of Henri Baruk and Frederik De Jong on the use of bulbocapnine to induce catatonia in animals— which manifestly did not have schizophrenia.[31]

Their studies attracted wide attention in the scientific world, even though not considered top-drawer science by colleagues.[32] (De Jong and Baruk are incorrectly credited with introducing the concept of "periodic catatonia"; see the Zurich dissertation in 1900 of August Müller, a Bleuler student.[33]) An early voice from the neuroscience side in the United States was neuropsychiatrist William Lorenz in Wisconsin, who argued in 1930 that "The catatonic shows more pronounced disorder at the physiological level than most other so-called functional disorders."[34]

In the United States, an opening gun in psychiatric criticism of the "catatonic schizophrenia" concept was an article by Morris Herman at Bellevue Hospital and colleagues in the New York State Medical Journal in 1942, which began, "It has not been stressed in the literature that catatonic states occur in conditions other than schizophrenia."[35]

By the mid-1950s, a general unhappiness about including catatonia in "schizophrenia" started to brew. In January 1956, Kurt Schneider, now professor of psychiatry in Heidelberg, said that recent findings, such as his colleague Gerd Huber's discovery with air encephalography (in 1953) that some catatonias were a result of brain atrophy, were causing the diagnosis to be rethought. (Catatonia was not Huber's word, but some of his "schizophrenic" patients clearly had catatonia.[36]) Schneider said, "Even aside from Kleist, people have long tried to separate the hyperkinetic psychoses from the schizophrenias. That is true above all for fatal catatonias and for those in which there is complete recovery, for the phasic often periodic catatonias, also for the postpartum catatonias. These catatonias create an impression, in comparison to the other schizophrenic pictures, of being more primary, corporeal, 'organic.' " Schneider said the stuporous catatonias might remain part of schizophrenia, but the hyperkinetic— read "agitated"—catatonias were a separate disorder.[37]

Still, the notion that catatonia was not a part of schizophrenia was unacceptable to many. At a meeting at the National Institute of Mental Health (NIMH) in 1956, on conducting drug trials, Ivan Bennett, the chief of psychiatric research in the

Veterans Administration system, had dismissed schizophrenia as a "wastebasket diagnosis." Vernon Kinross-Wright, a well-known advocate of heavy doses of neuroleptics, rushed to the defense of "schizophrenia": "If you go to any back ward of any state hospital you can find people who have been standing on one leg for many years. There aren't too many of these people, but I think that everyone would agree that they are schizophrenics." Ironically, Kinross-Wright had selected a classic symptom of catatonia as evidence of the reality of the diagnosis of "schizophrenia."[38]

Yet *pace* Kinross-Wright, the differential effects of treatment were now causing people to question the very existence of "schizophrenia." Sodium Amytal was effective in "catatonic" schizophrenia but not in the other subtypes. Insulin coma therapy appeared effective in "paranoid schizophrenia," but not in the catatonic version. And the recent neuroleptic drugs were proving their value in "hebephrenic schizophrenia," yet were only second-line treatments in the catatonic variety.[39] As roguish psychiatrist Nathan Kline, who combined asylum-based research with a Park Avenue practice for the psychoneuroses, told a meeting at the University of Texas Medical Branch in Galveston in 1955: "One of the great problems is the classification of schizophrenia. . . . I think that we are due for a pharmacological approach; that the fact that these patients do respond and other patients don't respond, may allow, eventually, for an alternative classification which may be more heuristic and productive of therapy."[40] Note how carefully he phrased this to a room where schizophrenia was still meat and drink.

The subtypes of schizophrenia began to seem less certain. A study conducted around 1959 at the University of Maryland compared the original diagnosis of "schizophrenia" with the diagnosis in a subsequent admission. Said sociologist John Clausen, "[f]or subtypes of schizophrenia there was agreement in only 15 percent of the cases."[41]

The link between catatonia and "schizophrenia" began to appear increasingly absurd. In 1967, Norman Jaffe at Edenvale Hospital in Johannesburg reported a patient with severe liver disease who became catatonic. He "was diagnosed as a catatonic schizophrenic. With improvement in hepatic function the catatonia disappeared." The "schizophrenia" vanished.[42]

In the early 1970s, the reliability of the diagnosis "schizophrenia" received a shattering reverse. A comparison of hospital statistics showed that schizophrenia was nine times more common in New York than in London.[43] Moreover, eight videotapes of selected patients were shown to panels of psychiatrists at the Psychiatric Institute in New York and the Maudsley Hospital in London: the diagnoses diverged wildly: in tape number 5, for example, virtually all the New York psychiatrists diagnosed "schizophrenia," whereas only half of the London psychiatrists did so. The report concluded that a difference in the frequency of diagnosis "no longer justifies pursuing the hypothesis that the patients in the two regions are different."[44]

After examining the records of 2,500 hospitalized patients with extended follow-up at the University of Iowa, James Morrison, in 1973, reported that 10 percent met criteria for catatonia at their index admission. Re-examining the records at a later date, 40 percent had, at some point, recovered completely after treatment with sedative hypnotics or with ECT.[45,46] Morrison argued that these patients could not be examples of schizophrenia, a disorder for which common neuroleptic treatments, at best, reduced the severity of the symptoms but did not relieve the illness.

In 1976, Alan Gelenberg at the Massachusetts General Hospital reprised in the *Lancet* the theme that catatonia was not a subtype of schizophrenia. He listed all the conditions in which it might occur. "Catatonia is not a rare phenomenon, does not automatically imply a 'functional' disorder, and certainly does not always indicate schizophrenia."[47] Herman van Praag, one of the founders of biological psychiatry (and subject to death threats from the psychotherapy-friendly Dutch when he took up the psychiatry chair at Utrecht), had little time for the diagnosis of schizophrenia, which he called in 1978 "an impossible concept." Among the diseases dragged together under that "umbrella label," he said, "There is catatonia, a psychotic clinical picture in which motor disorders dominate, such as stereotypies, stupor, grimacing, etc."[48]

A near-fatal thrust to the concept of "catatonic schizophrenia" occurred in that same year, 1976, with Richard Abrams' and Michael Alan Taylor's study of 55 patients with catatonic symptoms seen over the course of 14 months in the inpatient psychiatric unit of Metropolitan Hospital in New York City. The authors were, at the time they did the study, members of the department of psychiatry of New York Medical College. Of the 55, only 4 "satisfied our research criteria for schizophrenia, whereas over two thirds had diagnosable affective disorders, usually mania."[49-51] Indeed, catatonia was far commoner in mood disorders than in madness. This well-executed study caused widespread reaction. The field had truly been sold a bill of goods with "catatonic schizophrenia." (When, in 2004, Stanley Caroff and co-workers surveyed the recent English-language studies of underlying diagnoses of patients with catatonic symptoms, in only 3 of the 11 studies did schizophrenia outnumber mood disorders.[52])

The challenge to catatonia as a type of schizophrenia continued in a 1986 report of 25 catatonic patients admitted to the Neurology Service of the Middlesbrough General Hospital in the UK, with only one patient meeting the criteria for schizophrenia while nine were diagnosed with major depression.[53] Five patients met criteria for primary neurologic diagnoses of encephalitis, tuberculous meningitis, multiple sclerosis, and epilepsy. ECT was effective in relieving catatonia in half the patients.

In 1987, James Lohr and Alexander Wisniewski at NIMH laid a heavy thumb on the independent-disease side of the scales in a book that has since become the standard guide to movement disorders in psychiatry and much of neurology. "In conclusion," they said, "we believe there is evidence that catatonia represents a distinct entity, but that it should be diagnosed on the basis of motor signs alone."[54]

These challenges questioned the connection of catatonia to schizophrenia. The increasing reports of deaths as a consequence of treating catatonia with potent neuroleptics stimulated interest in effective treatments and forced the separation of catatonia from schizophrenia.

11

CATATONIA IN DSM-III AND AFTER

A consensus is emerging that schizophrenia is an ill-defined disorder, an image in the mind of the beholder, without verification by tests or by response to treatment. It is a curse-word applied when the patient frightens the doctor. In a defined "catatonic," if the doctor THINKS the patient is psychotic, he labels him schizophrenic and prescribes neuroleptics. I know of no specific finding that would verify the label of schizophrenia.[1]
—Max Fink

The scandal of the perpetuation of schizophrenia and its many subtypes played out in the official diagnostic manual of American psychiatry, the *Diagnostic and Statistical Manual of Mental Disorders* (DSM). For centuries, the desire to record the causes of death led to multiple attempts at disease classification. As sanitaria housed ever increasing numbers of patients in the twentieth century, political and budgetary reasons led to detailed descriptions of the populations that went beyond counting the numbers of idiots and lunatics. For much of history, patients were categorized as idiots (the mentally deficient) and lunatics (the behaviorally psychotic). The model of the classification of species by Linnaeus prompted more detailed identifications, seeking ways to better predict courses of illness and outcomes. The psychopathologists Kahlbaum, Kraepelin, Griesinger, Bleuler, and Jaspers offered detailed classification schemes based on patient behaviors, thoughts, and moods with some attention to course and outcome. It was thus German psychiatry that led us into the twentieth century.

In 1917, during the First World War, the need to identify those soldiers who failed to meet conscription standards and the many who were being cared for in the Veterans Administration facilities led to an administrative classification of psychiatric illnesses by the American Medico-Psychological Association. This, then, led to a similar classification during the Second World War, and that is where our story begins.

AGONIZING OVER THE DSM

In 1946, under the leadership of psychoanalyst William C. Menninger, the Army published its own "Nomenclature of Psychiatric Disorders and Reactions," as Technical Bulletin "Medical 203."[2] Heavily psychoanalytic in inspiration, "Medical 203" became the basis of subsequent illness classifications by the American Psychiatric Association (APA). A prompt for the APA was the World Health Organization (WHO)'s addition of a section on psychiatric illnesses to its sixth *International Classification of Diseases*

(ICD) in 1949. Ten categories for psychosis/neurosis and seven for disorders of character, behavior, and intelligence were proposed.

These initiatives prompted the APA to publish its first diagnostic and statistical manual in 1952, subsequently known as DSM-I. Following Adolf Meyer's psychobiological view of mental illness, the labeled conditions were identified as *reactions* to psychological, social, and biological stressors, not as systemic or brain disorders. Pressures to amplify this code and make it more clinically relevant led to a revision, as DSM-II in 1968, again presenting the illnesses as reactions to psychological and situational stressors. In both DSM-I and DSM-II, catatonia is cited solely as a type of schizophrenia (295.2 *schizophrenia, catatonic type*).

Proposals by the WHO to revise ICD-9 in 1975 prompted the APA to update the DSM. Robert Spitzer of Columbia University organized the revisions by appointing committees of academic researchers to specify explicit diagnostic criteria for more than 300 diagnoses. They devised a complex numeric system and avoided considering hypotheses as to causes of the conditions. The DSM-III classification went beyond the needs of statistical epidemiology, seeking also to identify populations for clinical and research uses. The diagnoses discarded the Meyerian model and presented diagnoses by symptoms and signs, with some attention to the clinical course.

The laboratory and clinical tests that were used in clinical medicine as verifiers of specific diagnoses were rejected on the excuse that no tests assured any of the diagnoses pictured by the academic clinicians. (They rejected the possibility that the response to tests, such as the dexamethasone suppression test as a sign of melancholic depression, might identify a more homogeneous population of psychiatric ill.) This decision weakened the classification and inhibited the search for confirming measures, leaving the DSM-III as a subjective, nonverifiable diagnostic scheme.[3]

DSM-III appeared in 1980, with catatonia again recognized only as a type of schizophrenia, designated 295.2. This marriage of catatonia with schizophrenia confused clinical practice. Catatonia patients did not meet the criteria for schizophrenia, with the expected disorders in thought, disorganized speech, and abnormal behaviors. The neuroleptic drugs commonly prescribed for schizophrenia not only did not relieve catatonia, but instead precipitated severe neurotoxic reactions that were often fatal, clustered as the "neuroleptic malignant syndrome (NMS)." Other treatments were ignored, and the single label of catatonia within schizophrenia became associated with lethal neurotoxic reactions, a barrier to effective patient care.

The repeated demonstration of catatonia among patients with mood disorders raised doubts whether catatonia should remain identified solely as a type of schizophrenia in the DSM-IV revision. As we have seen, by this time, many examples of catatonia were recognized outside of schizophrenia, increasing the need for an independent category, one that acknowledged the unique characteristics of catatonia.

The argument for an independent class of catatonia was widely presented by catatonia scholars with two supports. Catatonia was recognized outside of schizophrenia, particularly among those with depressed and manic mood disorders,[4,5] as the toxic response to neuroleptic drugs[6] and as a systemic response in diverse medical and neurological disorders.[7] Motor signs are central to catatonia but are only incidental in patients with schizophrenia.[8]

A second argument was the specific relief of catatonia by the rapid induction of seizures (ECT). The signs of catatonia are quickly lifted by three to six seizures, regardless of associated systemic conditions or whether the accompanying behaviors are of psychiatric or systemic medical origin. In other types of schizophrenia—paranoid, hebephrenic, undifferentiated, residual, and simple—ECT offers little benefit, supporting the uniqueness of the catatonia type.

In 1991, in an article in the journal *Integrative Psychiatry*, Max Fink and Michael Taylor recommended the divorce of Kraepelin's marriage of catatonia with schizophrenia and urged that catatonia be recognized as an independent syndrome warranting a home of its own in the psychiatric classification.[9,10] The suggestion was reviewed by Pierre Pichot,[11] the doyen of Parisian psychiatry and by Robert Spitzer,[12] the organizer of DSM-III.

Pichot cited the proposal as "drastic," although he observed that many authors had reported catatonia outside schizophrenia and cited examples of "catatonism" and "catatoniform" variations among manic-depressive and organic syndrome patients. After much mental wiggling he proposed that "the catatonic syndrome be treated in the same way as the depressive disorder is now treated . . . adding to the chapter 'Mood Disorders' a 'catatonic form' (in the same way as the present 'form with psychotic features' characterized by hallucinations and delusions)."

Spitzer had limited clinical experience with hospitalized mentally ill. In discussing catatonia in an earlier venue in 1975, he had written that "These symptoms are very rare nowadays, and should only be considered present when they are obvious."[13] He complained of the lack of an acceptable definition of catatonia, citing the numerous signs that are recognized in the syndrome and the lack of agreement as to how many signs for how long characterized its presence. "A consensus definition of diagnostic criteria for the catatonic syndrome, with guidelines for determining the threshold for the presence of symptoms, requires input from the growing number of investigators."

How common is the disorder, and could it be considered independent of other conditions? He complained that no data were presented to support the notion of a "primary catatonia" and asked "what disorders are sometimes present with a catatonic syndrome? The answer would seem to be: schizophrenia, mood disorders (both manic and depressive episodes), and systemic illness. For those disorders, it would be appropriate to have a diagnostic *modifier* which would note the presence of a catatonic syndrome."

Donald Klein, a member of the DSM-IV Affective Disorders Committee, wrote to Max Fink: "I would have no trouble using 'with catatonic features' as a modifier for affective and schizophrenic disorders."[14] John Rush, Chairman of the DSM-IV Affective Disorders Committee, made a similar suggestion in a note to Allen Frances, chairman of the DSM-IV commission: "The data regarding catatonia and ECT seems pretty convincing to me (we even use it in practice.) . . . The problem for DSM-IV . . . is where to put it (i.e., it is not always an affective disorder). . . . *the choice seems logically to be (a) ignore it, (b) emphasize in the text of both schizophrenia and affective disorders, or (c) create a new category akin to schizoaffective that is neither in the Schizophrenia nor Mood Disorders sections.*" In a footnote Rush favored option (c).[15]

The DSM-IV commission members and the academic community considered the designation of a modifier in the fifth digit for catatonia for the primary diagnoses. Catatonia would be recognized by secondary coding as xxx.xN, with catatonia listed as a feature within each main psychiatric class. Such a designation was rejected in the final formulation.

The published 1994 DSM-IV retained the class of *schizophrenia, catatonic type* and added an independent class of "*catatonia secondary to a general medical condition*" (293.89). It also added "catatonic features" as a "specifier" (meaning no diagnostic code) for mood disorders.[16] At the presentation of the *DSM-IV* classification to members of the APA at its meeting in Los Angeles, Spitzer met Max Fink outside the meeting hall and thumped Fink's chest, saying that Fink would be satisfied by the addition of a class of "catatonia secondary to a medical condition (293.89)" as closest to an independent class for catatonia that he (Spitzer) could accept. This notation recognized catatonia as a unique entity outside schizophrenia.[17] A goodly part of this decision was the lack of an acceptable definition for catatonia and of how many signs and of what duration identified the syndrome, and the lack of consensus on how best to treat the syndrome once it was recognized.

SEARCHING FOR DATA TO SATISFY SPITZER

Catatonia scholars were pleased that catatonia was acknowledged as an independent syndrome, hoping that such a designation would encourage its early recognition and the prescription of effective catatonia treatments, and increase interest in its study. Indeed, the number of publications indexed as "catatonia" in the National Library of Medicine PubMed did increase sharply (Figure 11.1). From 1975 to 1994, the citations averaged less than 38 per year; from 1995 to 2004, citations increased to 60 per year; and from 2005 to 2016, increased further to more than 100 per year.[18]

Scholars sought to provide answers to the questions raised by the DSM commissioners with studies of how catatonia is best diagnosed and treated and its

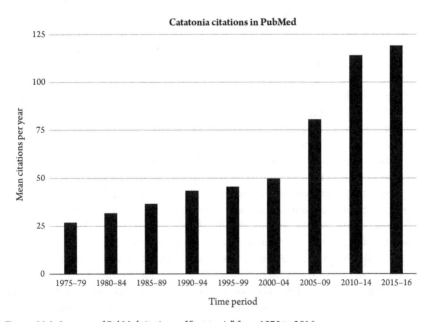

Figure 11.1 Increase of *PubMed* citations of "catatonia" from 1975 to 2016.

associations with other psychiatric and medical disorders. A catatonia rating scale with 27 items had been published by Lohr and Wisniewski in 1987.[19] It was soon followed by other scales varying between 21 and 40 signs.[20] At University Hospital at Stony Brook, Fink, Andrew Francis, and their colleagues developed a catatonia rating scale and an examination listing 23 signs of catatonia. The items were derived from the 17 signs identified by Kahlbaum, with additions from Kraepelin[21] and items suggested in other reports.[22] The various scales were increasingly applied, and, in 2011, Pascal Sienaert and his colleagues in Kortenberg, Belgium, favored the ease and use of the Stony Brook rating scales compared to others.[23]

The Stony Brook University Hospital records over the preceding six years were examined for patients coded at discharge as "schizophrenia, catatonic type."[24] Twenty records were found with chart diagnoses of schizophrenia, manic-depression, and neurotoxicity. Two-thirds of the patients were relieved by ECT. Some had been treated with lorazepam, but these treatments were not particularly effective, mainly (in retrospect) because the dosing had been too low.

To determine the incidence of catatonia, all admissions to the psychiatry, neurology, and psychiatry-emergency room services in six months in 1992 were examined for the presence of nine catatonia signs using the catatonia screening scale.[25] Two or more signs warranted a full evaluation using the 23-item rating scale. Of 215 patients surveyed, 15 (7 percent) met the criteria for catatonia, and all presented with at least three signs (average 6.6).

The Stony Brook catatonia clinical inpatient study group included these 15 patients plus 13 other catatonic patients admitted just before or after the screening period of the study. Of the 28 patients, 15 (54 percent) met criteria for affective disorders, 6 (21 percent) for systemic medical disorders, 2 (8 percent) for schizophrenia, and 1 for an atypical psychosis. The systemic illnesses were NMS in three, and one each with seizures after closed head injury, anticholinergic delirium, and steroid-induced stupor. The catatonia patients were younger and more likely to have comorbid mania than the inpatient population from which they were identified. In one patient, no other systemic illness was discerned and the label of *Catatonia NOS* (not otherwise specified) was assigned.

The measured incidence of catatonia is consistent with other studies. Rosebush and her colleagues found catatonia in 9 percent (12 of 140) of patients admitted to their university psychiatric facility.[26] Gabor Ungvari and his colleagues reported an incidence of 8 percent (18 of 212).[27,28] David Healy, using the Stony Brook catatonia rating scale, reported more than 13 percent of patients met criteria for catatonia among 114 patients assessed in India and 112 examined in Wales.[29] Other surveys identified incidences from 3.5 to 17 percent, with a mean of 9.8 percent.[30] In each survey, schizophrenia diagnoses constituted a minority of the sample, with the majority suffering affective disorders.

In the long-stay Long Island Pilgrim Psychiatric Hospital, 42 chronically hospitalized patients were assessed with individual rating scales for catatonia, parkinsonism, tardive dyskinesia, and akathisia by the Stony Brook researchers.[31] The catatonia rating scale successfully distinguished catatonia from other motor symptoms. Rigidity was the one catatonic sign overlapping with other motor syndromes. Catatonia among the chronic mentally ill had a similar distribution as among those with the acute syndrome.

An intravenous challenge test dose of 1 or 2 mg lorazepam to verify the presence of catatonia was developed. The severity of the catatonia signs was reduced within 15 minutes in 16/21 patients (76 percent). All catatonia patients were treated with increasing doses of lorazepam, with all but five responding well. The prescription of 3 mg/day, increased rapidly by 3 mg increments to 30 mg/day was their regimen. Of the nonresponders to lorazepam, four consented and were treated successfully with ECT; three recovered within 3 days and one required 11 days.[32]

Thus, Spitzer's demand for reliable data was satisfied. These experiences became the basis for a catatonia identification and treatment protocol published in 1996 that has since been widely adopted. Catatonia is identified by the presence of two or more signs lasting for 24 hours or longer. A reduction of the catatonia scores by 50 percent within a few minutes of an intravenous challenge of lorazepam is considered verification. Increasing daily doses of lorazepam (up to 30 mg/day in some studies) are prescribed with the expectation that 80 percent will recover. Treatment with ECT is usually successful for those who do not respond to lorazepam. For patients with the more malignant febrile illnesses, daily ECT may be necessary. Such a protocol is remarkably effective for the full relief of catatonia, regardless of accompanying signs of illness.[33,34]

THE CONTINUING ARGUMENT POST-DSM-IV

The DSM-IV addition of the code for catatonia secondary to a medical condition (293.89) aroused little professional interest. As mentioned, catatonia scholars argued about whether the proper treatment of NMS as a form of malignant catatonia should be with benzodiazepines and induced seizures, or whether, as a result of neuroleptic-induced dopamine blockade, it should be treated by the withdrawal of neuroleptics, and prescription of dopamine agonists (bromocriptine), and muscle relaxants (dantrolene). Discussions were active at meetings of the APA and international associations. Many opined that the NMS was a specific toxic form of malignant catatonia.[35-38] The evidence seemed to go largely in that direction.

As an aside, one wonders why, on the basis of such overwhelming evidence, the treatment of catatonia with lorazepam and ECT was not immediately accepted. Two forces inhibited the rate at which NMS was recognized and successfully treated. The Federal Bureau of Narcotics and Dangerous Drugs' classification of the benzodiazepines as scheduled drugs restricted availability and gave an aura of risk to the high doses that were being prescribed for catatonia. Pharmacists questioned the dosage in prescriptions, raising fears among clinicians that they were taking undue risks in following the guidelines in the published case material. A second inhibition was the limited availability of ECT treatment facilities with therapists knowledgeable of the special needs to relieve catatonia. As experience with ECT in catatonia was limited, many treating doctors assumed that the treatment parameters recommended for geriatric depression were appropriate for patients with malignant catatonia. In many instances, the weakened parameters recommended to treat elderly depressed patients were applied and were unsuccessful. Catatonia patients, particularly those with the malignant forms, require higher energy dosing and more frequent, often daily, treatments for efficacy.[39]

DSM-5 REVISION

The APA announced in 2008 that it was preparing an update of DSM-IV; it assigned catatonia to the Psychosis Work Group.[40] By this time, a literature supporting catatonia as an independent entity had developed, and there was a groundswell of arguments asking that the catatonia type of schizophrenia (295.2) be deleted and that catatonia be designated by a single code as a distinct, definable, and treatable syndrome. The questions were many.

How should catatonia be assigned in the classification? As a type of schizophrenia, as a variation of other identified illnesses, or as an independent disorder? Should catatonia be deleted as a sign of schizophrenia? Since multiple forms of catatonia had been identified, should catatonia be classified in subtypes, such as retarded, delirious, malignant, and not otherwise specified (NOS), or as a single independent entity?[41]

In the *Schizophrenia Bulletin*, in 2009, Max Fink, Edward Shorter, and Michael Taylor challenged the Kraepelinian definition of catatonia.[42] Catatonia was noted to be more common among patients with mood disorders and neurotoxic syndromes than among those with schizophrenia. The article also said that catatonia was characterized by the *precipitation* of the neurotoxic syndrome by neuroleptic drug treatments and by the unique *response* of catatonia to benzodiazepines and induced seizures; these were responses not shared by schizophrenia.

The article was discussed in three reviews. Patricia Rosebush and Michael Mazurek endorsed the suggestion of an independent classification and seconded the special efficacy of benzodiazepines in relieving catatonia.[43] They hesitated to delete the connection to schizophrenia, citing the failure of these treatments in long-term chronically ill catatonic patients.

A similar argument that benzodiazepines were poorly effective in long-term psychotic Chinese patients with catatonia, supporting catatonia as a type of schizophrenia, was made by Gabor Ungvari, Stanley Caroff, and Jozsef Gerevich.[44] But neither Rosebush nor Ungvari had treated their severely ill with the high benzodiazepine dosages necessary in severe catatonia, especially when accompanied by psychosis. Nor did they treat their patients with induced seizures. Their argument against a single class for catatonia came down to incomplete treatment studies and their loyalty to the Kraepelin tradition.

Stephan Heckers and his Work Group colleagues Rajiv Tandon and Juan Bustillo noted that catatonia appeared in multiple sections of DSM-IV: as a distinct condition among medical disorders, a subtype of schizophrenia, an episode specifier for mood disorders, and as NMS.[45] The latter was seen as a form of catatonia by some scholars. With these opportunities, the authors asked whether it was necessary to change the classification as put forth by Max Fink in the DSM-IV sourcebook.[46]

They considered reasons for change. On the plus side, current teaching of the mental status examination de-emphasizes psychomotor behavior, and a more prominent position for catatonia could pave the way for better recognition, thus facilitating proper treatment that requires early intervention with benzodiazepines. It would also caution clinicians not to prescribe neuroleptics as these induce a neurotoxic syndrome. And third, better recognition of catatonia would catalyze neural and genetic research.[47]

On the minus side, they noted that most patients with catatonia do not meet criteria for schizophrenia: "not all is schizophrenia, but some is." They concluded that it would be problematic for catatonia to be conceived as an independent diagnostic class. If catatonia is taken out of the psychosis section, where among the 17 classes should it be inserted? (This point ignored the objection that there is actually no such clinical entity as "schizophrenia.")

Following these arguments, the Work Group considered the replacement of the codes for the "schizophrenia subtype" and "secondary to a medical illness" by the more radical use of specifiers (which don't have codes) for each of the major diagnostic classes. Yet such a noncoded term would surely decrease recognition of catatonia and its classification. This suggestion was strongly opposed by 34 catatonia scholars in a public letter in the *Journal of ECT* who argued that a better option was the retention of the 293.89 code, with revision of its description to broadly encompass the catatonia syndrome without imputing a link to primary psychiatric or general medical conditions.[48] A unique and broadly defined code would foster recognition of the catatonia syndrome and permit research on nosology, treatment, and outcome. These goals would not be met by the DSM-5 plan for noncoded modifiers.[49]

A letter by Stephan Heckers to the catatonia scholars dated June 7, 2012, listed the many recommendations for catatonia: deletion of catatonia as a type of schizophrenia (295.2), creation of a new class of Catatonia Not Elsewhere Classified (298.99), retention of the code 293.89 from DSM-IV, and a catatonia specifier code xxx.x5 to be added for 10 primary diagnoses, with the catatonia signs originally configured as five clusters adopted from DSM-IV. This complexity was widely discussed among the catatonia scholars. It was a case of too many cooks. The proposal was much too complex for what was needed: a simple recognition of catatonia as an identifiable, verifiable, and treatable syndrome, akin to the status of neurosyphilis.[50]

PUBLICATION OF DSM-5

DSM-5 was published in May 2013, affirming catatonia as an identifiable syndrome much along the lines recommended by the catatonia scholars. It deleted the class of schizophrenia, catatonic type (295.2); continued the class of catatonia secondary to a systemic medical condition (293.89); offered a new class of "unspecified catatonia" (781.89); and included a "catatonia specifier" coded as xxx.x5 for 10 principal disorders including depressions, bipolar disorders, and schizophrenia types. This variety of labels reflected the conflicts within the work group seeking to respond to the catatonia scholars but unable to discard the ties of the syndrome to Kraepelin. The Work Group members defended these recommendations in detailed reviews in April 2013.[51,52]

The divorce of catatonia from schizophrenia favorably recognizes catatonia as an independent clinical entity. It leads to the earlier prescription of effective treatments with resulting lower rates of chronic illness and death. Many variants of catatonia with unique effective treatments are now recognized as Kahlbaum's stupor, malignant catatonia (encompassing NMS), delirious mania, self-injurious behaviors among those with autism, and others.[53] Once considered rare, catatonia is now reported in about 10 percent of the populations admitted to psychiatric hospital units, assuring earlier recognition and more effective treatments.[54]

The connection of the catatonia scholars to the DSM-5 Psychosis Work Group was through Stephan Heckers, the chairman of Psychiatry at Vanderbilt University. Earlier, he had twice described delirious mania as a form of catatonia, citing its effective response to benzodiazepines and ECT.[55,56] That he accepted catatonia as an independent, treatable syndrome is seen in his retrospective chart review published at the beginning of 2015. After examining 339 hospital charts, two or more signs of catatonia were recorded in 300 patients, with 232 validated by positive relief with lorazepam treatment or ECT. The mean lorazepam dose was 6 mg/day with 84 percent responding. ECT was applied in 20 percent, with 42 of 45 (93 percent) responding.[57] This independent verification of catatonia as an acute identifiable and treatable syndrome was most welcome.

Present understanding distinguishes the Kraepelin and Kahlbaum forms of the illness, with the former tied to chronicity and poor responsiveness and the latter accepted as the expression of diverse, acute, treatable illnesses. Recognizing the many expressions of catatonia as variations of a systemic syndrome and not mainly a behavioral syndrome suggests that catatonia is best considered in the dictionary of medical disorders and not limited to psychiatric disorders.[58]

12

NEW FACES OF CATATONIA?

According to an old story, there are three types of baseball umpires. The first says: "I call them [balls and strikes] as they are"; the second says: "I call them as I see them"; and the third says: "What I call them is what they become."
—Frederick Grinnell, 1992[1]

Just to recap: The recognition of the neuroleptic malignant syndrome (NMS) as a form of the Kahlbaum disease led to effective treatments that strongly influenced the fate of patients suffering this lethal illness. The patients did not look like the typical case of catatonia—the mute, posturing, rigid, staring, negativistic subject with poor self-care. They were acutely ill, febrile, and toxic. Periods of excitement alternated with stupor. Such patients were labeled with the eponymic names of Bell's mania and Stauder's delirium, without discussing a connection to catatonia.[2] Their excitement leads to the automatic prescription of potent neuroleptics, commonly haloperidol, often precipitating the malignant neurotoxic syndrome.

To the 17 signs of catatonia described by Kahlbaum, Kraepelin had added *automatic obedience* and *perseveration*. Other writers added still other behaviors that make up the catalogs of up to 30 signs that are identified in rating scales for catatonia. The signs identified by Kahlbaum make up the core of each scale and diagnosis.[3]

The immediate relief of catatonia by injections of sodium Amytal described in 1929–30 quickly became the prescribed response to the recognition of the syndrome. In the training of physicians in the 1940s, in-house residents routinely carried ampoules of Amytal and vials of sterile water on their rounds, injecting the sedative in excited, mute, or negativistic patients. Patients responded quickly, reducing the number of catatonia cases in most clinical facilities so much so that a neurologist, in 1981, bemoaned the rarity of catatonia.[4]

The report by Gregory Fricchione in 1983, that intravenous lorazepam was a useful alternative to amobarbital to relieve catatonia, was quickly verified and widely adopted.[5] Lorazepam and diazepam became the challenges used to verify the diagnosis and also the core treatment for NMS and other forms of catatonia. By 1996, the intravenous lorazepam challenge test was increasingly used to verify the presence of catatonia.[6,7] In Europe, other authors used the oral administration of zolpidem for the same purpose.[8] That is the story to date. Now, we need a larger context for it.

THE MEDICAL MODEL OF DIAGNOSIS

These events are consistent with the philosophy of a medical model of diagnosis, the methodology that is the basis for the identification of a systemic illness.[9,10] The steps are the *identification* of a form of illness, *verification* by systemic signs and clinical or laboratory tests, and *validation* by the response to specific treatment. The methodology is initially credited to Thomas Sydenham in the seventeenth century, who identified a form of chorea using patient history, signs of illness, and the response to treatments.[11] The present version *defines* an illness by history, symptoms, and course of illness, narrowed by specific clinical signs. Examination and tests seek to identify or *verify* the most likely diagnosis, which is then *validated* by the relief afforded by specific treatments. The model is widely used in clinical medicine to identify the cornucopia of described diseases but is only occasionally applied in psychiatric illnesses. Neurosyphilis and lately NMS are examples of the successful application defining a syndrome by symptoms and course, verified by signs and tests, and validated by successful treatments. The Washington University physicians Eli Robins and Sam Guze used this model to develop the Research Diagnostic Criteria for psychiatric illnesses in 1970.[12]

The medical model was applied to catatonia. As catatonia was divorced from schizophrenia, various systemic syndromes met the criteria for catatonia and were "lumped" together by Fink and Taylor as variants of catatonia.[13,14] The presence of two or more catatonia signs for 24 hours and relief by the test of intravenous lorazepam (or other benzodiazepine or zolpidem) verified the syndrome as probable catatonia. The remission following treatment with a benzodiazepine and ECT validated the diagnosis. Earlier, the Kahlbaum variant, delirious mania, excited catatonia, neurotoxic syndromes, and malignant catatonia were described based on the medical model of disease. Additional illnesses now recognized as treatable forms of catatonia are anti-N-methyl-D-aspartate receptor encephalitis, self-injurious behaviors in mental retardation and autism, and selective and akinetic mutisms.[15] Recognition as forms of catatonia encourages the prescription of effective catatonia treatments and leads to better outcomes than viewing these syndromes as unique and unrelated to catatonia.

ANTI-N-METHYL-D-ASPARTATE RECEPTOR ENCEPHALITIS

Limbic encephalitis, an acute autoimmune neurological disorder, is a newly demarcated clinical syndrome described in the 1960s as a "paraneoplastic condition"—a self-poisoning systemic disorder associated with tumors. More than 80 different autoimmune disorders are described in the medical literature.[16] Tissue receptors, one of which is the N-methyl-D-aspartate receptor (NMDAR), are part of the body's defensive physiology and are seen as abnormal in these conditions. The pathophysiology is poorly understood, and the treatments are empiric and of limited efficacy.

A case report in 2007 in the *New England Journal of Medicine* described a 26-year-old woman admitted for headache, behavioral changes, abnormal limb movements, and mutism of seven weeks' duration. After extensive laboratory examinations, a positive serum anti-NMDAR encephalitis test was reported. Throughout her illness, she had been somnolent, mute, and negativistic, with repetitive movements of her arms and mouth, but these were neither recognized nor treated as catatonia. An ovarian teratoma was found, surgically removed under anesthesia, and an encephalitis syndrome dominated by catatonia resolved within a day. Was the removal of the tumor or the anesthesia the key link in the therapeutic chain? The rapidity of the resolution and her course favor the likelihood that the catatonia syndrome was relieved by the anesthesia.[17]

A 16-year-old boy was in protracted stupor, with psychomotor retardation, mutism, posturing, and stereotypical movement. He refused to eat and drink and was episodically agitated.[18] A positive blood test supported the anti-NMDAR diagnosis. The presence of catatonia was not recognized, and no consideration given to its treatments. Instead, haloperidol and other antipsychotic agents were prescribed, worsening the symptoms. After seven months of nursing care, the illness abated. The experience was trumpeted as a clinical lesson in the *American Journal of Psychiatry* in 2011, despite the clinicians' failure to recognize catatonia or to consider its treatment. These shortcomings were severely criticized by Dirk Dhossche and his colleagues.[19]

In a report of 100 cases of encephalitis with positive NMDAR serum tests, catatonia signs in the abnormal behaviors included "unresponsiveness with catatonic features," a febrile course, followed by "reduction in verbal output and echolalia to frank mutism," accompanied by "periods of agitation and catatonia," in which "patients resist eye opening but show . . . no response to painful stimuli." These signs of catatonia were not recognized, nor were effective treatments discussed.[20]

Case reports increasingly dot the literature, with most patients being female and with resolution after resection of ovarian teratomas when found. But the syndrome is also reported in males and among many patients without evidence of tumors.[21] The presumed connection to tumors sends patients to whole-body searches, but the syndrome is also accepted as a diagnosis on the positive laboratory test without finding a tumor.[22]

The heightened enthusiasm for this diagnosis is reflected in an editorial in the *British Journal of Psychiatry* in April 2012, calling for laboratory tests for anti-NMDAR encephalitis in "all individuals with a first presentation of psychosis, or people with psychosis and features of autonomic disturbance, movement disorder, disorientation, seizures, hyponatraemia or rapid deterioration . . . with the possibility of antibody-mediated encephalitis in mind." The recommendation continues: "This assessment should include, as a minimum, a neurological and cognitive examination and early serum testing for antibodies against the NMDA receptor and voltage-gated potassium channel. All patients testing positive for these serum antibodies should be referred to neurological centres with expertise in managing these cases."[23] The association with catatonia and its treatments is not mentioned.

By 2016, catatonia had been recognized in eight patients with anti-NMDAR encephalitis and successfully treated with ECT.[24–27] Identifying catatonia in anti-NMDAR encephalitis offers prompt, effective treatment.

The enthusiasm for this diagnosis is illustrated by a rapidly increasing case report literature. The first references to anti-NMDAR encephalitis were cited in Medline in 2007. By July 2014, the number had increased to 230 citations; by December 2015, to 333; and in July 2017, to 874. The number of essays co-authored by Josef Dalmau, the holder of the patent for the laboratory test, were 27 by September 2011, 50 by July 2014, and 101 by July 2017.

SELF-INJURIOUS BEHAVIORS IN MENTAL
RETARDATION AND AUTISM

The self-injurious behaviors (SIB) common in autism are another form of catatonia. Autism, a disorder of socialization and speech with an onset in early childhood, surfaced in the German literature in the 1920s[28] and was then popularized by Leo Kanner in 1943[29] and by Hans Asperger in 1944.[30] These writers described children with delayed maturation, poor socialization, and a plethora of repetitive behaviors. Much debate ensued as to the distinctions between childhood autism, mental retardation, and childhood schizophrenia. Common to descriptions of autism are the catatonia signs of mutism, echolalia, echopraxia, odd hand postures, freezing of ongoing movements, rigidities, forced vocalizations, stereotypy, and insensitivity to pain. Although we lack systematic studies identifying and treating catatonia in autism, case reports in the literature indicate relief for even the most severely ill when catatonia treatments are applied.

Self-injury in children has long been a concern of pediatric medicine.[31] In 1887, J. Langdon Down, London physician and the virtual founder of the study of developmental disabilities, wrote of puberty, "It is important . . . to be on guard against any concealed suicidal impulse, and to note its slightest indication, as the tendency in such cases is to melancholia and in some instances temptation to self-inflicted injury."[32] Theodor Ziehen, professor in Halle and among the pioneers of pediatric psychiatry in Germany, noted in 1915 "the remarkable self-mutilations without suicidal intent, which occasionally take place among abnormal children, for example among the schizophrenic."[33] Complicating the analysis is that SIB—a term that came into common medical use only in 1966—often was described under other labels that are unfamiliar today and lost in the literature.[34]

One of the earliest descriptions of SIB in the context of catatonia comes from an Athenian physician, G. G. Caryophylis, who interned in Paris and published a case study in a French journal in 1892.[35] A 13-year-old boy from a prominent Athenian family "was already attending school when he began refusing to eat." He stopped speaking and then: "Whenever he was constrained, the patient simulated contractions, did contortions of every kind, tore out his hair, grabbed his larynx to strangle himself, and struck his head against the wall. He spent most of the time stretched out on a sofa mute and staring at the ceiling, insensible to all the caresses of his sisters and the injunctions of his parents." Dr. Caryophylis restored him to health in a private clinic through "forced suggestion." The negativism (refusal to eat), mutism, stereotypies, and stupor of catatonia shine through.

French medical dissertations, a thesis required for the MD degree, are a valuable source of information. In 1892, Lucie G, age 17, was admitted to the Evreux asylum with symptoms of psychosis that also included negativism, refusal to eat, and periods of violent agitation.[36] "She demonstrated voluntary self-mutilations, trying to tear off a fingernail and to remove the tip of her left breast." In the course of a decade-long illness trajectory, she developed stupor and posturing, "able to remain indefinitely on a couch or standing without moving."

When the medical student Mlle. Hollaender at the University of Geneva interned at the private psychiatric clinic Bel-Air in that city around 1908, she encountered quite a bit of SIB among the catatonic child and juvenile patients.[37] Malvine B, age 8, when still at home had experienced "attacks of agitation." "She threw objects out of the window, rolled objects on the table, on the ground. During these attacks she spoke a great deal and insulted, grabbed and hit her mother. . . . She often declared that she wanted to commit suicide and once threw herself off her bed, injuring her forehead." Admitted to the clinic in January 1908, "she sometimes [dating from two months ago] makes nervous movements with her mouth and arms . . . . [Later that month] the girl has a moment of agitation: she leaps on a sofa, wants to throw herself onto the floor and tries to strangle herself."

Another subject, a Russian boy of 13, would occasionally "jump entirely into the air." "[He displays] tics in his hands, eyes and head. He frequently makes movements with his hands as though 'to chase someone.'" Later, he holds his body stiffly, "his neck in slight opisthotonos . . . His gaze is constantly fixed on the ceiling at the same point. In bed, he stares at the same spot." He walks in small steps with an "affected" gait. "All of his movements are slow and repetitive. He gives the impression of an automaton," passing his handkerchief 15 times across his nose after sneezing. He develops mutism, stereotypies, grimacing, and stupor. Mlle. Hollaender uses the adjective "catatonic." By April 1907, he had begun head-banging, which clearly qualified as SIB in the context of catatonia.

In the *Diagnostic and Statistical Manual of Mental Disorders* (DSM) classifications, the self-injury syndrome is included as "stereotypical movement disorder," a diagnosis presented as an independent disease entity. Outside the DSM world, however, where the para-Freudian assumptions of North American child psychiatry are less firmly rooted, clinicians note the association between catatonia and SIB. In 1986, the German nosologist Karl Leonhard, originator of the concept of "bipolar disorder," noted "auto-aggressivity" in children with catatonia. Leonhard, whose experience in pediatrics was considerable, wrote, "Aggressivity is, in the genesis of negativistic catatonia in early childhood, connected with autoaggressivity. . . . The drive can be so powerful that a caregiver must be stationed next to the patient almost continually, if autoaggressivity is to be prevented. The patients strike their faces with their fists, smash their heads against hard objects, even bite themselves. Some patients have scars in their faces or elsewhere on the body, because they have caused themselves serious harm." He further relates that "a few days later I saw the girl who had knocked off my glasses. Now she forcefully hits her face, with the right hand, with the left hand, at times with both hands simultaneously."[38]

In 1981, Mahendra asked "where have all the catatonics gone?"[39] Yet attention to catatonia in psychiatry was increasing; sporadic reports of its association with pediatric self-injury and affective illness began to appear, including successful treatment with ECT. In 1983, Carr et al. presented a 12-year-old girl with acute mania and self-injury consisting of flinging her body against hard surfaces, who achieved comprehensive symptom remission with seven ECT treatments.[40] Two years later, Black et al. reported an 11-year-old boy with major depression and head-banging self-injury similarly alleviated by 12 ECT treatments.[41] In 1996, Cizadlo and Wheaton presented an 8-year-old girl suffering from major depression with catatonic features who further engaged in hand–head SIB, yet who achieved affective and behavioral stabilization with 19 ECT treatments.[42]

Shifting toward individuals with autism spectrum disorders, Wing and Shah's large UK population-based study revealed the intriguing presence of catatonia in up to

17 percent of autistic adolescents and young adults,[43] a figure that was subsequently reported at 12 percent in a 2006 Swedish study,[44] and at 18 percent in a Midwestern US study of autistic individuals.[45]

Additional case reports of catatonia in autistic patients relieved with ECT began to appear, and, in 2008, Wachtel et al. presented an 18-year-old girl with classic Kahlbaum catatonia admitted in a rigid and stuporous state, completely dependent on gastrostomy tube feeding, but additionally having flurries of extreme self-injury toward her head and body that had already caused multiple bony ossifications, traumatic cataract formation, bilateral retinal detachment, and complete loss of sight in one eye. The young woman's classic catatonic symptoms disappeared with ECT, along with the self-injurious behavior that had perplexed her clinicians for more than 15 years.[46] The same year, Chung and Varghese reported an 11-year-old girl with psychosis, catatonia, and self-injury including head-banging, self-scratching, and self-cutting, again alleviated by ECT.[47] Multiple autistic patients with catatonia and concomitant extreme self-injury subsequently appear in the literature. Many of these patients presented with additional affective, psychotic, and tic disorders and demonstrated profound, life-altering symptom reduction with ECT.[48–54]

Among patients referred for ECT at University Hospital at Stony Brook was a 14-year-old mentally retarded boy with persistent self-injurious behavior. He required helmet, gloves, and restraints to keep him from seriously injuring his head. The referring physician asked whether ECT was an option. Fink had successfully treated other mentally retarded patients, despite the widespread professional and public belief that such patients already had brain damage and that ECT would further their disability.[55] With parental consent, a trial of ECT was begun, and, within two weeks, the restraints were no longer needed and he was allowed the freedom of the hospital unit. Over the next half year, continuation ECT sustained him in his community residence without the return of the self-injurious behaviors.[56]

Such patient experiences across multiple clinical sites led to the view that repetitive self-injury without operant, or purposeful, function is a movement disorder, best characterized along the spectrum of agitated catatonic behavior and with direct implications for the utility of ECT. Multiple patients have achieved relief from horrendous self-injury after enduring years of failed behavioral and medication trials. Many had been confined to extensive protective equipment and had already incurred irreparable tissue injury. Parents and caregivers have been astounded by the nearly miraculous abolition of self-injury,[57] with one father remarking that recognition of repetitive self-injury along the catatonic spectrum, with subsequent implementation of ECT, "released [his son] from the shackles of hell."[58] Fink officially included repetitive self-injury in autism along the catatonic spectrum in the 2013 update to his authoritative 2003 catatonia textbook.[59]

Patients previously identified as suffering from mental retardation are now discussed as suffering autism or autism spectrum disorders. Such patients often exhibit persistent repetitive movements, screaming or hitting themselves. Such self-injurious behaviors cause much damage. Restraints, antipsychotic and other medications, and deconditioning procedures are poorly effective. Courses of ECT markedly reduce repetitive behaviors, and many young patients have been returned to home and community.[60] They do require continuation ECT, however. The success of these treatments has encouraged broader acceptance of ECT among child and adolescent psychiatrists.

THE SELECTIVE MUTISMS

The syndrome of selective mutism is a condition in children and adolescents who become mute while interacting with family and friends. Mutism is persistent, often in a withdrawn, posturing, rigid adolescent. The condition is commonly appreciated as an anxiety disorder despite the presence of characteristic signs of catatonia, with its treatments ignored. Administered the panoply of verbal and chemical treatments for anxiety, the patients languish in prolonged illness. Other severe mutisms seen in neurological units are labeled *akinetic mutism* and the *locked-in syndrome*. No effective treatments are discussed for these patients.

The disorder described as "pervasive refusal syndrome" that became popular in the UK in 1991 meets the criteria for catatonia.[61] Four girls between the ages of 9 and 14 suffered "a profound and pervasive refusal to eat, drink, walk, talk or care of themselves in any way over a period of several months." They required nasogastric tube feeding and spent such prolonged periods in bed that they "occasionally requir[e] manipulations of the joints under general anesthetic to prevent contractures." After extended hospital care and family and individual psychotherapies, they eventually recovered. There was a Danish report of a 12-year-old boy who withdrew into prolonged stupor after an acute illness and required tube feeding and intensive nursing care, gradually responding after 34 months. At follow-up at age 20 he was pursuing a normal independent life.[62]

An 8-year-old girl stopped eating and drinking after a viral infection and was hospitalized for more than a year before being returned to her family in partial remission; the report was discussed by Donald Klein, who asked whether the patient met criteria for catatonia and whether not testing and treating for catatonia was unethical.[63] The authors offered a complex rejoinder without explaining the failure to test with barbiturates or benzodiazepines.[64]

Later, Fink was consulted by the Irish child psychiatrist Dr. Fiona McNicholas about an 11-year-old prepubertal girl who developed symptoms of asthma, abdominal pain, and insomnia. She refused to attend school or to eat or drink, became withdrawn and mute, and required nasogastric feeding and hospital care. After many months, Fink viewed a video of her behavior. Mutism, negativism, and posturing confirmed catatonia. Lorazepam testing and treatment was recommended. The parents refused medication treatments but participated in family therapy. At first the girl participated, but, in time, she refused. After 18 months of hospital care, as the date for her return home was imminent, she began to speak, eat, and care for herself. Over the next six years, she completed her schooling and went on to university.[65]

Fewer than 30 additional cases are cited in the literature, with a 3:1 ratio of girls to boys. Each of the reported cases required prolonged hospital care.

Another mutism, labeled *akinetic mutism*, is described in neurologic texts: patients who lie inert and mute, appear alert, and regard the clinician only by moving their eyes. They may follow the movement of objects or be diverted by sound. Neither voluntary movements nor restlessness nor negativism are seen. A painful stimulus may produce reflex withdrawal or no movement. Patients have to be fed and are incontinent of urine and feces.[66] They appear lifeless and may be mistaken for dead.[67] The condition has since been described under such names as "coma vigil," "apallic syndrome," "stiff-man syndrome," "locked-in syndrome," and "stupor of unknown etiology." The terms "vegetative state" and "minimally conscious state" are also used.

One newly labeled catatonia syndrome is that of "pediatric cerebellar mutism syndrome," a benzodiazepine-responsive mutism associated with cerebellar surgery.[68] The symptoms of each of these syndromes differ little from those of the more severe forms of inhibited catatonia. Whether the patient is seen as having a form of akinetic mutism on a neurologic service or as catatonia on a psychiatric or medical service, the difference is in the eyes of the beholder and not in any specific characteristic behavior.[69]

Patients in chronic stupors or catatonia-like states form a portion of many chronic neurological medical services. When first seen, each patient is thoroughly examined for brainstem lesions, and, when found, may be relieved medically or surgically. But in many cases, lesions are not found, and it is in such instances that the question arises whether the signs meet the criteria for catatonia and offer the opportunity for its successful treatment.

A 22-year-old woman, lying mute in stupor, not moving to sound or pinprick, is seen in a bed filled with furry animal figures on the neurology service of a university hospital. Her illness began a month earlier, with acute malaise and somnolence followed by headaches and abnormal movements, and then a seizure. Extensive medical and neurologic examinations identified no systemic cause; treatments for epilepsy were prescribed, with the chart diagnosis of "stupor of unknown etiology." Plans for transfer to a long stay at a neurologic center were under way. An intravenous lorazepam test elicited eye opening, hoarse verbalization, and movements to pick up an animal figure and to smile. Over the next few days, increasing dosages of lorazepam resulted in some speech, and sitting, standing, and walking. With family consent, ECT was begun, and, after four treatments, the patient was fully responsive, able to feed and care for herself, and talking responsively. Within two weeks she was discharged to her home as recovered.[70]

13

TREATMENTS OF CATATONIA

Diseases desperate grown, by desperate appliance are relieved.
—Hamlet, Act IV, Scene 3, line 9

Between 1932 and 1933, John Romano, later a distinguished Rochester psychiatrist but at the time a medical student, served as an extern at the Milwaukee County Asylum for Chronic Mental Disease. Conditions were as bad as one might imagine. "The patient population was exclusively that of chronically ill persons." Many of the patients had been diagnosed with dementia praecox. He later said, "I recall walking on hospital floors where one would find row after row of patients sitting on chairs placed against the walls of large rooms, sometimes rocking, nodding, or performing peculiar mannerisms of hand-to-hand, hand-to-face, hand-to-body rubbing. . . . Others would be standing immobile or would shuffle or walk, at times with peculiar or bizarre gaits. Most were silent or would mumble, and occasionally there would be explosive verbal outbursts on the part of one or more patients, at times followed by physical injury to themselves or to those about them."[1] The description is chilling, except that what Romano was describing was largely not dementia praecox but catatonia. And his encounter with these rows of rocking men, inaccessible to treatment, is all the more poignant because in 1929–30 the first effective treatment for catatonia was introduced at the University of Wisconsin in Madison, a stone's throw from Milwaukee: the barbiturate sodium Amytal.

EARLY THERAPIES

The early pharmacology of catatonia was a grab-bag. In 1877, William O'Neill, a physician in Greenock, Scotland, had best results in stopping the nightly stupors (and waxy flexibility and muscle rigidity) of Miss G, "a country girl of eighteen years of age," with a mixture of valerianate of zinc and *Cannabis indica*.[2] Valerian is a time-tested remedy in psychopharmacology, as is *C. indica*, which was even marketed in England in the years between the wars as a commercial preparation, Indonad.[3] It is unsurprising that "catalepsy," Dr. O'Neill's diagnosis, would be responsive to these agents as catalepsy is responsive to so many different remedies.

And the narcotics? Opium, though a powerful antimelancholic, does not have a record of success in the treatment of catatonia, and Kahlbaum found it useless.[4] Cocaine has a considerable history in the treatment of catatonic stupor, especially in Central Europe. In what has been called "the first chemical treatment of catatonia,"

Hans Berger, professor of psychiatry at the University of Jena—who originated electroencephalography later in the 1920s—initiated in 1921 the treatment of stupor with cocaine. Eight of eleven cases roused from their stupor and "gave information." He said he had already tried cocaine 20 years previously but had published a notice in an obscure journal that excited little attention. Yet relief in these eight patients was short-lived. "In all cases I observed that the improvement was only very temporary, and often the time in which the patients gave information lasted only 1–2 hours. Thus, a practical therapeutic application of these cocaine injections is not realistic."[5] Still, the article attracted considerable notice, and one Italian psychiatrist referred to the procedure as "decatatonization."[6]

The 1920s saw various attempts to relieve stupor with cocaine. The capstone was research in 1927, by August Jacobi at the provincial asylum in Göttingen, in 24 stuporous patients with various underlying diagnoses. (In one of the earliest instances of self-experimentation in psychiatry, Jacobi first injected cocaine into himself and a colleague.) Using much higher doses than Berger (50 mg was Berger's highest, Jacobi's lowest), Jacobi determined that cocaine produced agitation of variable duration in the place of stupor and that it did not really have a therapeutic effect. He recommended against incorporating cocaine into the pharmacopoeia of catatonia. Yet he did make one interesting observation: "The possibility exists of gaining with cocaine an insight into the otherwise inaccessible psychic life of the patients."[7] Psychoanalysis was spreading. Insight into psychic life was very à la page.

Research moved on to carbon dioxide. In 1918, Arthur Loevenhart, 38, a physician and professor of pharmacology at the University of Wisconsin, and William F. Lorenz, 34, director of the Wisconsin Psychiatric Research Institute, then at Mendota, in the course of research on the physiology of oxygen in the brain, demonstrated that mild doses of sodium cyanide stimulated a particular brain center.[8] They noted by chance that a dementia praecox patient who had been mute for several months started speaking again after a sodium cyanide injection.[9] They did not pursue this finding.

Then, in 1929, with Lorenz now in charge of the new neuropsychiatry department at the Wisconsin medical school, they returned again to this agenda, but abandoned cyanide after unsatisfactory results. What else might they try to stimulate the stuporous patient? They hit upon a mixture of carbon dioxide and oxygen, given that one member of the team, an anesthetist, was familiar with using carbon dioxide as a respiratory stimulant. The results were on the whole positive: "The most favorable and striking reactions occurred in those patients who had been mute and mentally inaccessible for long periods of time." The patients passed from deep stupor to the ability to "carry on conversation." After a period of 2–25 minutes, the patients would then relapse to their previous state. The research, they concluded, "permits a period of contact with the individual which offers opportunities for further physiological and psychological investigations."[10]

The carbon dioxide gauntlet was picked up quickly. In 1931, Karl H. Langenstrass, a Tübingen graduate of 1919 who had emigrated to the United States and worked at St. Elizabeths Hospital in the District of Columbia, and Ethel Friedman-Buchman, a Berne medical graduate of 1924, who would later become a staff psychiatrist at Allentown State Hospital in Pennsylvania, published in German a note on treating stupor in manic-depressive illness and dementia praecox. They induced fevers (fever-therapy) with injections of a mixed vaccine from the Parke-Davis Company, combined with carbon dioxide inhalation and psychotherapy. The results were impressive: of nine patients, they obtained lasting recoveries in four.[11] (Buchman was among the earliest female investigators in the United States in biological psychiatry.) In 1931, Langenstrass reported on his own, in English, on the four recovered patients. The cases were translated from the German version: "Case 4: The patient had been in stupor for ten years. One hour after the inhalation treatment he sat in a wheelchair and read a newspaper for the first time in a decade. For two months he worked well about the grounds; then he was transferred to the laundry, and made good. He is now working on the farm, and the manager says he is one of the best helpers he has had."[12]

In 1934 Leland Hinsie, 41, at Columbia University threw a wet blanket on the treatments. Hinsie, a psychoanalyst, was assistant director of the New York State Psychiatric Institute and author of *Dictionary of Psychiatry*.[13] Hinsie and colleagues, using an oxygen-carbon dioxide mixture, treated "catatonic schizophrenia" in four groups of five patients each, in various settings: an oxygen chamber for two and a half months [*sic*], an oxygen dormitory, and so forth, and found that few improved or recovered. "The present technique of administering carbon dioxide creates intense anxiety in the patient and leads to states of great resistance," they noted.[14]

One might quibble whether these extreme experimental conditions prejudiced the results. The Hinsie work put an end to mixed carbon dioxide-oxygen treatment. Yet, not fully. In an article in 1942 on catatonia apart from schizophrenia, Morris Herman and researchers in New York City mentioned casually, "Contact may be obtained by the inhalation of a mixture of CO_2 and O_2."[15]

There were other early efforts to treat catatonia, such as inducing "protein shock" and fever with vaccines, including typhoid. But none of these efforts caught on because sodium Amytal intervened.[16]

SODIUM AMYTAL: DISCOVERED

In the 1920s, a new class of medications—the barbiturates—became popular as sedatives. They were introduced into medicine in 1903, and amobarbital, patented by Eli Lilly in 1924 and marketed as intravenous sodium Amytal, came to be a prized preparation because it had a shorter half-life than the earlier barbiturates and could be used as a hypnotic with little sedation the following day. So widespread had the use of the barbiturates as sleeping potions become that one asylum psychiatrist in Rotterdam said in 1930 that the use of narcotic-sedatives is now so common "that you can almost speak of a massive exercise in experimental psychopathology that humanity is making on itself."[17]

The first effort to treat catatonia with barbiturates was undertaken by Henri Claude, the professor of psychiatry, and Henri Baruk, then an asylum staffer (*chef de clinique*), in Paris, in 1928. They treated eight controls and five catatonic patients with the combination barbiturate Somnifen (aprobarbital and substituents). The controls became more relaxed, and the drug had nonspecific effects on the treatment group.[18] The authors viewed the work as inconclusive, and it was forgotten.

In 1923, Lorenz asked young William Bleckwenn, 28, who had trained at Bellevue Hospital in New York City and at the Wisconsin Psychiatric Institute, to join the staff in the University of Wisconsin's neuropsychiatry program. Bleckwenn later said that in those years he and colleagues had administered "more than 10,000 intravenous injections" of barbiturates for hypnosis, mainly Amytal. He referred to the technique as "a method of chemical psychoanalysis."[19]

One technique that Bleckwenn and Lorenz pioneered did not put agitated patients to sleep with Amytal but used it to induce periods of clarity in stuporous and agitated catatonic patients. Particularly in stupor, Amytal seemed to have a paradoxical effect—rather than sedating, it awakened. The neuropsychiatry team at Wisconsin issued three reports on this technique at meetings in 1929, which then were published in 1930 or 1931.

Before the Milwaukee Neuro-Psychiatric Society on November 12, 1929, Bleckwenn described their early results in inducing intervals of normality in patients with chronic catatonic symptoms, some of whom had been in stupors for months and years. The case histories were very brief, yet clearly here lay a new advance. The paper was submitted to the American Medical Association's *Archives of Neurology and Psychiatry* early in 1930 and published later that year.[20]

Lorenz gave the first detailed report on the technique on December 6, 1929, at the dedication of the New York State Psychiatric Institute. He presented a single case, a woman, 27, unhappily married, who had been admitted to a state hospital, then transferred to the University's Psychiatric Institute in Madison "in a state of catatonic stupor," with extreme muscular rigidity, negativism, and her body folded into a fetal posture. They gave her half a gram of Amytal dissolved in 10 cc of distilled water. She thereupon went into a state of deep narcosis for about seven hours. "She was then aroused by speech and she responded to conversation, asked for food and drink. She continued in this aroused mental state for four hours," then dropped off to sleep again, at which point her catatonic symptoms reappeared. They proceeded to treat her repeatedly with Amytal. "The most striking and, in some respects, pleasant behavior has been the voluntary request for food. This patient ordered a large meal, all of which she ate with apparent relish." (Previously, stuporous patients had often been tube fed.) And, during her stupor, she had actually been paying attention to current events. "She inquired as to the progress of a football game which was being played between Wisconsin and Purdue. This game was actually in progress on the Saturday afternoon when she was aroused for the first time. . . . It seemed everything said or done in her presence was clearly known to her."[21] This single case report was quite striking but did not elicit much attention.

Then on December 27–28, 1929, at a meeting in New York of the Association for Research in Nervous and Mental Diseases, Bleckwenn reported on the use of sodium Amytal in 15 cases of catatonia. In the course of the team's work on Amytal in the induction of sleep, he said, "a case of catatonic excitement was treated. As the narcosis was being induced the patient had a period of about two minutes during which he seemed quite normal and discussed his illness and future plans. Following the initial period of sleep, which lasted about four hours, he again seemed quite rational for a period of two hours." This immediately recalled the success that his colleagues Loevenhart and Lorenz had had with sodium-cyanide and carbon dioxide-oxygen anesthesia. "Now an entirely different drug, apparently a cortical depressant, is more effective in the production of this phenomenon."

Eleven of the fifteen patients had responded to the Amytal treatment. "Catatonic patients can be aroused from their stupor states for intervals of from two to fourteen hours during which, if previously tube-fed, they eat ravenously, show spontaneity, ask and answer questions with consistent emotional reactions." The older barbiturates, he noted, also had the same effect (though later authors did not always agree with this and found Amytal singularly effective). Repeated injections returned some of the patients to "normal," Bleckwenn said. A woman, 36, had been tube-fed for two years and lay continuously in a fetal position, during which she developed flexion contractures. "Following sodium Amytal injections, she has returned to a normal level. She is completely oriented, recalls outstanding facts during the past two years,—'my revival with the gas' as she puts it." They were attempting to stretch out her contractures. "Recently she was able to walk, with assistance."[22] Bleckwenn presented this key paper in 1929, but it was published only in 1931. He also took black-and-white films of four of his patients with catatonia and the relief afforded by Amytal. The film is available for public viewing from the archives of the National Library of Medicine.[23]

The major debut of the Amytal treatment of catatonia came in the *Journal of the American Medical Association* in October 1930. It is unclear why Lorenz was not a co-author, given that he headed the neuropsychiatry service and had clearly been involved in the research. Possibly he wanted to give his younger colleague a career boost, in the way that Kahlbaum had done with Hecker. Bleckwenn included one catatonia vignette, plus the news that "some twenty cases of catatonia of the stuporous, cataleptic and negativistic types have been treated." In the vignette, a medical student, 20, had developed agitation, psychosis, negativism with food refusal, and "bizarre gesticulations and facial grimaces." "He was given sodium iso-amylethyl barbiturate [Amytal] and just as he was going to sleep said that he realized he was having a terrible time and hoped to recover so as to enter school at the beginning of the next semester." After his initial sleep, he awoke "quite normal for about four hours, during which time he discussed current topics, his illness, school and his future plans." He then fell asleep again and returned to his excited state upon reawakening. But the staff continued the injections; he gradually improved, was transferred to a sanatorium, and at discharge did not return to school but began working for a florist "and seems perfectly adjusted at present."[24] This would be a typical recovery from catatonia: the veil is lifted, no traces remain, and the patient is perfectly normal, either until the next episode, or permanently.

Interestingly, with Amytal, we have for the first time a genuinely American story. It was Eli Lilly, an Indianapolis drug company, that synthesized and patented Amytal. And it was doctors at the University of Wisconsin and the University of Iowa (see the following section) who introduced it to the clinic. In the UK, the first article on Amytal in catatonia did not appear until 1939.[25] German science was envenomed in Nazi rule; France, just emerging from the Depression, was about to be invaded, and Europe would be scientifically *hors de combat* for the next decade. Yankee inventiveness and energy came to the fore.

SODIUM AMYTAL BECOMES THE TREATMENT OF CHOICE FOR CATATONIA

The Wisconsin results were so spectacular that Amytal came quickly into use elsewhere. In 1931, Erich Lindemann, at the Psychopathic Hospital of the State University of Iowa—a German-trained investigator who went on to Harvard to become a major figure in American psychiatry—reported a trial of 24 patients with a variety of diagnoses including catatonia and four controls. The Iowa investigators didn't think the Wisconsin results could be explained on the basis of narcosis alone, so they gave small doses of Amytal "not leading to any narcosis or sleep at all." The normals experienced "a feeling of serenity and well-being, a desire to communicate and to speak about problems of personal matters usually not spoken of to strangers." (This experience gave Amytal the reputation as a "truth drug." "There was the feeling of being unable to guard against saying things which one does not want to and an inability to refuse to answer questions even if they refer to very intimate matters.")

As for the Iowa patients: "The outstanding change was an increase in ability or willingness to communicate thought content and memories. Catatonic patients who had been mute for months became communicative and gave valuable material about their trends of thought. . . . Catatonic patients lost their rigidity and their cataleptic symptoms. . . . Sleep and narcosis are not necessary conditions for the production of the mental changes discovered by previous authors."[26]

In 1932, Lindemann reported further details. In a male, 38, "Whenever he was approached with the request to state what was worrying him, he would begin to produce inarticulate, barking sounds which could not be understood. . . . Finally he was given sodium Amytal, and under the influence of the drug he related with many tears that as a boy he had sexual plays with animals" and "feared that God would punish him for bestiality. . . . A marked feeling of guilt had developed; shame and embarrassment prevented him from speaking." The patient was permanently relieved by the Amytal "and soon afterward was discharged as recovered." By now, 30 patients were treated at the Psychopathic Hospital. In all, Lindemann found "a striking change from a resistive, seclusive attitude to friendly and emotionally warm communication, with a feeling of wellbeing and desire to retain the condition produced by the drug." Amytal did not, however, affect the content of the delusions and hallucinations, but at least they could be rationally discussed with the clinicians rather than hidden away.[27]

Now the trials tumbled forth. In 1933, Carl Phillip Wagner, at the exclusive Hartford Retreat in Connecticut, found that Amytal worked well for the negativism of catatonia and for psychosis. Of the 37 patients with a variety of diagnoses, they reported 9 "complete recoveries" and 17 instances of slow improvement. In the discussion, Walter Freeman, of St. Elizabeths Hospital in the District of Columbia (the Freeman of lobotomy fame) offered: "We have been using sodium Amytal for the purpose of bringing our catatonic patients back into contact with reality. In their catatonic state they are inaccessible and one cannot carry out any satisfactory therapeutic procedure beyond physical ones. Sodium Amytal renders them accessible, so that they can discuss their problems."[28]

These comments reflect the belief of the day that psychotherapy represented the principal treatment of psychiatry and that Amytal was useful because it made possible psychotherapy with these catatonic, withdrawn individuals. In 1946, Paul Hoch at Columbia University called Amytal "a form of short psychotherapy."[29]

The effectiveness of Amytal in catatonic stupor ("schizophrenia") reverberated down the decades. For Seymour Kety, a neurophysiologist who got science going at the fledgling National Institute of Mental Health in the 1950s, witnessing an Amytal treatment was a life-changing experience. He later said, "It was in the studies on schizophrenia that I first saw the temporary but remarkable restoration in the thinking and affect of some schizophrenics under the influence of sodium Amytal narcosis. I was impressed that a drug could produce such dramatic effects, which suggested that biochemical processes on which a drug could act were responsible for the psychic symptoms."[30] Kety went on to direct such research, changing the face of biological psychiatry.

Even into the 1990s, sodium Amytal remained a mainstay in the treatment of catatonia. In 1992, W. Vaughn McCall and colleagues at the Bowman Gray School of Medicine in Winston-Salem, North Carolina, determined that Amytal beat placebo in the treatment of mutism.[31] In another publication that year, McCall said, "All catatonic presentations should be assumed to have a favorable prognosis."[32]

CONVULSIVE THERAPY

At Bellevue Hospital in the 1940s, as Max Fink recalls: "Patients who were posturing, mute and not feeding would quickly respond [to Amytal] and talk and begin eating. A few hours later they would be back in their posturing, back in their mute state. I didn't realize it at the time, but those patients were all later treated with ECT."[33]

There is a long history of treating psychosis with electricity. On May 25, 1788, George Wilkinson of Edinburgh was called to the bedside of Miss A. Crawford, 28, who, two weeks previously "was seized at two o'clock in the morning, while in bed, with a rigidity and stiffness of the whole body. At four she became totally insensible." She recovered hours later. But the fits resumed, "their accession being always sudden. A universal spasm, producing a rigidity of the whole frame, took place in a moment, and deprived her of the power of speech and recollection." She exhibited what other writers had described as a "death-like sleep." She also showed gegenhalten , though it would be a century before the term was coined: "The position of her fingers, hands, and arms, was altered with difficulty." And waxy flexibility: "They preserved every form of flexure they acquired."

Now it was June 7: "Her fits again returned . . . and I was sent for in great haste [a week later], and found her sitting in her chair, perfectly sensible, but with her jaw completely locked, her face somewhat distorted, her head drawn backwards, and the muscles of her neck rigid and inflexible."

He diagnosed "catalepsy." "I determined to try the effects of electricity," said Wilkinson. He procured a primitive sparking device and proceeded over the weeks ahead to treat her jaw, her spine, and her mouth, "which had been closed eighteen hours [and] opened almost instantaneously, and she regained her speech." Six weeks later, she was well again.[34] This is an early example of the successful use of electricity in the treatment of catatonia, but it is not ECT; that treatment is effective by the repeated induction of grand mal seizures.

If Amytal launched the modern era of psychopharmacology, the convulsive therapies launched the definitive treatment of catatonia. Amytal often offered temporary relief, with the patient relapsing into a stupor until the next treatment—though many patients did recover definitively. With ECT, relief occurs rapidly, after six induced seizures or so, and remains in effect for a much longer period, often permanently.

Inducing grand mal seizures to relieve catatonia began in Budapest on January 23, 1934. Ladislas Meduna, 38, after a decade of neuropathology research at the Budapest

Neurological Research Institute, gave intramuscular injections of camphor to induce grand mal seizures in schizophrenic patients. In his neuropathology studies, he observed that the brain glia concentrations were diminished in schizophrenic patients and increased in the epileptic. Was it possible that a paucity of glia was the pathology of schizophrenia, and would inducing seizures increase gliosis and relieve psychosis?[35] He left the research institute and moved to the chronic mental illness hospital at Lipótmezö, where he was able to treat severely ill patients.

By good fortune, as Gabor Gazdag and collaborators determined in a later review of the charts of these patients, 7 of Meduna's first 11 patients had catatonia, which Meduna considered "schizophrenia."[36] He announced that he had discovered a means of considerably relieving a disease hitherto considered untreatable. Meduna then switched from camphor as the epileptogen to a cardiac stimulant, intravenous pentylenetetrazol—marketed as Cardiazol in Europe, Metrazol in the United States—which induced seizures even more efficiently. In 1935, Meduna reported his experience with 43 patients, gaining remission in 19. And, in 1937, he described his overall experience with 110 patients, half of whom had responded well to his induction of seizures.[37] Meduna was widely disbelieved in Budapest, where the official doctrine insisted that schizophrenia was untreatable and genetic in origin; in the mid-1930s, he emigrated to Chicago, where he spent the rest of his years in scientific productivity.[38] This was the beginning of "chemical convulsive therapy."

ECT FOR CATATONIA

In 1938, Ugo Cerletti, professor of psychiatry at the Rome University Psychiatric Hospital, demonstrated that electricity induced brain seizures instantaneously, without the anxiety-provoking latency period that accompanied chemical convulsive therapy. Cerletti had no particular interest in catatonia, but did notice that many of his "schizophrenia" patients, as well as those with melancholic depression, responded well to the new treatment, and, from 1938 on, ECT made its way into the world as the most powerful treatment that psychiatry had to offer[39]—as indeed it still is today.

ECT quickly established itself in the treatment of catatonia, known then as "catatonic schizophrenia." The story continues to have a heavily Central European cast.

Lothar Kalinowsky, whose mother was Jewish, had fled Hitler's Germany in 1933 for Mussolini's Italy, and then, in 1940, traveled farther via London to New York City. Kalinowsky had been present at Cerletti's early trials, appreciated the effectiveness of ECT, and became in New York the treatment's most distinguished apostle. He divided his time between Pilgrim State Hospital on Long Island and the New York State Psychiatric Institute on the Upper West Side of Manhattan. And it was at Pilgrim State, in 1943, that Kalinowsky conducted what were the first large trials of ECT in catatonia ("catatonic schizophrenia"). Of 200 patients with schizophrenia, the main finding was that the earlier the treatment was initiated, the higher the recovery rate (67 percent of those ill for less than 6 months recovered or were much improved after a course of ECT). Kalinowsky did comment in passing on catatonic schizophrenia, though offered no numbers: "Convulsive treatment is successful in breaking up the motor symptoms of all cases of catatonic stupor; however, their schizophrenic residue offers a poor outlook. More favorable results are obtained in patients with catatonic excitement; or in those patients whose symptomology [*sic*] shifts between stupor and excitement." This alternation is one of the core symptoms of catatonia, and Kalinowsky saw that inducing seizures relieves the illness. "Of 200 patients a year later, 57 percent were still in remission, 23 percent improved, and 20 percent unimproved."[40]

In 1948, Donald M. Hamilton and James H. Wall at the New York Hospital, Westchester Division, in White Plains, reported on 100 women said to be "schizophrenic" as a result of sexual problems: "Of the 100 patients, almost two-thirds were precipitated into mental illness by factors concerned with sexual function." This was, of course, the heyday of psychoanalysis. Yet, in addition to inpatient psychotherapy, these 100 women also received ECT "to improve the patients' contact with the environment so that they might become more responsive to other therapeutic procedures." Whatever problems these women actually had, some were afflicted with catatonia. Of the 54 catatonic patients, 57 percent recovered; of the paranoid, 30 percent; of the hebephrenic, only 2 of them went home, neither recovered.[41]

In the mid-1970s, two large university studies established the efficacy of ECT in "catatonic schizophrenia," as opposed to other kinds of schizophrenia. In 1973, Donn A. Wells at the University of Rochester reported that, of 276 patients with schizophrenia treated with ECT in the years 1960–69, 55 percent of those with catatonic schizophrenia had a "good" result, as did 40 percent of those with "schizoaffective schizophrenia" and 34 percent of those with paranoid schizophrenia.[42]

But it was really the studies on the "Iowa 500"—a review of records of patients admitted to the Iowa Psychopathic Hospital since it opened in 1920—that provided strong evidence that there was something about catatonia that responded selectively to ECT. Of 250 patients with a diagnosis of catatonic schizophrenia, catatonic syndrome, or dementia praecox, catatonic type, at discharge, 40 percent of those treated with ECT had a "complete recovery without relapse," as did 27 percent of those treated with ECT plus a neuroleptic, and 16 percent of those treated with "milieu therapy." Of those treated with neuroleptic only, none had a superior result, and the best outcome was recovery followed by relapse (and worse).[43] Here was an early warning that neuroleptic medications were not the treatment of choice for catatonia. Morrison's studies restored ECT for catatonia to the psychiatric radar. (Iowa was a veritable font of catatonia data: in 1993, Barbara M. Rohland and collaborators found that in 26 of 28 catatonia patients (93 percent) admitted between 1989 and 1992, the syndrome resolved with ECT.[44])

ECT FOR DELIRIOUS MANIA AND MALIGNANT CATATONIA

It is widely overlooked that, in 1947, Angel Dominguez Borreguero, director of the provincial mental hospital of Salamanca in Spain, reported the treatment of "mortal catatonia" with ECT. He had begun the procedure in 1945, and, by 1946, had successfully treated four cases. All survived. He concluded with justified pride, "As we have determined, Stauder's mortal catatonia is not necessarily mortal. . . . Are we justified in continuing to use this appellation? In our opinion, this designation of Stauder's is inapplicable [inactual] . . . because of its curability with electroshock, as we have seen."[45] This path-breaking report remains virtually unknown, however, possibly because of unfamiliarity with the Spanish language or a reluctance to accept as important an accomplishment from Franco's Spain.

Credit for introducing ECT in the treatment of fatal catatonia has gone to a group of clinicians in Vienna, a city still renowned as a world medical hub despite the horrors of the war. In 1948, Ottokar ("Otto") Arnold, 31, at the Steinhof mental hospital in Vienna, confirmed the effectiveness of the treatment of delirious mania and fatal catatonia with ECT. At first, he did not understand the importance of treating the patients in the first day or two after the appearance of symptoms of potential lethal catatonia, and, of his 15 patients in the 1946–47 period whom he treated with ECT, all died. (The three who were treated early received only a single stimulus, not sufficient to preserve their lives. It is to Arnold's credit as a scientist that he had the courage to publish these discouraging results.[46]) The following two-year period was almost as bad: collaborating with a junior psychiatrist at the Steinhof, in 1947–48 Arnold administered ECT to 18 patients, of whom 15 died. Before 1949, Arnold had not yet had his epiphany about the importance of early treatment. But of the 16 lethal catatonia patients seen at the University *Klinik* (not at the Steinhof) in 1949–50, 10 were treated immediately on day 1–2 and then daily, and all survived. Five who were treated later on days 3–4 survived, too; all who were treated after day 5 died. Arnold used the "shock-block" method that Anton von Braunmühl introduced for ECT in 1940, customarily three stimulated seizures at 15-minute intervals, followed by further treatments at lengthening intervals.[47] For Arnold, there were two take-home messages: ECT was the only possible treatment of fatal catatonia, nothing else was effective, there were no counterindications, and early treatment was absolutely essential.[48] (Arnold went on to become in 1979 a full professor of psychiatry.[49])

Just as Otto Arnold was figuring out the correct administration of ECT for lethal catatonia in 1949 in Vienna, in 1949 Ottar Lingjaerde, director of the Lier mental hospital in Norway, was doing the same thing. Until he got it right, said Lingjaerde, every one of their 50 lethal catatonia patients seen before 1949 died. Then, in 1949, Lingjaerde instituted a new treatment program consisting of cortisone and "intensive shock therapy," meaning 1–2 seizures per day. Lingjaerde, too, emphasized the importance of immediate treatment. Of the 19 patients with "acute delirium," or fatal catatonia, seen from 1949 to 1954, only one died.[50] (These years saw a soon to be abandoned vogue for the use of corticosteroids in the treatment of catatonia.)

The Borreguero, Arnold, and Lingjaerde reports were of great importance in developing the effective treatment of delirious mania. Unfortunately, almost all appeared in local or regional psychiatry journals and had trouble reaching an international audience.

In 1967, Frederik Tolsma, chief of the Rotterdam Municipal Mental Hospital, said of the "acute pernicious psychoses": "The most efficacious therapy is still treatment with electroshock series in block form as indicated by Arnold. All the cases recently treated by us have stayed alive."[51]

Ironically, after the 1960s, public opinion in Germany turned against convulsive therapy; ECT for deadly catatonia, where the Germans had previously led, became politically infeasible. In 1982, Heinz Häfner, a senior German figure, admitted that an "inappropriate reticence" about ECT obliged them to use neuroleptics for deadly catatonia and that two of these patients had died. Now, however, his service in Mannheim had gone over to ECT.[52] In 1985, the Health Ministry of the German province of Hesse ordered psychiatric hospitals to abstain entirely from ECT, with the result that fatal catatonia patients were transferred by ambulance to neighboring provinces where the procedure was still available, leading to "substantial resistance from hospital personnel" and critical articles about ECT in the local press.[53] So, the German chapter in this story began to close.

14

L'ENVOI

O Freunde, nicht diese Töne,
sondern lasst uns angenehmere
anstimmen, und freudenvollere.
—Friedrich Schiller[1]

Catatonia is an identifiable and verifiable syndrome of abnormal motor and psychic changes, acute in onset, disruptive of living, often malignant with fatal outcome, and yet eminently recognizable and fully treatable today. It is an unheralded behavior in the classification of illnesses that has undergone a remarkable recognition in the immediate past few decades.

Catatonia was demarcated in 1874 among hospitalized patients in a German private psychiatric clinic by the psychopathologist Karl Kahlbaum. Within a few decades, the syndrome was co-opted and misidentified by Emil Kraepelin as a feature of his poorly defined and poorly treatable syndrome of dementia praecox. Alas, his writings were so authoritative that for more than a century catatonia remained buried within his disorder.

Two effective treatments of catatonia were discovered, sodium Amytal in 1929–30 and the induction of grand mal seizures in 1934, that developed into the present electroconvulsive therapy, the definitive treatment of catatonia. These treatments were remarkably effective, and, for a time, catatonia was considered a solved psychiatric problem, with little professional or public interest. It was a piece of the schizophrenia puzzle!

Once the cascade of new psychotropic drugs—and the new third edition of the *Diagnostic and Statistical Manual of Mental Disorders* (DSM) in 1980—stimulated fresh thinking about matching agents to illnesses, the position of catatonia as a marker of schizophrenia was weakened. American authors identified catatonia among patients with disorders in mood and as a neurotoxic syndrome that resulted from treatment with neuroleptic drugs. Debates as to whether the toxic syndrome was best relieved by dopamine agonists and muscle relaxants or by sedatives and electroshock converged on the point: catatonia was an independent and treatable syndrome. By the 1990s, catatonia was increasingly recognized as a unique disorder in the psychiatric glossary, a recognition that was finalized in the 2013 publication of the American Psychiatric Association's DSM-5.

Catatonia is readily identified today by motor behaviors itemized in rating scales, verified by a benzodiazepine or sedative relief test, and validated by its remission within a few weeks with applications of its known treatments. It is a unique syndrome in modern psychiatry, its story matched only by that of neurosyphilis, the infectious disease that is identifiable by skin, ocular, behavioral, and neurological signs; verified by positive serology tests; and treatable by the antibiotic penicillin.

Like syphilis, catatonia has many expressions. A widely recognized retarded form of mutism, stupor, posturing, catalepsy, repetitive acts, and psychosis is cited here as Kahlbaum's catatonia. An excited delirious mania with frenzy, cited as Bell's mania and Stauder's lethal catatonia, is another variant. Malignant, often fatal, febrile catatonias are described secondary to neuroleptic or serotonin drug toxicities. Self-injurious behaviors are common among adolescents with autism and mental retardation.

Other not yet acknowledged syndromes with catatonia characteristics and responsive to catatonia treatments are anti-N-methyl-D-aspartate receptor (NMDAR) encephalitis, the Gilles de la Tourette syndrome, various mutisms, and obsessive-compulsive disorders. Among hospital neurology services, patients with persistent stupors of unknown etiology and akinetic mutisms are relieved when recognized and treated as catatonia. Thus, the disorder is not uncommon.

Little is known about catatonia's pathophysiology. Its recognition as a distinct syndrome that can be positively identified and systematically studied is recent. Kraepelin's authority kept catatonia as a type of schizophrenia during most of the twentieth century, and any possible test findings were lost within the morass of that syndrome. In the early days of electrophysiology, attempts to identify an electroencephalographic (EEG) pattern for catatonic schizophrenia failed. SPECT testing was done before and after relief, but no distinct pattern was discerned. Some studies report low serum iron levels and elevated creatine phosphokinase levels in patients with malignant catatonia.[2–5]

When catatonia is now recognized and benzodiazepines in adequate dosing prescribed, more than 80 percent of the patients recover rapidly. For those who fail to respond to sedatives, the response to induced seizures is almost universally successful. In their 2003 textbook *Catatonia*, Fink and Taylor reviewed the reports of failed responses of catatonia to ECT[6] Each failed effort was explicable by clinicians' errors. Neuroleptic medications were continued in the belief that catatonia was schizophrenia, sustaining the pathology of the neuroleptic malignant syndrome. Dosing of benzodiazepines was inadequate, the practitioners fearing impairment of breathing with the high doses recommended or that the patients would become tolerant and drug dependent. Believing that the technical criteria for treating catatonia with ECT were the same as for patients with major depression, practitioners elicited ineffective seizures, using unilateral electrode placements and minimal-energy dosing. Treatments were administered twice weekly, neglecting the reality that the severe forms of catatonia are life-threatening illnesses that require more frequent stimuli, often daily.[7] In some instances, consent was withdrawn at the first sign of relief, relapse quickly followed, encouraging the erroneous conclusion that the treatment had failed.

Catatonia's association with schizophrenia has been a catastrophic misbelief in medical history, leading to its teaching as a *psychiatric* emotional disorder and blocking interest in the syndrome as a *systemic bodily* disorder. The psychological elements in catatonia—the role of fear and terror—do not necessarily mean that catatonia is psychiatric in nature. Our present understanding takes catatonia out of the psychiatric curriculum. It is best recognized and treated by physicians, pediatricians, neurologists, and specialists in infectious diseases and emergency medicine,[8] not by psychologists and psychiatrists whose practices in outpatient clinics and private offices cater to the ambulant wounded. It is time to revise the teaching curricula in medical schools and residency training programs to bring catatonia within the systemic medical realm and out of the psychiatric dictionary.

The unfortunate association of catatonia with schizophrenia is worsened by psychiatry's rejection of the physical examination and today's reliance on verbal inquiries and visual observation of behavior for a clinical diagnosis. Catatonia signs are best observed and tested as responses to simple commands, but patients do require "hands-on" examination. For much of the twentieth century, the explanations for psychiatric illnesses were based on ephemeral concepts of "mind," rejecting the role of the brain and systemic functions. In the twenty-first century, with the shift to recognizing the role of the brain in behavior disorders, the interest changed from the clinician to the laboratory scientist, often equating animal physiology and behavior to that of humans.[9]

Catatonia does not result from a structural defect in a body organ, nor is it associated with an identifiable physiologic dysfunction, although vegetative symptoms are a common accompaniment. It is not the consequence of a recognized brain lesion. It occurs in the context of systemic medical illnesses and is frequently associated with manic-depressive disease. After catatonia is relieved, we see no residuals. Before modern treatments were known, patients with prolonged catatonia occasionally resolved spontaneously. Catatonia is a disorder of the whole organism, arising suddenly and vanishing without a trace. It is similar to crying, an inherited behavior that expresses a strong emotion.

Catatonia is not a disorder in thought or emotion, although such accompaniments are common. Some authors consider catatonia an "end-state" whole-body response to imminent doom, a behavior inherited from ancestral encounters with carnivores, an adaptation that remains an inherent feature of living.[10] This image makes catatonia an atavism.

Catatonia is associated with fear and has been likened to the animal defense of tonic immobility, the relic of the flight-and-fight defenses of living in a predatory environment. Mutism, negativism, posturing, and rigidity are adaptations that disappear when the stress is relieved. Catatonia is seen in patients with autism or mental retardation who develop self-injurious behaviors.[11] Its pathophysiology has received little attention, although consideration has been given to the neurology of the frontal lobes.[12,13]

Neuroscientists commonly seek to understand behavior disorders by brain imaging and genetic profiling of clusters of patients identified by imprecise DSM criteria, hoping that modern computer programs will bring out useful patterns by the analyses of "big data."[14] The problem is that DSM diagnoses are vastly heterogeneous, and the lack of solid phenotypes does not bode well for the search for genetic markers or characteristic brain images for any psychiatric illness. Identifying populations by catatonia criteria—acute onset of illness, measurable and scorable motor behaviors, and validation by the relief accorded by barbiturates and benzodiazepines or by induced seizures—is an opportunity to specify homogeneous patient samples for neuroscience and biological studies.

The discovery of the syndrome of catatonia as an acute, identifiable, verifiable, and treatable behavior disease is an unheralded accomplishment in medical science. The story is largely unknown. The mistaken marriage with the ill-defined concept of schizophrenia and the ready availability of immediate relief by injections of barbiturates hid the syndrome behind a curtain of nonrecognition for a century. It took the lethal effects of neuroleptic drugs to bring catatonia from behind this curtain to gain recognition as an independent syndrome relieved in a remarkable manner by inducing grand mal seizures. The causes of the syndrome, the changes in systemic and brain physiology, the unprecedented responses to the benzodiazepines and to induced seizures challenge physician-clinicians to recognize and relieve catatonia and challenge neuroscientists and body physiologists to understand the somatic changes.

We have noted the overlap of catatonia and melancholia with numerous cases exhibiting the motor signs of catatonia and the mood signs of melancholia.[15,16] More severely ill melancholics are mute or repeatedly exhibit stereotypic wailing and retarded movement, refusal of food, unusual posturing, and stupor. Many patients have positive findings on both melancholia and catatonia rating scales. Most striking is the remarkable responsivity of both syndromes to relief by induced seizures. The more severely ill are relieved of life-threatening symptoms with 1–3 properly elicited seizures. Such overlap encourages the search for other commonalities. In melancholia, abnormal neuroendocrine functions of cortisol and thyroid have been well-documented, as has their normalization with induced seizures. Similar studies of neuroendocrine functions have not been done in catatonia, offering a challenge and opportunity to neuroscientists and clinicians. We have decried the rejection of the neuroendocrine findings in melancholia by clinicians,[17] and we hope that the increasing interest in catatonia and the ability to identify more homogeneous population samples of catatonia patients will encourage neuroendocrine studies. These will surely offer better understanding of catatonia's pathophysiology. We are also impressed with the role of fear in catatonia, and anticipate that, as catatonia is increasingly recognized as a singular entity, hormone studies that have identified changes in conditions of fear and flight will test the significance of this image.

The rapid progress in our understanding of catatonia is a remarkable and unheralded achievement of modern clinical science. Its understanding also focuses attention on electoshock, the widely stigmatized science that merits greater public recognition and research attention.

Karl Kahlbaum and his followers recognized that their understanding of catatonia was comparable to that of neurosyphilis, as distinct systemic syndromes of identifiable behaviors. They lacked effective treatment, so that many of their patients became chronically ill and many died. Kahlbaum would be very pleased today with the increasing recognition accorded his syndrome and the widespread success in its relief. He would have been dismayed and discouraged when Emil Kraepelin, in 1899, the year of Kahlbaum's death, tied catatonia to the singular, nonverifiable, and untreatable illness whose victims were supposedly doomed to dementia. Kahlbaum would take pleasure in today's acceptance of catatonia as a response to a systemic illness of many causes and many origins, much as he had envisioned it.

NOTES

Prelims

1. WP Berrington. A Psycho-Pharmacological Study of Schizophrenia. J Ment Sci. 1939;85: 406-488, 439

Chapter 1

1. Döblin A. *Berlin Alexanderplatz*, trans. Eugene Jolas (1929 New York: Continuum; 1999: 595.
2. Communication from a mother to the authors, September 6, 2016. On the therapeutic effects of ball playing in catatonia, see Straus EW et al. Pseudoreversibility of catatonic stupor. *AJP*. 1955;111:680–685, 682–683.
3. Lee JWY et al. Catatonia in a psychiatric intensive care facility: incidence and response to benzodiazepines. *Ann Clin Psychiatry*. 2000;12:89–96. One group puts the range at 7–17 percent of patients hospitalized with acute psychiatric disorders. See also Caroff SC et al. Epidemiology, in Caroff et al. eds., *Catatonia: From Psychopathology to Neurobiology*. Washington DC: American Psychiatric Press; 2004: 15–31, 16–17. Another study gives the prevalence among inpatients at 8–19 percent. Al Sayegh A et al. Prevalence of catatonic signs in acute psychiatric patients in Scotland. *Psychiatrist*. 2010;34:479–484. For further data on incidence, see Chapter 13.
4. Wilson JE, Niu K, Heckers SZ. The diagnostic criteria and structure of catatonia. *Schizophrenia Res.* 2015;164:256–262, 256.
5. Faculty wore long white coats, denoting their more responsible status. In the past half-century, these traditions of wearing clothes to denote status have disappeared.
6. Fricchione GL, Kaufman LD, Gruber BL, Fink M. Electroconvulsive therapy and cyclophosphamide in combination for severe neuropsychiatric lupus with catatonia. *Am J Med.* 1990;88:442–443.
7. Kahlbaum K. *Die Katatonie, oder das Spannungsirresein*. Berlin: Hirschwald; 1874: 87.
8. See Moskowitz AK. 'Scared stiff': catatonia as an evolutionary-based fear response. *Psychol Rev.* 2004;111:984–1002.
9. Victor Peralta and colleagues propose thinking of the Kahlbaum syndrome as a third psychosis, alongside schizophrenia and mood disorders. This has the advantage of detaching psychotic catatonia from schizophrenia, the disadvantage of failing to distinguish between catatonia as Kahlbaum conceived it and the catatonic syndrome that may be present in numerous other psychiatric and medical illnesses. On manifest Parkinson's disease (clinically established PD) as opposed to the red flags of parkinsonism (clinically probable PD), see Postuma RB et al. MDS clinical diagnostic criteria for Parkinson's disease, *Movement Dis.* 2015;30:1591–1599.

10. Fink M, Taylor MA. The many varieties of catatonia. *Eur Arch Psych Clin Neurosci.* 2001;257(Suppl. 1):1/8–1/13. Bernard Pauleikhoff sees the catatonic syndrome in various diseases as quite different from endogeneous catatonia. Katatoniforme Syndrome bei körperlich begründbaren Psychosen sind zu unterscheiden von der endogenen Katatonie. Pauleikhoff B. Die Katatonie (1868–1968), *Fortschritte der Neurologie und Psychiatrie.* 1969;37:461–496.

11. Fink M, Taylor MA. *Catatonia: A Clinicians's Guide to Diagnosis and Treatment.* New York: Cambridge University Press; 2003; *Melancholia: The Diagnosis, Pathophysiology, and Treatment of Depressive Illness.* New York: Cambridge University Press; 2006.

12. Michael Alan Taylor to Edward Shorter, personal communication, May 23, 2013.

13. Skae D. The Morisonian Lectures on insanity for 1873, Lecture II. *J Ment Sci.* 1874;19:491–507, 498.

14. Kahlbaum's work was not translated into English until its centenary in 1973.

15. Claretie J. *La Vie à Paris.* Paris: Havard; 1881: 28, 134. Claretie was doubtless much under the influence of Charcot's student, Paul Richer, who published in 1881 his massive *Études Cliniques de l'Hystéro-épilepsie ou Grande Hystérie.* Paris: Delahaye; 1881; see 367–368 on the *état cataleptique,* part of the stages of *la grande hystérie.* (In retrospect, proceedings at the Salpêtrière under the influence of Charcot's doctrine of hysteria were a grand exercise in medical suggestion. and medical credulousness). The tuning fork story; the striking of which threw everyone into catalepsy, is at p. 373.

16. McKinney WT Jr. Interview, in Thomas Ban, ed., *An Oral History of Neuropsychopharmacology.* Brentwood, TN: ACNP; 2011: VII, 359.

17. Shorter E. *What Psychiatry Left Out of the DSM-5.* New York: Routledge; 2015.

Chapter 2

1. Tissot S-A. *Traité des Nerfs et de Leurs Maladies: De la Catalepsie, de l'Extase.* Lausanne: Grasset; 1789, 18–19.

2. Bülbül F et al. Persistent catatonia for 1.5 years finally resolved with electroconvulsive therapy. *JECT.* 2013;29:e1.

3. On the history of catalepsy in classical times, see Puel T. *De la Catalepsie.* Paris: Baillière; 1856, 7–16.

4. Puel, *De la Catalepsie* (1856), 29–32; males, 68; females, 80. Gender not given in 2.

5. This story, which originally appeared in the *Annales de la Ville de Toulouse* (1687), was reprinted by the Parisian surgeon Pierre Dionis, *De la Catalepsie: Maladie Rare et Extraordinaire* (1718); this appeared as an separately paginated appendix to Dionis P. *Dissertation sur la Mort Subite et sur la Catalepsie.* Paris: d'Houry; 1718, 112–115.

6. Tissot, *Traité des Nerfs et de Leurs Maladies* (1789), 11–17.

7. Paré A. *Oeuvres,* 8th ed. Paris: Buon; 1628, 975.

8. Medicus FC. *Geschichte periodischer Krankheiten.* Karlsruhe: Macklor; 1764, 16–17.

9. Hirschel LE. *Gedanken von der Starrsucht oder Catalepsis.* Berlin: Mylius; 1769, 5–6.

10. Mezler FX. Beobachtung einer Starrsucht (Catalepsis). *Medicinisch-Chirurgische Zeitung* (Salzburg). 1794;1:139–141.

11. See Shorter E. *From Paralysis to Fatigue: A History of Psychosomatic Illness in the Modern Era.* New York: Free Press; 1992, 136–146.

12. Bourdin C-E. *Traité de la Catalepsie.* Paris: De Just; 1841, vii.

13. Pinel P. *Nosographie Philosophique*, vol. III (first published 1803); 4th ed. Paris: Brosson; 1810, III, 65–68. For an overview of the nosological place of ecstasy, see the discussion in *AMP*, 3rd ser, 1 (1855), at 528–550.

14. A Constant Observer [John Haslam?], *Sketches in Bedlam, or Characteristic Traits of Insanity.* London: Sherwood; 1823, 155–157.

15. Monro H. On the nomenclature of the various forms of insanity. *Asylum Journal of Mental Science.* 1856;2:286–305, 302–303. This shortly became the *Journal of Mental Science*, which in turn became the *British Journal of Psychiatry.*

16. Case of John B, Wellcome Medical Records Archive, Holloway House collection, ms 5162, p. 180.

17. Quoted in Birnbaum K. *Psychopathologische Dokumente.* Berlin: Springer; 1920, 271.

18. De Lorde A. *La Dormeuse.* Paris: Librairie Théatr'ale; 1901.

19. Guislain J. *Traité sur les Phrénopathies.* Brussels: Etabl Encyclograph; 1833, 34, 258, 260.

20. Straus EW, Griffith RM. Pseudoreversibility of catatonic stupor. *AJP.* 1955;111:680–685, 682.

21. Puel, *Catalepsie* (1856), 108–109.

22. Michael Trimble to Max Fink (July 1, 2017), authors quote from the English translation of Johann Wolfgang von Goethe's *Faust, Part I*, trans. A. S. Kline (2003), Act I, scene 3, lines 1224–1237.

23. Oxford psychiatrist Ivor Jones later challenged this distinction as being without a difference; Jones I. Observations on schizophrenic stereotypies. *Comprehens Psychiatry.* 1965;6:323–335.

24. Bucknill JC, Tuke DH. *A Manual of Psychological Medicine.* Philadelphia: Blanchard; 1858, 304; this part of the volume was written by Bucknill.

25. Falret J-P. *Des Maladies Mentales.* Paris: Baillière; 1864, XL.

26. We quote from the later, revised version of Ésquirol's *démence* essay published in 1838), the original appeared in 1814. Esquirol, De la Démence, in Esquirol, ed., *Des Maladies Mentales.* Paris: Baillière; 1838, II: 222–223.

27. Kraepelin E. *Psychiatrie*, 8th ed. Leipzig: Barth; 1915, IV: 1836.

28. Rosenthal M. Ueber Katalepsie (Starrsucht), *Allgemeine Wiener Medizinische Zeitung.* April 13, 1869;14:113–114; two installments followed.

29. Hufeland CW. *Enchiridion Medicum* (1836), 6th ed. Berlin: Jonas; 1842, 168–169.

30. Skae D. The Morisonian Lectures on insanity for 1873, Lecture IV, *J Ment Sci.* 1874;20:200–211, 204–205.

31. Reil JC. *Rhapsodien über die Anwendung der psychischen Curmethode auf Geisteszerrüttungen* (1803, reprint, Amsterdam: Bonset; 1968, 127.

32. Friedreich JB. *Skizze einer allgemeinen Diagnostik der psychischen Krankheiten.* Würzburg: Strecker; 1829, 75.

33. Guislain J., *Leçons Orales sur les Phrénopathies.* Ghent: Hebbelynck; 1852, 273.

34. Guislain, *Leçons Orales sur les Phrénopathies* (1852), 270.

35. Guislain, *Leçons Orales sur les Phrénopathies* (1852), 273; see also his *Phrénopathies* (1833), 240–241, where he describes automatisme in slightly different terms.

36. Dagonet H. *Traité Élémentaire et Pratique des Maladies Mentales.* Paris: Baillière; 1862, 368.

37. Mazars de Cazelles F. Sur une Catalepsie Occasionnée par la Terreur, *Journal de Médecine, Chirurgie, Pharmacie.* Jan. 1762;15:131–143, 135.

38. It is not true, as some have claimed, that the term *stupidité* was introduced by the classifier François Boissier de Sauvages in his *Nosologia Methodica Sistens Morborum.* Amsterdam: De

Tournes; 1763, 377; he assigned it to what he called in a later edition of 1771 maladies imaginaires. Boissier, *Oeuvres Diverses*. Paris: Costard; 1771, I, 330. In 1763, the term was already in wide use. Vogel RA. *Definitiones Generum Morborum*. Göttingen: Schulz; 1764, 20.

39. Chiarugi V. *Della Pazzia in Genere, E in Specie*. Florence: Carlieri; 1794, vol. 3, 108; see also pp. 149, 183.

40. As stated, we quote from the later, revised version of Ésquirol's *démence* essay, published in 1838), the original appeared in 1814; this particular patient was admitted to Charenton in 1836. See Esquirol, De la Démence, in Esquirol, ed., *Des Maladies Mentales*. Paris: Baillière; 1838, II, 225–228.

41. Georget E-J. *De la Folie*. Paris: Crevot; 1820, 115–117.

42. Étoc-Demazy G-F. *De la Stupidité chez les Aliénés*. Paris: Medical Dissertation; 1833, 22–23.

43. See Shorter E. *What Psychiatry Left Out of the DSM-5: Historical Mental Disorders Today*. New York: Routledge; 2015, 68–75.

44. Baillarger J. De l'État Mental Désigné chez les Aliénés Sous le Nom de Stupidité, *AMP*. 1843;1:76–103, 79.

45. Delasiauve L. Du Diagnostic Différentiel de la Lypémanie, *AMP*. 1851;3:380–442. The entire *stupidité* literature is reviewed by Chaslin P. *La Confusion Mentale Primitive*. Paris: Asselin; 1895, 10–54.

46. Victor Sauze describes a brief case in the Répertoire d'observations inédites, *AMP*. 1853;2(5):344–345.

47. Earle P. *A Visit to Thirteen Asylums for the Insane in Europe*. Philadelphia: Dobson; 1841, 132.

48. Crichton-Browne J. Acute dementia. *West Riding Lunatic Asylum Medical Reports*. 1874;4:265–290, 265–274.

49. Hoffmann F. Ueber die Eintheilung der Geisteskrankheiten in Siegburg. *AZP*. 1862;19:367–391, 388.

50. Kraepelin E. *Compendium der Psychiatrie*. Leipzig: Abel; 1883; this is the first edition of Kraepelin's textbook.

51. Crichton-Browne, *Acute Dementia*. 1874, 265–290, 265–274.

52. Inevitably, a concept as deeply entrenched as *stupidité* would not extinguish entirely, and Henri Baruk discusses it in his *Traité de Psychiatrie*. Paris: Masson; 1959, I, 73–74.

53. Guislain, *Phrénopathies* (1833), 226–227.

54. Kraepelin E. *Psychiatrie: ein Lehrbuch für Studierende und Aerzte*, 8th ed. Leipzig: Barth; 1913, III (2), 950.

55. Guislain, *Phrénopathies* (1852), 260–261.

56. Rosebush PI et al. Catatonia and its treatment, *Schizophrenia Bull*. 2010;36:239–242.

57. Perfect W. *Select Cases in the Different Species of Insanity*. Rochester: Gillman; 1787, 251–255.

58. Morel B-A. *Études Cliniques: Traité Théorique et Pratique des Maladies Mentales*. Paris: Masson; 1853, II, 292.

59. Kelp FAL. Melancholia Cataleptica (II). *Correspondenz-Blatt der deutschen Gesellschaft für Psychiatrie und gerichtliche Psychologie*. 1864;11:321–323.

60. The original source was Mende, *Zeitschrift für die Staatsarzneikunde*, 1821, quoted in Griesinger W. *Die Pathologie und Therapie der psychischen Krankheiten*, 2nd ed. Stuttgart: Krabbe; 1861, 262–263.

61. Esquirol, De la Manie (1818), in *Des Maladies Mentales* (1838), II, 146.

62. Calmeil L. Manie, in *Dictionnaire de Médecine ou Répertoire Général des Sciences Médicales*, 2nd ed., vol. 19. Paris: Béchet; 1839, 117–141, 133.

63. Whyte R. *Observations on the Nature, Causes, and Cure of those Disorders Which Have Been Commonly Called Nervous, Hypochondriac, or Hysteric*, 2nd ed. Edinburgh: Becket; 1765, 235–237.

64. Morel B-A. *Études Cliniques: Traité Théorique et Pratique des Maladies Mentales*. Paris: Masson; 1853, II, 281.

65. Delasiauve L-J-F. *Traité de l'Épilepsie*. Paris: Masson; 1854, 263.

66. Delasiauve, *Du Diagnostic Différentiel de la Lypémanie* (1851), 380–442, 427.

67. See Taylor MA, Fink M. *Melancholia: The Diagnosis, Pathophysiology, and Treatment of Depressive Illness*. New York: Cambridge University Press; 2006, 30–32, 181–183.

68. Auenbrugger L. *Von der Stillen Wuth oder dem Triebe zum Selbstmorde*. Dessau: Verlagskasse; 1783, 52–55.

69. Morel B-A. *Études Cliniques: Traité Théorique et Pratique des Maladies Mentales*. Paris: Masson; 1852, I, 432–433.

70. Griesinger, *Die Pathologie und Therapie der psychischen Krankheiten* (1861), 251–252.

71. Maudsley H. *The Physiology and Pathology of the Mind*. New York: Appleton; 1867, 336–337.

72. Schüle H. *Klinische Psychiatrie*, 3rd ed. Leipzig: Vogel; 1886, 214.

73. In present day therapeutics, both catatonia and melancholia are syndromes that are remarkably sensitive to induced seizures (electroshock); patients are relieved within a few seizures of the morbid signs of both syndromes.

74. Calmet AA. *Dissertations sur les Apparitions des Anges, des Démons et des Esprits*. Paris: De Bure; 1746, 268–269, 451.

75. Reynell R. The case of a cataleptic woman. In Martyn J, ed., *Philosophical Transactions, 1732–1744*, vol. 9. London: Innys; 1747, 216–218.

76. Spedding J et al. eds., *The Works of Francis Bacon*, vol. X. Boston: Taggard; 1864, 151.

77. Linas J-A. Catalepsie. In A Dechambre, ed., *Dictionnaire Encyclopédique des Sciences Médicales*, ser 1. Paris: Asselin; 1874, XIII, 59–90, 82.

78. Maubray J. *The Female Physician, Containing all the Diseases Incident to That Sex*. London: Holland; 1724, 405–406.

79. See, on this aspect of premodern medicine, Shorter E. *Doctors and Their Patients: A Social History*. New Brunswick; NJ: Transaction Publishers; 1991, 26–54.

80. Pfendler GF. *Quelques Observations pour Servir à l'Histoire de la Léthargie*. Paris: Medical Thesis; 1833, 11–12; Pfendler, a professor of chemistry in Vienna, gained a Paris degree in medicine. Yet, in Vienna, he clearly was involved in the practice of medicine.

81. Pfendler, *Quelques Observations pour Servir à l'Histoire de la Léthargie* (1833), 13.

82. Dezeimeris JE. *Dictionnaire Historique de la Médecine*, vol. 4. Paris: Béchet; 1839, 264–265; Pfendler, *Quelques Observations pour Servir à l'Histoire de la Léthargie* (1833), 14.

83. Calmeil L. Catalepsie. In *Dictionnaire de Médecine ou Répertoire Général des Sciences Médicales*, 2nd ed., vol. 6. Paris: Béchet; 1834, 479–489, 483.

84. Janet P, Raymond F. *Les Obsessions et la Psychasthénie*. Paris: Alcan; 1903 II, 138.

85. Conolly J. Hysteria. In J Forbes et al. *Cyclopaedia of Practical Medicine*. London: Sherwood; 1833, II, 560.

86. Macculloch JA. *The Childhood of Fiction: A Study of Folk Tales and Primitive Thought*. Ann Arbor: Gryphon; 1971, 86–87.

87. See Critchley M. Periodic hypersomnia and megaphagia in adolescent males. *Brain.* 1962;85:627–657.

88. Regnard P. *Sorcellerie, Magnétisme, Morphinisme.* Paris: Plon; 1887, 213–214.

Chapter 3

1. Hirshfeld A. *The Electric Life of Michael Faraday.* New York: Walker & Co.; 2006.

2. Kahlbaum, perhaps the second-most important psychiatrist in Germany after Kraepelin, has not fared well at the hands of his biographers. Under H.-P. Lauschke's pen, for example, Allenberg becomes Allenstein. In Memoriam C-L Kahlbaum. *Psychiatr Neurol Med Psychol.* 1979;31:217–233. No rigorous archive-based biography of Kahlbaum exists.

3. Arndt E. Ueber die Geschichte der Katatonie. *Centralblatt für Nervenheilkunde und Psychiatrie.* 1902;25:81–121, 93.

4. Kahlbaum K. *Die Gruppirung der psychischen Krankheiten und die Eintheilung der Seelenstörungen.* Danzig: Kafemann; 1863. *Gruppirung,* as the old German spelling, is correct.

5. Kahlbaum gives a clear overview of his system in *Die Gruppirung der psychischen,* 133–135.

6. Munsche H et al. Eighteenth century classification of mental illness: Linnaeus, de Sauvages, Vogel, and Cullen. *Cogn Behav Neurol.* 2012;25:224–239, 227.

7. Guislain J. *Traité des Phrenopathies.* Brussels: Etabl. Encyclograph; 1833, 184, 216–217.

8. See, on this Shorter E. *What Psychiatry Left Out of the DSM-5: Historical Mental Disorders Today.* New York: Routledge; 2015, 147–153.

9. Bericht über die Psychiatrische Section der Versammlung deutscher Naturforscher und Aerzte und die Sitzung des deutschen Vereins der Irrenärzte in Innsbruck im September 1869. *Archiv für Psychiatrie und Nervenkrankheiten.* 1869;2:502.

10. Dr Kahlbaum, Klinische Mitteilung. *AZP.* 1869;26:719.

11. Note on 13. ordentliche Versammlung des psychiatrischen Vereines zu Berlin am 15. März 1872, *AZP.* 1873;29:455.

12. Arndt R. Ueber Tetanie und Psychose. In Bericht über die psychiatrische Section der Naturforscherversammlung zu Leipzig im August 1872. *AZP.* 1874;30:53–62, Hecker's comment in discussion, p. 60.

13. Wilmanns K. Ewald Hecker. In Theodor Kirchhoff, ed., *Deutsche Irrenärzte,* vol. II. Berlin: Springer; 1924, 208.

14. See the respective monographs in Kirchhoff, *Deutsche Irrenärzte,* vol. II.

15. Kahlbaum K. Ueber Heboïdophrenie. *AZP.* 1890;48:461–474, 462.

16. Hecker E. Karl Ludwig Kahlbaum. *Psychiatrische Wochenschrift.* July 11899;1:125–128, 128; for Hecker's second use of Katatonie in 1871, see his Zur Begründung des klinischen Standpunktes in der Psychiatrie. *Archiv für pathologische Anatomie und Physiologie und für klinische Medicin.* 1871;52:203–218, 217.

17. Hecker E. Die Hebephrenie. *Archiv für pathologische Anatomie und Physiologie und für klinische Medicin.* 1871;52:394–429, 395–396, 405, 420.

18. Hecker, Die Hebephrenie (1871), 412–413.

19. Ilberg G. Das Jugendirresein. *(Volkmann) Sammlung Klinischer Vorträge, NF, Innere Medicin,* No. 67. Leipzig: Breitkopf; 1898, 1287–1308, 1297.

20. Z [Theodor Ziehen]. Necrolog: Karl Ludwig Kahlbaum. *Monatsschrift für Psychiatrie und Neurologie.* 1899;5:479–480.

21. Schüle H. Ueber das Delirium acutum. *AZP.* 1867;42:316–351.

22. See Arndt E. Ueber die Geschichte der Katatonie (1902), 90–91, on how motor symptoms were a concept in discussion in the 1860s and '70s.

23. Kahlbaum K. *Die Katatonie, oder das Spannungsirresein: eine klinische Form psychischer Krankheit.* Berlin: Hirschwald; 1874, vi, xii–xiii.

24. Kahlbaum, *Die Katatonie* (1874), vi. Karl Kleist emphasized Kahlbaum's originality in making this contrast: Die gegenwärtigen Strömungen in der Psychiatrie. *AZP.* 1925;82:1–41, 2.

25. Kahlbaum, *Die Katatonie* (1874), 4.

26. Kahlbaum, *Die Katatonie* (1874), 6.

27. Kahlbaum, *Die Katatonie* (1874), 23.

28. Kahlbaum, *Die Katatonie* (1874), 6–10

29. Rogers DM. *Motor Disorder in Psychiatry.* Chichester: Wiley; 1992, 28.

30. Kahlbaum K. Die klinisch-diagnostischen Gesichtspunkte der Psychopathologie. *(Volkmann) Sammlung klinischer Vorträge.* 1878;126:1127–1146, 1141.

31. Kahlbaum, *Die Katatonie* (1874), 25, 93.

32. Warnock J. A case of catalepsy, with prolonged silence, alternating with verbigeration. *J Ment Sci.* 1895;41:82–86.

33. Kraepelin E. *Psychiatrie: Ein kurzes Lehrbuch für Studirende und Aerzte,* 4th ed. Leipzig: Abel; 1893, 149.

34. Kahlbaum, *Die Katatonie* (1874), 30–31.

35. Kahlbaum, *Die Katatonie* (1874), 31.

36. Kandinsky V. *Kritische und klinische Betrachtungen im Gebiete der Sinnestäuschungen.* Berlin: Friedländer; 1885, 18.

37. Norman HJ. *Mental Disorders.* Edinburgh: Livingstone; 1928, 86.

38. Kraepelin E. *Compendium der Psychiatrie.* Leipzig: Abel; 1883, 211.

39. See, for example, Weygandt W. Idiotie und Dementia praecox. *Zeitschrift für die Erforschung und Bearbeitung des jugendlichen Schwachsinns.* 1907;1:311–332, 314.

40. Kraepelin E. *Psychiatrie: Ein Lehrbuch für Studirende und Aerzte,* 5th ed. 1896, 196.

41. Kleist K. Gegenhalten (motorischer Negativismus), Zwangsgreifen und Thalamus opticus. *Monatsschrift für Psychiatrie und Neurologie.* 1927;65:317–396.

42. Kahlbaum, *Die Katatonie* (1874), 36–53.

43. Calmeil L. Aliénés. In *Dictionnaire de Médecine ou Répertoire Générale des Sciences Médicales,* 2nd ed., vol. 2. Paris: Béchet; 1833, 151–203, 196.

44. Schüle H. Klinische Beiträge zur Katatonie. *AZP.* 1901;58:221–242, 222,

45. Brosius CM. Die Katatonie. *AZP.* 1877;35:770–802, 775–776.

46. Jensen J. Katatonie. In JG Ersch et al. eds., *Allgemeine Encyclopädie der Wissenschaft und Künste,* vol. 34 (2). Leipzig: Brockhaus; 1883, 259–274, 261. The essay was written in 1881.

47. Neisser C. Discussion. *AZP.* 1908;65:473.

48. Neisser C. *Ueber die Katatonie: ein Beitrag zur klinischen Psychiatrie.* Stuttgart: Enke; 1887, 4.

49. As early as 1886, Heinrich Schüle describes echolalia in catatonia; see *Klinische Psychiatrie,* 3rd ed. Leipzig: Vogel; 1886, 209.

50. Ilberg G. Das Jugendirresein. *Volkmann Sammlung Klinischer Vorträge, NF, Innere Medicin,* no. 67. Leipzig: Breitkopf; 1898, 1287–1308, 1299

51. Ilberg, Das Jugendirresein (1898), 1303–1305.

52. Sommer R. *Lehrbuch der psychopathologischen Untersuchungs-Methoden.* Berlin: Urban; 1899, 93.

53. Westphal C. Ueber die Verrücktheit. *AZP.* 1878;34:252–257, 256. Westphal did, however, believe that Kahlbaum's differentiation between mania and catatonic agitation was important. See also, later that year, Westphal C. Kahlbaum's Katatonie. *AZP.* 1878;34:753–756. By 1907, however, Westphal had evidently changed his mind, treating catatonia as independent (at least of dementia praecox) and finding pupillary irregularities in catatonic stupor. Westphal. Über bisher nicht beschriebene Pupillenerscheinungen im katatonischen Stupor. *AZP.* 1907;64:694–701.

54. Schüle H. *Handbuch der Geisteskrankheiten.* Leipzig: Vogel; 1878, 512–513.

55. Schüle H. 1878, 524; *Die Dysphrenia Neuralgica.* Karlsruhe: Müller; 1867.

56. Schüle, 524. Schüle later maintains that catatonia is not a separate disease but assents to Kahlbaum's stage theory. Schüle. Zur Katatonie-Frage. *AZP.* 1898;54:515–552, 516.

57. Mendel EE. *Die Manie.* Berlin: Urban; 1881.

58. Discussion, *AZP,* 37 (1881), 570.

59. Wernicke C. *Grundriss der Psychiatrie.* Leipzig: Thieme; 1900, 428–429.

60. Wernicke C. *Krankenvorstellungen aus der psychiatrischen Klinik in Breslau.* Breslau: Schletter; 1899, 45–48.

61. Burgmair W et al. eds., *Emil Kraepelin, vol. IV: Kraepelin in Dorpat, 1886–1891.* Munich: Belleville; 2003, 155.

62. Roller CF. Motorische Störungen beim einfachen Irresein. *AZP.* 1886;42:1–60; Roller said that some of his patients were cataleptic (27–30).

63. Freusberg A. Ueber motorische Symptome bei einfachen Psychosen. *Archiv für Psychiatrie und Nervenkrankheiten.* 1886;17:757–794, 786–787.

64. At this meeting, Heinrich Schüle's paper on catatonia was read in his absence and only the discussion was printed; Session of November 7, 1897. *AZP.* 1898;55:60–67.

65. Session of November 7, 1897, 62–67; the meeting of the Südwestdeutscher psychiatrischer Verein took place in November 1897.

66. Session of November 7, 1897, 62–67.

67. Mairet A. Folie de la puberté, II. *AMP.* 1889;47:34–47, 40.

68. Séglas J, Chaslin P. La catatonie. *Archives de Neurologie.* 1888;15:254–266, 420–433; 188;16:52–65; the article was translated into English as T. [*sic*] Séglas and Ph. Chaslin, Katatonia. *Brain.* 1889;12:191–232, 212–213.

69. Raymond F, Janet P. Les Obsessions. Paris: Alcan; 1903, II: case no. 13, 26–27; case no. 224, 492–495, case no. 229, 503–504.

70. Dide M, Guiraud P. *Psychiatrie du Médecin Praticien.* Paris: Masson; 1922, 42–45.

71. Clouston TS. *Clinical Lectures on Mental Diseases.* London: Churchill; 1883, 233.

72. Wellcome Medical Records Archive, Holloway House Collection, no. 432.

73. Wellcome Medical Records Archive, Holloway House Collection, no. 460.

74. Wellcome Medical Records Archive, Holloway House Collection, no. 454.

75. Goodall G. Observations upon "katatonia." *J Ment Sci.* 1892;38:227–233, 228.

76. Kiernan JG. Katatonia, a clinical form of insanity. *Am J Insanity.* 1877;34:59–91, 71, 86.

77. Hammond WA. *A Treatise on Insanity.* New York: Appleton; 1883, 579–584.

78. Peterson F, Langdon CH. Katatonia. *Proc Am Medico-Psychol Assoc.* 1897: 278–299, 297–298.

79. Meyer A. Discussion. In ST Orton, "Some neurologic concepts applied to catatonia." *Arch Neurol Psychiatry.* 1930;23:114–129, 127; the talk was given in May 1929.

80. For this story, see Fields A. *Katharine Dexter McCormick: Pioneer for Women's Rights.* Westport: Praeger; 2003.

Chapter 4

1. Schneider K., Kraepelin und die gegenwärtige Psychiatrie/ *Fortschritte der Neurologie und Psychiatrie.* 1956;24:1–7, 1.

2. This analysis borrows from Schröder P. Ueber katatone Symptome. *Zeitschrift für die gesamte Neurologie und Psychiatrie.* 1922;29:75–76.

3. Edward Hare raised this possibility in Schizophrenia as a recent disease. *BJP.* 1988;153:521–531.

4. Morel B-A. *Études Cliniques: Traité Théorique et Pratique des Maladies Mentales.* Nancy: Grimblot; 1852, I, 361.

5. On evolving concepts of adolescent insanity in the nineteenth century, see Shorter E. *What Psychiatry Left Out of the DSM-5: Historical Mental Disorders Today.* New York: Routledge; 2015, 101–107.

6. Charpentier R. *Les Démences Précoces.* Paris: Leve; 1890.

7. Pick A. Ueber primäre chronische Demenz (sog. Dementia praecox) im jugendlichen Alter. *Prager Medizinische Wochenschrift.* 1891;16:312–315; here Pick also offers a comprehensive overview of the previous literature.

8. Kraepelin E. *Psychiatrie: Ein kurzes Lehrbuch für Studirende und Aerzte,* 4th ed. Leipzig: Abel; 1893, 435–445, 435.

9. Meyer M. Emil Kraepelin, M.D., 1856–1926. In FG Ebaugh, ed., *The Collected Papers of Adolf Meyer.* Baltimore: Johns Hopkins University Press; 1951, III, 526.

10. Burgmair W et al. eds., *Emil Kraepelin vol. I: Persönliches Selbstzeugnisse.* Munich: Belleville; 2000, 77–78.

11. Engstrom EJ. *Clinical Psychiatry in Imperial Germany: A History of Psychiatric Practice.* Ithaca: Cornell University Press; 2003, 124–125.

12. Wirth W. Emil Kraepelin zum Gedächtnis! *Archiv für die gesamte Psychologie.* 1927;58:III.

13. Walser HH ed. *August Forel: Briefe, Correspondance, 1864–1927.* Berne: Huber; 1968, 166–167.

14. Kraepelin E. *Compendium der Psychiatrie zum Gebrauche für Studirende und Aerzte,* 1st ed. Leipzig: Abel; 1883, 222–227.

15. Burgmair W et al. eds., *Emil Kraepelin, Briefe I, 1868–1886.* Munich: Belleville; 2002, 333.

16. Kraepelin, *Psychiatrie,* 1st ed. (1883), 121

17. Kraepelin E. *Psychiatrie: Ein kurzes Lehrbuch für Studirende und Aerzte,* 2nd ed. Leipzig: Abel; 1887, 337–339.

18. Kraepelin E. *Psychiatrie: Ein kurzes Lehrbuch für Studirende und Aerzte,* 3rd ed. Leipzig: Abel; 1889, 332–336.

19. Kraepelin, *Psychiatrie,* 3rd ed. (1889), 335.

20. Behr A. *Die Frage der 'Katatonie' oder des Irreseins mit Spannung.* Dorpat: Medical dissertation; 1891, 56–58.

21. Kraepelin E. Ueber Katalepsie. *AZP.* 1892;48:170–172, 171.

22. Kraepelin E. *Lebenserinnerungen.* Berlin: Springer; 1919/1983, 49.

23. Daraszkiewicz L. *Ueber Hebephrenie, insbesondere deren schwere Form.* Dorpat: Medical dissertation; 1892.

24. Kraepelin, *Lebenserinnerungen* (1919/1983), 70–74.

25. Kraepelin, *Psychiatrie*, 4th ed. (1893), 438, 442.

26. Kraepelin E. Fragestellungen der klinischen Psychiatrie. *Zentralblatt für Nervenheilkunde.* 1905;28:573–590 (also quoted in Pauleikhoff, Die Katatonie (1969), 463.

27. Kraepelin E. Die Abgrenzung der Paranoia. *AZP.* 1894;50:1081–1082.

28. Kraepelin, *Psychiatrie*, 4th ed. (1893), 442.

29. Nissl F. Ueber die Entwicklung der Psychiatrie in den letzten 50 Jahren. *Verhandlungen des naturhistorisch-medizinischen Vereins, NF.* 1908;8:510–524, 521.

30. Kraepelin E. *Psychiatrie: Ein Lehrbuch für Studirende und Aerzte,* 5th ed. Leipzig: Barth; 1896, v. In 1897, in a talk to the German Psychiatric Society, Kraepelin gave an exact description of his research techniques, explaining how each patient received a one-pager (*Zählkarte*), which permitted the patient to be followed and gave an overview for the purposes of sorting patients into categories. Of course, this raised, in a collegial setting, the issue of course as opposed to a momentary clinical snapshot. And from this overview emerged, in particular, the importance of the underlying disease process of dementia (*Verblödungsprocesse*). Kraepelin did not overclaim discoveries of psychopathology at this point and was content to say: The more we can differentiate in the clinical pictures the essential phenomena from the incidental, the more we come closer to the goal of constructing etiologically similar groups. Kraepelin E. Ziele und Wege der klinischen Psychiatrie. *AZP.* 1897;53:840–848, 843, 847.

31. Kraepelin E. Ueber Remissionen bei Katatonie. *AZP.* 1896;52:1126–1127. The meeting, as noted, occurred in 1895.

32. Kraepelin, *Psychiatrie*, 5th ed. (1896), 458.

33. Kraepelin, *Psychiatrie*, 5th ed. (1896), 429, 436, 439.

34. Kraepelin E. Zur Diagnose und Prognose der Dementia praecox. *AZP.* 1899;56:254–263, 258–259.

35. Neisser C. Discussion. *AZP.* 1908;65:474.

36. Aschaffenburg G. Die Katatoniefrage. *AZP.* 1898;54:1004–1026, 1017.

37. Kraepelin, Zur Diagnose und Prognose (1899), 254–263, 257.

38. Kraepelin E. *Psychiatrie: Ein Lehrbuch für Studirende und Aerzte,* 6th ed. Leipzig: Barth; 1899, II, 149, 159–160, 163–164, 175, 182–183.

39. See Engstrom's informative discussion, *Psychiatry in Imperial Germany* (2003), 135–145.

40. Kraepelin E. *Psychiatrie: Ein Lehrbuch für Studierende und Aerzte,* 7th ed. Leipzig: Barth; 1904, II, 224. Note that in this edition the spelling of Studierende became modernized.

41. Kraepelin E. *Psychiatrie: Ein Lehrbuch für Studierende und Aerzte,* 8th ed. Leipzig: Barth; 5 vols. 1909–1915; III (2) (1913), 687. Kraepelin distinguished *Zerfahrenheit* from oral *Entgleisungen* (derailments), III, 738.

42. Kraepelin, *Psychiatrie*, 7th ed. (1902), I, 279, 301. Note that volume I appeared in 1903, volume II in 1904.

43. Kraepelin, *Psychiatrie* 8th ed. (1909–1915), vol. I, 528; see fig. 22 on 527.

44. Hoch P. Discussion. In J Zubin, ed., *Field Studies in Mental Disorders.* New York: Grune & Stratton; 1961, 119; the conference was in February 1959.

45. Stransky E. *Ms Autobiography,* p. 272, archived in Institut für Geschichte der Medizin in Vienna, HS 2.065.

46. Henderson DK. *The Evolution of Psychiatry in Scotland.* Edinburgh: Livingstone; 1964, 173.

47. Kraepelin, *Psychiatrie*, 8th ed. (1913), vol. III, 944.

48. Kraepelin, *Psychiatrie*, 8th ed. (1913), 809.

49. Kraepelin, *Psychiatrie*, 8th ed. (1913), 810.
50. Kraepelin, *Psychiatrie*, 8th ed. (1913), 810
51. Kraepelin, *Psychiatrie*, 8th ed. (1913), 819–820, 825. On dilated pupils in catatonia and their restoration to normal following ECT, see Arias LM et al. Catatonic pupil in the setting of electroconvulsive therapy. *J ECT*. December 7 2016(Epub ahead of print).
52. Kraepelin, *Psychiatrie*, 8th ed., vol. I (1909), 366.
53. Kraepelin E. Die Erscheinungsformen des Irreseins. *Zeitschrift für die gesamte Neurologie und Psychiatrie*. 1920;62:1–29, 28.
54. Kraepelin, *Psychiatrie*, 8th ed., vol. II (1910), 537–538.
55. Kraepelin, *Psychiatrie*, 8th ed., vol. III (1913), 1292–1293.

Chapter 5

1. Bumke O. Die Auflösung der Dementia Praecox. *Klinische Wochenschrift*. March 11, 1924:437–440, 438.
2. Gay P. *Freud: A Life for Our Time*. New York: Norton; 1988, 200.
3. Bleuler E. Die Kritiken der Schizophrenien. *Zeitschrift für die gesamte Neurologie und Psychiatrie*. 1914;22:19–44, 32.
4. Müller A. *Periodische Katatonien*. Zurich: Medical dissertation; 1900.
5. Vereinsberichte. *Correspondenzblatt Schweizer Aerzte*. 1900;30:541.
6. Bleuler E. Dementia praecox. *J Ment Pathol*. 1902;3:113–120.
7. Bleuler E. Die Kritiken der Schizophrenien. *Zeitschrift für die gesamte Neurologie und Psychiatrie*. 1914;22:19–44; Schizophrenia and dementia praecox differ only in inclusiveness [*Grenzbereinigungen*] without principal significance (p. 19).
8. Bleuler E. Die Prognose der Dementia praecox (Schizophreniegruppe). *AZP*. 1908;65: 436–464, 436.
9. Bleuler E, Jung CG. Komplexe und Krankheitsursachen bei Dementia praecox. 1908; *Zentralblatt für Nervenheilkunde und Psychiatrie* 19:220–227, 222.
10. Clemens Neisser clearly affirms Kraepelin's opposition to primary–secondary in Discussion. *AZP*. 1908;65: 475.
11. Lehmann HE. Schizophrenia: Introduction and History. In AM Freedman et al. eds., *Comprehensive Textbook of Psychiatry*, 2nd ed. Baltimore: Williams & Wilkins; 1975, vol. I, 851–860, 853.
12. Bleuler E. Die Prognose der Dementia praecox (Schizophreniegruppe). *AZP* 1908;65, 436–464; longer quotes from pp. 445, 447, 450, 453, 454, 464.
13. Bleuler, Die Prognose (1908), 453.
14. Bleuler E. Freudsche Mechanismen in der Symptomatologie von Psychosen. *Psychiatrisch-Neurologische Wochenschrift*. 1906;34:316–318.
15. Wilmanns K. Die Schizophrenie. *Zeitschrift für die gesamte Neurologie und Psychiatrie*. 1922;78:325–372, 330.
16. Wernicke C. *Grundriss der Psychiatrie in klinischen Vorlesungen*. Leipzig: Thieme; 1900, 113.
17. Bleuler, Discussion, *AZP* (1908), 480.
18. See Shorter E. *From Paralysis to Fatigue: A History of Psychosomatic Illness in the Modern Era*. New York: Free Press; 1992, 159–165.
19. Maatz A, Hoff P. The birth of schizophrenia or a very modern Bleuler: a close reading of Eugen Bleuler's 'Die Prognose der Dementia praecox' and a re-consideration of his contribution to psychiatry. *History of Psychiatry*. 2014;25:431–440, 437.

20. Neisser C. Discussion of Bleuler 'Schizophrenia' paper. *AZP*. 1908;65:476. Karl Heilbronner in Utrecht seconded this opinion.

21. Bleuler E. Zur Theorie des schizophrenen Negativismus. *Psychiatrisch-Neurologische Wochenschrift*. July 30, 1910;12:171–176, 184–187, 189–191, 195–198. See esp. 185.

22. Bleuler, Zur Theorie des schizophrenen Negativismus (1910), 191–192, 196.

23. See Hamilton M, ed. *Fish's Clinical Psychopathology*, 2nd ed. Bristol: Wright; 1974, 98–99.

24. Weygandt W. *Atlas und Grundriss der Psychiatrie*. Munich: Lehmann; 1902, 376, 379.

25. Aschaffenburg G. *Handbuch der Psychiatrie, Allgemeiner Teil*, published in 11 vols. (1912–1927), Spezieller Teil in 18 vols. (1911–1927).

26. Stransky, *Autobiographie*, 288, 333–335 in Vienna, Institut für Geschichte der Medizin, HS 2.065; Zur Kenntnis gewisser erworbener Blödsinnsformen. *Jahrbücher für Psychiatrie und Neurologie*. 1903;24:1–149; Stransky E. *Ueber Sprachverwirrtheit*. Halle: Marhold; 1905; Stransky E. Bemerkungen zur Prognose der Dementia praecox und über die intrapsychische Ataxie. *Neurologisches Centralblatt*. 1909;28:1297–1299. Bleuler acknowledged earlier that he had somehow neglected to cite Stransky's seminal 1905 work on confused speech (*Sprachverwirrtheit*), which laid out the concept of intrapsychic ataxia. See also Bleuler, Die Kritiken der Schizophrenien (1914), 19–44, 42, where he apologizes for overlooking Stransky's work.

27. Bleuler M. Preface. In E Bleuler ed., *Dementia Praecox oder Gruppe der Schizophrenien*. Tübingen: Diskord ed.; 1911/1988, vii.

28. Bleuler, *Schizophrenien* (1911), 278; Kraepelin, *Psychiatrie*, 6th ed. (1899), vol. II, 200. Bleuler said he attached no particular importance to these discrepant figures (p. 278), yet that may have been a political effort to avoid huge disagreements between himself and the older (by one year) Kraepelin.

29. Müller M. *Erinnerungen: Erlebte Psychiatriegeschichte, 1920–1960*. Berlin: Springer; 1982, 32.

30. Bleuler, *Dementia Praecox oder Gruppe der Schizophrenien* (1911/1988), 9.

31. Bleuler, *Schizophrenien* (1911), 5.

32. Bleuler, *Schizophrenien* (1911), 43–44.

33. Bleuler, *Schizophrenien* (1911), 304.

34. Bleuler E. Das autistische Denken. *Jahrbuch für psychoanalytische und psychopathologische Forschungen*. 1912;4(1): 1–39, 18.

35. Hoch P. Discussion. In J Zubin ed., *Field Studies in the Mental Disorders*. New York: Grune & Stratton; 1961, 119.

36. Bleuler, *Schizophrenien* (1911), 228–229.

37. Bleuler, *Schizophrenien* (1911), 149.

38. Kraepelin E. *Psychiatrie*, 7th ed. Leipzig: Barth; 1903, vol. I, 291.

39. Bleuler, *Schizophrenien* (1911), 169, 177.

40. Bleuler, *Schizophrenien* (1911), 191–192.

41. Bleuler E. *Lehrbuch der Psychiatrie*. Berlin: Springer; 1916, 110.

42. Bleuler, *Lehrbuch der Psychiatrie* (1916), 324.

43. Wilmanns K. Die Schizophrenie. *Zeitschrift für die gesamte Neurologie und Psychiatrie*. 1922;78:325–372, 330.

44. Zubin J. Discussion. In J Zubin ed., *Field Studies in the Mental Disorders*. New York: Grune & Stratton; 1961, 202; the conference took place in 1959.

Chapter 6

1. de Sanctis S. Sopra alcune varietà della demenza precoce. *Rivista sperimentale di freniatria.* 1906;32:141–165, 142.

2. Taylor MA, Shorter E, Vaidya N, Fink M The failure of the schizophrenia concept and the argument for its replacement by hebephrenia: applying the medical model for disease recognition. *Acta Psychiatr Scand.* 2010;122:73–183.

3. See the correspondence in Burgmair W et al. eds. *Kraepelin in Heidelberg, 1891–1903.* Munich: Belleville; 2005, vol. 5 of the series of Kraepelin letters edited by Burgmair.

4. Aschaffenburg G. Die Katatoniefrage. *AZP.* 1898;54:1004–1026, 1006, 1013–1014.

5. Ilberg G. Das Jugendirresein. In *[Volkmann] Sammlung klinischer Vorträge, NF, Innere Medicin.* Leipzig: Breitkopf; 1898, 1286–1308, 1290.

6. In Burgmair et al. ed., *Kraepelin in Heidelberg,* vol. 5, 276.

7. Wilmanns K. Zur Differentialdiagnostik der 'funktionellen' Psychosen. *Centralblatt für Nervenheilkunde und Psychiatrie.* 1907;30:569–588.

8. Wilmanns K. Die Schizophrenie. *Zeitschrift für die gesamte Neurologie und Psychiatrie.* 1922;78:325–372, 328.

9. Burgmair W et al. eds., *Emil Kraepelin in München I.* Munich: Belleville; 2006, 296; vol. VI of Emil Kraepelin papers.

10. Wilmanns K. Zur Differentialdiagnostik der 'funktionellen' Psychosen. *Centralblatt für Nervenheilkunde und Psychiatrie.* 1907;30:569–588, 572,

11. Gaupp R. Zur prognostischen Bedeutung der katatonischen Erscheinungen. *Centralblatt für Nervenheilkunde und Psychiatrie.* 1903;26:680–683,

12. Jaspers K. *Allgemeine Psychopathologie.* Berlin: Springer; 1913, 114.

13. Mayer-Gross W. Die Klinik. In K Wilmanns, ed., *Die Schizophrenie.* Berlin: Springer; 1932, 293–605; see 391–418 on *katatone Bilder;* this is vol. 9 (part 5) of O Bumke, ed., *Handbuch der Geisteskrankheiten.*

14. Pappenheim M. Discussion. *AZP.* 1908;65:470–471.

15. Ziehen T. Les psychoses de la puberté. In A Ritti, ed., *Section de Psychiatrie: Comptes Rendus,* XIIIe Congrès International de Médecine, Paris, 1900. Paris: Masson; 1901, 10–29, 28.

16. Ziehen T. *Die Geisteskrankheiten,* 2nd ed. Berlin: Reuther; 1915; 2nd ed., Berlin: Reuther; 1920, 249.

17. There is some evidence that Nijinsky's psychotic illness, whatever its nature, had a catatonic overlay. He shows signs of negativism (*Ne me touchez pas*) and of alternating between muteness and agitation. See Acocella J. ed. *The Diary of Vaslav Nijinsky,* unexpurgated ed. New York: Farrar Straus and Giroux; 1999, xliii, xliv.

18. Binswanger O et al. eds. *Lehrbuch der Psychiatrie.* Jena: Fischer; 1904, 48–50; 6th ed.; 1923. By this sixth edition, Alfred Hoche at Freiburg had grudgingly come to accept the concept of schizophrenia.

19. Richard von Krafft-Ebing R. *Lehrbuch der Psychiatrie,* 1879; 7th ed., 1903; Reprint edition, Saarbrücken: VDM Verlag Dr Müller; 2007, 373–377.

20. See, for example, Reiter PJ. Extrapyramidal motor-disturbances in dementia praecox. *APS.* 1926;1:287–310, 293, 296.

21. On Urstein's life, see Marcinowski F, Urstein M. Forgotten Polish contributor to German psychiatry. *Psychiatr Pol.* 2014;48:195–204; it is surprising that a challenger to the Kraepelinian synthesis of Urstein's importance should have been forgotten.

22. Urstein M. *Die Dementia praecox und Ihre Stellung zum Manisch-Depressiven Irresein.* Berlin: Urban; 1909; Urstein M. *Manisch-depressives und periodisches Irresein als Erscheinungsformen der Katatonie.* Berlin: Urban; 1912.

23. Dreyfus GL. Kritische Bemerkungen zu M. Urstein's Buch: "Die Dementia praecox und ihre Stellung zum manisch-depressiven Irresein." *Centralblatt für Nervenheilkunde und Psychiatrie.* 1910;33:9–19, 16.

24. Urstein, *Katatonie* (1912), 647, 650.

25. Bumke O. Die Auflösung der Dementia praecox. *Klinische Wochenschrift.* March 11, 1924;3:437–440, 440.

26. See his textbook, Bumke O. *Lehrbuch der Geisteskrankheiten* (1917), 2nd ed. Munich: Bergmann; 1924.

27. Lange J. *Katatonische Erscheinungen im Rahmen manischer Erkrankungen.* Berlin: Springer; 1922, 15.

28. Kraepelin E. *Klinische Psychiatrie,* 9th ed., vol. I. Leipzig: Barth; 1927; this is vol. II of Kraepelin and Lange, *Psychiatrie.* A second volume of *Klinische Psychiatrie* never appeared.

29. Lange J. *Allgemeine Psychiatrie,* 9th ed. Leipzig: Barth; 1927, 617.

30. Meduna LJ. *Oneirophrenia: The Confusional State.* Urbana: University of Illinois Press; 1950, 20.

31. Ilberg G. Das Jugendirresein. In [*Volkmann*] *Sammlung klinischer Vorträge, NF, Innere Medicin.* Leipzig: Breitkopf; 1898, 1286–1308, 1302–1303.

32. Séglas J. Démence Précoce et Catatonie. *Nouvelle Iconographie de la Salpêtrière.* 1902;15:330–348, 338.

33. Albrecht P. Zur Symptomatologie der Dementia praecox. *AZP.* 1905;62:659–686, 669.

34. Freyhan F. Discussion. In RL Spitzer, DF Klein, eds., *Critical Issues in Psychiatric Diagnosis.* New York: Raven; 1978, 107.

35. Bostroem A. Katatone Störungen. In O Bumke, ed., *Handbuch der Geisteskrankheiten,* part II (2). Berlin: Springer; 1928, 134–206, 135.

36. Schneider K. Über Wesen und Bedeutung katatonischer Symptome. *Zeitschrift für die gesamte Neurologie und Psychiatrie.* 1914;22:486–505.

37. Schneider K. Kraepelin und die gegenwärtige Psychiatrie. *Fortschritte der Neurologie und Psychiatrie.* 1956;24:1–7, 6.

38. Schneider, *Über Wesen* (1914), 486.

39. Chaslin P. *La Confusion Mentale Primitive.* Paris: Asselin; 1895, 78–79; he does discuss Kraepelin's *la démence précoce* at pp. 126, 176–177.

40. For an overview, see Shorter E. *Historical Dictionary of Psychiatry.* New York: Oxford University Press; 2005, 107–108, 208.

41. Séglas J, Chaslin P. La Catatonie. *Archives de Neurologie.* 1888;15:254–266, 420–433; 16: 52–65, 64; in an English translation of their article, they suggested the insanity of tonicity as a translation for *Spannungsirresein,* a more exact term than tension insanity. Yet, perhaps because of unfamiliarity, it didn't catch on. See Séglas and Chaslin, Katatonia. *Brain.* 1889;12:191–232, 213.

42. Roubinovitch J. *Des Variétés Cliniques de la Folie en France et en Allemagne.* Paris; Doin; 1896, 183.

43. Manheimer M. *Les Troubles Mentaux de l'Enfance.* Paris: Medical dissertation; 1899, 112–113.

44. See Parent AV. Letter from France: the question of dementia praecox in France. *Am J Insanity.* 1905;61:501–519.

45. Charpentier E. *Les Démences Précoces*. Paris: Leve; 1890, 11.

46. Sérieux P. La nouvelle classification des maladies mentales du Professeur Kraepelin. *Revue de Psychiatrie*. 1900;3:103–125.

47. Sérieux P. La Démence précoce. *Revue de Psychiatrie*. 1902;5:241–266, 265.

48. Séglas J. Démence précoce et catatonie. *Nouvelle Iconographie de la Salpêtrière*. 1902;15: 330–348, 344, 346.

49. Leroy R. Disparition trois semaines avant la mort, par tuberculose aiguë, de tout symptome catatonique chez une jeune malade présentée autrefois à la Société. *Bulletin de la Société Clinique de Médecine Mentale*. 1922;10:88–91.

50. For an overview of Henri Baruk's lifetime work on catatonia, see his *Traité de Psychiatrie*. Paris: Masson; 1959, vol. I, 563–683, quotes from pp. 602, 605.

51. Claude H, Baruk H. L'épreuve du somnifène dans la catatonie. *L'Encéphale*. 1928;8: 724–730.

52. de Jong H, Baruk H. *La Catatonie Experimentale par la Bulbocapnine*. Paris: Masson; 1930.

53. Baruk, *Traité* (1959), vol. I, 701, 705.

54. Delay J et al. Le choc amphétaminique. *AMP*. 1947;105:271.

55. Séglas and Chaslin, Katatonia (1889), 191–232.

56. Hack Tuke D. *Dictionary of Psychological Medicine*. London: Churchill; 1892, vol. I, 184–185.

57. Neisser, ibid, I, 724–725.

58. Bruce LC, Peebles AMS. Clinical and experimental observations on katatonia. *J Ment Sci*. 1903;49:614–628.

59. Ion RM, Beer MD. The British reaction to dementia praecox, 1893–1913. *History of Psychiatry*. 2002;13; part I:285–304; part II, 419–431.

60. Henderson DK. Catatonia as a type of mental reaction. *J Ment Sci*. 1916;62:556–572. On Henderson's fame as a psychiatrist, see the entry in Trail RR ed., *Lives of the Fellows of the Royal College of Physicians in London*, vol. IV. London: The College; 1968, 188–190.

61. Norman HJ. *Mental Disorders*. Edinburgh: Livingstone; 1928, 84–85.

62. Mayer-Gross W, Slater E, Roth M. *Clinical Psychiatry*. London: Cassell; 1954, 248–252.

63. Noll R. *American Madness: The Rise and Fall of Dementia Praecox*. Cambridge: Harvard University Press; 2011, 248.

64. Noll, *American Madness* (2011), 286.

65. Bleuler E. *Dementia Praecox or the Group of Schizophrenias*. New York: International Universities Press; 1950.

66. Sprague GP. Primary dementia. *Am J Insanity*. 1901;57:215–219, 217.

67. Kirby GH. The catatonic syndrome and its relations to manic-depressive insanity. *J Nerv Mental Dis*. 1913;40:694–704, 703.

68. Hoch A. *Benign Stupors: A Study of a New Manic-Depressive Reaction Type*. New York: Macmillan; 1921, 234–236.

69. Rachlin HL. A follow-up study of Hoch's benign stupor cases. *AJP*. 1935;92:531–558, 555, 557.

70. Main DC. Catatonic dementia praecox: physiotherapeutics, and results obtained in a series of twenty cases. *AJP*. 1923;79:473–483, 476.

71. See Arieti S. Schizophrenia: the manifest symptomatology. In S Arieti, ed., *American Handbook of Psychiatry*. New York: Basic Books; 1959, vol. I, 455–484.

72. Peters UH. Die deutsche Schizophrenielehre und die psychiatrische Emigration. *Fortschritte der Neurologie und Psychiatrie*. 1988;56:347–360, 348.

73. Boisen AT. Types of dementia praecox: a study in psychiatric classification. *Psychiatry.* 1938;1:233–236.

74. American Medico-Psychological Association and the National Committee for Mental Hygiene. *Statistical Manual for the Use of Institutions for the Insane.* New York: NCMH; 1918, 25.

75. American Psychiatric Association and the National Committee for Mental Hygiene. *Statistical Manual for the Use of Hospitals for Mental Diseases,* 7th ed. New York: NCMH; 1936, 21.

76. Logie HB, ed. *National Conference on Nomenclature of Disease, A Standard Classified Nomenclature of Disease.* New York: Commonwealth Fund; 1933, 88,

77. Peters CP. Concepts of schizophrenia after Kraepelin and Bleuler. In JG Howells, ed., *The Concept of Schizophrenia: Historical Perspectives.* Washington DC: American Psychiatric Press; 1991, 93–107, 98.

78. Straus EW, Griffith RM. Pseudoreversibility of catatonic stupor. *AJP.* 1955;111: 680–685, 683.

79. These are reviewed in Stengel E. *Bulletin of the World Health Organization.* 1959;21: 601–663; the statistics include annexes 1–3.

80. World Health Organization. *Manual of the International Statistical Classification of Diseases, Injuries, and Causes of Death, Sixth Revision, Adopted 1948.* Geneva: WHO; 1948, vol. II, 61, 389.

81. World Health Organization. *Manual of the International Statistical Classification of Diseases, Injuries, and Causes of Death, Seventh Revision Conference, 1955.* Geneva: WHO; 1957, vol. I, 115.

82. World Health Organization. *Manual of the International Statistical Classification of Diseases, Injuries, and Causes of Death, Ninth Revision Conference, 1975.* Geneva: WHO; 1977, vol. I, 183–184,

83. National Center for Health Statistics. *The International Classification of Diseases, 9th Revision, Clinical Modification: ICD 9 CM.* Washington DC: NCHS; 1978, 213–214, 219.

84. World Health Organization. *The ICD-10 Classification of Mental and Behavioural Disorders: Clinical Descriptions and Diagnostic Guidelines.* Geneva: WHO; 1992, 91–92.

85. Ladislas Meduna to ATW Simeons, April 10, 1946, in Meduna Collection, box I, University of Illinois Archives, Champagne-Urbana.

Chapter 7

1. Hirschel LE. *Gedanken von der Starrsucht.* Berlin: Mylius; 1769, 11.

2. For a quintessential expression of these views, see Mayer-Gross W. Klinik, section on Katatone Bilder. In K Wilmanns, ed., *Die Schizophrenie.* Berlin: Springer; 1932, 391–418; this volume appeared in the series O Bumke, ed., *Handbuch der Geisteskrankheiten,* vol. 9 (p. 5).

3. Jaspers K. *Allgemeine Psychopathologie.* Berlin: Springer; 1910, 281.

4. von Economo C. Encephalitis lethargica. *Wiener Klinische Wochenschrift.* May 10, 1917;30:582–585.

5. See Vilensky JA. *Encephalitis Lethargica: During and After the Epidemic.* New York: Oxford University Press; 2011.

6. This subject is quite overdue for a historian, but see Kroker K. Epidemic encephalitis and American neurology. *Bulletin of the History of Medicine.* 2004;78:108–147.

7. Berze J, Gruhle HW. *Psychologie der Schizophrenie.* Berlin: Springer; 1929, 76–77.

8. Roller C. Motorische Störungen beim einfachen Irresein. *AZP.* 1886;42:1–60.

9. Lehmann FF. Zur Pathologie der katatonen Symptome. *AZP.* 1898;55:276–301.

10. See the report of the meeting of Ostdeutscher Irrenärzte in Breslau in November 1892, in *AZP.* 1895;51:206.

11. Pfuhlmann B et al. The different conceptions of catatonia: historical overview and critical discussion. *Eur Arch Psychiatry Clin Neurosci.* 2001;251(suppl 1): S4–S7, S5.

12. Wernicke C. *Grundriss der Psychiatrie.* Leipzig: Thieme; 1900, 113.

13. Kleist K. *Untersuchungen zur Kenntnis der psychomotorischen Bewegungsstörungen bei Geisteskranken.* Leipzig: Klinkhardt; 1908, 144–145.

14. Kleist K. Schreckpsychosen. *AZP.* 1918;74:432–510.

15. Kleist K. Berichte über endogene Verblödungen: Klinischer Teil. *AZP.* 1919;75: 242–245, 243.

16. Kleist K et al. Katatonie und Degenerationspsychosen. *AZP.* 1936;104:124–127, 124.

17. Kleist K. Die Auffassung der Schizophrenien als psychische Systemerkrankung (Heredodegenerationen). *Klinische Wochenschrift.* 1923;2:962–963.

18. Kleist K et al. Die Katatonie auf Grund katamnestischer Untersuchungen, III. Teil. *Zeitschrift für die gesamte Neurologie und Psychiatrie.* 1940;168:535–586. 584.

19. Kleist K. Die Katatonien. *Nervenarzt.* 1943;16:1–10.

20. Kleist K. Gegenhalten (motorischer Negativismus), Zwangsgreifen und Thalamus opticus. *Monatsschrift für Psychiatrie und Neurologie.* 1927;65:317–396.

21. Kleist, Die Katatonien (1943), 1–10, 2.

22. Kleist K. Katatonie und Degenerationspsychosen. *AZP.* 1936;126. By contrast, see the less nuanced account of Kleist's life in the Nazi years in Neumärker K-J et al. Karl Kleist (1879–1960): a pioneer of neuropsychiatry. *History of Psychiatry.* 2003;14:411–458, 443.

23. Weitbrecht HJ. *Psychiatrie im Grundriss.* Berlin: Springer; 1963, 394.

24. Kleist K. Schizophrenic symptoms and cerebral pathology. *BJP.* 1960;106:246–255.

25. Her habilitation, *Die phasischen Psychosen nach ihrem Erscheinungs-und Erbbild,* was accepted by the Frankfurt faculty in 1947, and published as a book of that same title in 1949 by the Barth Verlag in Leipzig. Meanwhile, in 1948, Karl Leonard introduced the unipolar-bipolar distinction in print in connection with manic-depressive insanity. Leonhard K. *Grundlagen der Psychiatrie.* Stuttgart: Klett; 1948, 88. He conceded priority to her. I am grateful to Dr. Siegfried Hoyer for a personal communication of May 12, 2003, about Neele's curriculum vitae.

26. Leonhard K. *Die defektschizophrenen Krankheitsbilder.* Leipzig: Thieme; 1936.

27. See Leonhard K. *Meine Person und meine Aufgaben im Leben.* Hildburghausen: Salier; 1995, 33.

28. Leonhard K. Die den striären Erkrankungen am meisten verwandten zwei Formen katatoner Endzustände und die Frage der Systemerkrankung bei Schizophrenie. *Archiv für Psychiatrie und Nervenkrankheiten.* 1935;103:101–121.

29. See Leonhard, Die defektschizophrenen Krankheitsbilder (1936), 111.

30. Leonhard K. *Aufteilung der endogenen Psychosen.* East-Berlin: Akademie-Verlag; 1957.

31. Leonhard, Aufteilung (1957), 184.

32. Leonhard, Aufteilung (1957), 243–273.

33. Gerald Stöber, a Leonhard follower at the University of Würzburg; in 2001, he held that periodic catatonia is an unequivocally genetically transmitted illness. Genetic predisposition and environmental causes in periodic and systematic catatonia. *Eur Arch Psych Clin Neurosci.* 2001;251(suppl 1):1/21–1/24, 1/21.

34. Leonhard, *Aufteilung* (1957), 276.

35. Urstein M. *Manisch-Depressives und Periodisches Irresein als Erscheinungsformen der Katatonie.* Berlin: Urban; 1912, 602.

36. Schneider, *Fortschritte* (1956), 4. Kurt Schneider, "Kraepelin und die gegenwärtige Psychiatrie," *Fortschritte der Neurologie und Psychiatrie,* 24 (1956), 1–7, 4.

37. Conrad K. Das Problem der 'nosologischen Einheit' in der Psychiatrie. *Nervenarzt.* 1959;30:488–494, 402.

38. Stengel E. Discussion. In Zubin, ed., *Field Studies* (1959/61), 60. Joseph Zubin, ed., *Field Studies in Mental Disorders* (New York: Grune & Stratton, 1961), 60; the conference was in Feb 1959.

39. Baruk H. *Traité de Psychiatrie.* Paris: Masson; 1959, I, 607.

40. Arndt R. Chorea und Psychose. *Archiv für Psychiatrie und Nervenkrankheiten.* 1868;1: 509–544, 530–531.

41. Benedikt M. Vorlesungen über chronische Nervenkrankheiten. *Wiener Medizinische Presse.* April 18, 1869;10:361–365, 364.

42. Kahlbaum K. *Die Katatonie, oder das Spannungsirresein.* Berlin: Hirschwald; 1874,44.

43. Brosius CM. Die Katatonie. 1877; *AZP*:770–802, 774.

44. Kraepelin E. *Psychiatrie,* 5th ed., Leipzig: Barth; 1896, 141, 184.

45. Jung CG. *Ueber die Psychologie der Dementia praecox.* Halle: Marhold; 1907, 1–41.

46. Bleuler E. *Die Schizophrenien* (1911). Tübingen: Diskord; 1988, 363.

47. Klaesi J. *Ueber die Bedeutung und Entstehung der Stereotypien.* Berlin: Karger; 1922, 5.

48. Étoc-Démazy G-F. *De la Stupidité.* Paris: Medical thesis; 1833, 16–17.

49. Baillarger J. De l'état désigné chez les aliénés sous le nom de stupidité. *AMP.* 1843;1:76–103, 81–84.

50. Delasiauve L. Essai de classification des maladies mentales. *Recueil des Travaux de la Société Libre d'Agriculture, Sciences, Arts et Belles-Lettres du Département de L'Eure, année 1843.* 1844;2(4):158–195, 174–175.

51. Delasiauve L. Du diagnostic différentiel de la lypémanie. *AMP.* 1851;3:380–442, 385–386; the reference in Delasiauve's text was to "In exitu," but this can only refer to Psalm 116, as quoted.

52. Dagonet H. *Traité Élémentaire et Pratique des Maladies Mentales.* Paris: Baillière; 1862, 362, 367.

53. Janet P. *L'Automatisme Psychologique.* Paris: Alcan; 1889, 30.

54. Masselon R. *Psychologie des Déments Précoces.* Paris: Medical thesis; 1902, 168.

55. Monod G. *Les Formes Frustes de la Démence Précoce.* Paris: Medical thesis; 1905, 28.

56. Braus O. *Akademische Erinnerungen eines alten Arztes an Berlins klinische Grössen.* Leipzig: Vogel; 1901, 162–163.

57. Georg Northoff, personal communication to Max Fink and Edward Shorter, December 31, 2016.

58. Kahlbaum, *Die Katatonie* (1874), 5.

59. Kahlbaum, *Die Katatonie* (1874), 27.

60. Kahlbaum, *Die Katatonie* (1874), 30.

61. Mazars de Cazelles F. Sur une catalepsie occasionnée par la terreur. *Journal de Médecine, Chirurgie, Pharmacie.* January 1762;15:131–143, 132–137.
62. Delasiauve LJF. *Traité de l'Épilepsie.* Paris: Masson; 1854, 155.
63. Morel B-A. *Traité Théorique et Pratique des Maladies Mentales.* Nancy: Raybois; 1852, I, 295–296.
64. Kirby GH. The catatonic syndrome and its relation to manic-depressive insanity. *JNMD.* 1913;40:694–704, 696, 699.
65. Hoch A. *Benign Stupors: A Study of a New Manic-Depressive Reaction Type.* New York: Macmillan; 1921, 240.
66. Wolff BC. Thought content in catatonic dementia praecox. *Psych Q.* 1932;6:504–512, 504.
67. Lindemann E. Psychological changes in normal and abnormal individuals under the influence of sodium Amytal. *AJP.* 1932;88:1083–1091, 1085; the paper was presented in 1931.
68. Perkins RJ. Catatonia: the ultimate response to fear? *Aust NZ J Psychiatry.* 1982;16:282–287.
69. Northoff G et al. The subjective experience in catatonia: systematic study of 24 catatonic patients. *Psychiatr Praxis.* 1996;23:69–73.
70. Northoff G et al. Major differences in subjective experience of akinetic states in catatonic and parkinsonian patients. *Cogn Neuropsychiatry.* 1998;3(3):161–178.
71. Moskowitz A. 'Scared stiff': catatonia as an evolutionary-based fear response. *Psycholog Rev.* 2004;111:984–1002.
72. Volchan E. Is there tonic immobility in humans? Biological evidence from victims of traumatic stress. *Biol Psychiatry.* 2011; doi:10.1016/j.biopsycho.2011.06.002.
73. Galliano G et al. Victim reactions during rape/sexual assault. *J Interpers Violence.* 1993;8:109–114.
74. Schauer M, Elbert T. Dissociation following traumatic stress: etiology and treatment. *Zeitschrift für Psychologie (Jrl Psychology).* 2010;218(2):109–127.
75. Marx BP, Forsyth JP, Lexington JM. Tonic immobility as an evolved predator defense. implications for sexual assault survivors. *Clin Psychol Sci Prac.* 2008;15:74–90.
76. Burgess AW, Holmstrom LL. Coping behavior of the rape victim. *Am J Psychiatry.* 1976;133:413–418.
77. Gallup GG. Tonic immobility: the role of fear and predation. *Psychol Rec.* (1977;1:41–61.
78. Sallin K et al. Resignation syndrome: catatonia? culture bound? *Front Behav Neurosci.* January 29, 2016;10:7. doi: 10.3389/fnbeh.2016.00007.
79. Kakooza-Mwesige A et al. Catatonia in Ugandan children with nodding syndrome and effects of treatment with lorazepam: a pilot study. *BMC Res Notes.* 28 Dec. 2015;8:825. doi: 10.1186/s13104-015-1805-5.
80. Dhossche D. Autonomic dysfunction in catatonia in autism: implications of a vagal theory. *Autism* 2012;2:e114. doi:10.4172/2165-7890.1000e114.
81. Fink M. Rediscovering catatonia: the biography of a treatable syndrome. *Acta Psychiatr Scand.* 2013;127(suppl 441):1–50.

Chapter 8

1. Arthur W. *Creatures of Accident.* New York: Hill & Wang; 2006, 232.
2. Kraepelin E. *Psychiatrie: Ein Lehrbuch für Studierende und Aerzte,* 8th ed., vol. III. Leipzig: Barth; 1913, 814–815.

3. Kraepelin, *Psychiatrie*, 8th ed. (1913), 1255.

4. Kraepelin, *Psychiatrie*, 8th ed. (1913).

5. Kraepelin, *Psychiatrie*, 8th ed. (1913), 1255–1256.

6. See Taylor MA. Clinical examination. In SN Caroff et al. eds., *Catatonia: From Psychopathology to Neurobiology*. Washington DC: American Psychiatric Press; 2004, 45–52, 48.

7. See Leroy R. Disparition trois semaines avant la mort, par tuberculose aiguë, de tout symptôme catatonique chez une jeune malade présentée autrefois à la Société. *Bulletin de la Société Clinique de Médecine Mentale*. 1922;10:88–91.

8. Jensen J. Katatonie. In JG Ersch et al. eds., *Allgemeine Encyklopädie der Wissenschaften und Künste*, 2nd section, vol. 34. Leipzig: Brockhaus; 1883, 259–274, 266.

9. Auenbrugger JL. *Von der stillen Wuth oder dem Triebe zum Selbstmorde*. Dessau: Buchhandlung der Gelehrten; 1783, 41–47.

10. Pinel P. *Traité Médico-Philosophique sur l'Aliénation Mentale*, 2nd ed. Paris: Brosson; 1809, 157–158.

11. Fodéré FE. *Traité du Délire*. Paris: Croullebois; 1817, vol. I, 397, 400–401.

12. Calmeil L. Aliénés. In *Dictionnaire de Médecine ou Répertoire Générale des Sciences Médicales*, 2nd ed., vol. 2. Paris: Béchet; 1833, 151–203 160–161.

13. Calmeil L. Manie. In *Dictionnaire de Médecine*, vol. 19 (1839), 117–141, 123. In modern psychiatric literature, one often sees Calmeil 1833 cited as the first reference to delirious mania. The proper date would, of course, be 1839, and it is not really the first reference. Fodéré 1817 with his maniacal fury would have priority.

14. Calmeil L. Monomanie. In *Dictionnaire*, vol. 20 (1839), 138–168, 150.

15. Fink M, Taylor MA. *Catatonia: A Clinician's Guide to Diagnosis and Treatment*. New York: Cambridge University Press; 2003, 189.

16. Fink, Taylor, *Catatonia* (2003), 93–96, 184, 187–189.

17. Morel B-A. *Traité Théorique et Pratique des Maladies Mentales*. Nancy: Raybois; 1853, vol. II, 319–320.

18. Delasiauve L. *Traité de L'Épilepsie*. Paris: Masson; 1854, 149–150.

19. Bell LV. On a form of disease resembling some advanced stages of mania and fever. *Am J Insanity*. 1849;6:97–127.

20. World Health Organization. *Manual of the International Classification of Diseases, Injuries, and Causes of Death, Ninth Revision Conference, 1975*. Geneva: WHO; 1978, 59.

21. Cullen W. *First Lines of the Practice of Physic* (1777), new ed., vol. IV. Edinburgh: Elliot; 1789, 154–155.

22. Haslam J. *Observations on Insanity*. London: Rivington; 1798, 43–44.

23. Haslam J. *Considerations on the Moral Management of Insane Persons*. London: Hunter; 1817, 38.

24. Haslam J. *A Letter to the Governors of Bethlem Hospital, part I*. London: Taylor; 1818, 40.

25. [Haslam J], *Sketches in Bedlam*. London: Sherwood; 1823, 5, 75, 182–184.

26. Weber H. On delirium or acute insanity during the decline of acute diseases, especially the delirium of collapse. *Medical-Chirurgical Society Transactions* (London). 1865;48:135–159, 136, 153

27. Maudsley H. *Physiology and Pathology of the Mind* (1867), 352.

28. Maudsley H. *Responsibility in Mental Disease*. New York: Appleton; 1874, 143, 153–154.

29. Bevan Lewis W. *A Text-Book of Mental Diseases*. London: Griffin; 1889, 172–173. Italics in the original.

30. Hack Tuke D. *A Dictionary of Psychological Medicine.* London: Churchill; 1892, vol. I, 32, 52–55; vol. II, 760, 770

31. Norman HJ. *Mental Disorders.* Edinburgh: Livingstone; 1928, 74–75.

32. Friedreich JB. *Skizze einer allgemeinen Diagnostik der psychischen Krankheiten.* Würzburg: Strecker; 1829, 38.

33. Schüle H. Ueber das Delirium acutum, *AZP.* 1867;42:316–351.

34. von Krafft-Ebing R. *Lehrbuch der Psychiatrie.* Stuttgart: Enke; 1879, vol. II, 45–47, 99–107.

35. Kraepelin E. *Compendium der Psychiatrie,* 1st ed. Leipzig: Abel; 1883, 25, 238.

36. Kraepelin E. *Psychiatrie,* 2nd ed. Leipzig: Abel; 1887, 270.

37. Kraepelin E. *Psychiatrie,* 4th ed. Leipzig: Abel; 1893, 256.

38. Kraepelin E. *Psychiatrie,* 7th ed. Leipzig: Barth; 1903, vol. I, 44.

39. Kraepelin E. *Psychiatrie,* 8th ed. Leipzig: Barth; 1910, vol. II (1), 260; Kraepelin also allowed the diagnosis of manic delirium in this edition, though he used a circumlocution: "In a further smaller group of [mania] cases, the manic attack proceeds with the clinical picture of a delirious condition, with deep, dreamlike clouding of consciousness and perilous, confused hallucinations and delusions." See vol. III (1913), 1255.

40. For a *mise au point,* see Huber's student Glatzel J. Die akute Katatonie, unter besonderer Berücksichtigung der akuten tödlichen Katatonie. *APS.* 1970;46:151–179.

41. Ladame C. Psychose aigüe idiopathique ou foudroyante. *Schweizer Archiv für Neurologie und Psychiatrie.* 1919;5:3–28.

42. Scheidegger W. Katatone Todesfälle in der Psychiatrischen Klinik von Zurich von 1900 bis 1928. *Zeitschrift für die gesamte Neurologie und Psychiatrie.* 1929;120:587–649. 647. In 1940, Rosemarie Locher studied 16 schizophrenia deaths in the years 1935–39 at the Waldau University Psychiatric Hospital in Berne. The deaths in schizophrenic patients— four of whom had been diagnosed with catatonia—were all quite sudden. Were the deaths directly caused by the psychiatric illness, or was catatonia merely ancillary to an underlying organic disease? Autopsy findings pointed to the latter result. In most of these patients, an immediate influence of the psychosis on the fatal outcome can be excluded through autopsy or microscopic analysis. Locher, Über den plötzlichen Tod bei Geisteskranken und die akuten, katatoniformen Zustandsbilder mit tödlichem Ausgang. *Monatsschrift für Psychiatrie und Neurologie.* 1940;103:278–307, 305.

43. Stefan H. Über den plötzlichen natürlichen Tod infolge hochgradiger Erregung und Erschöpfung bei akuten Psychosen ohne wesentliche anatomisch nachweisbare Ursache. *Deutsche Medizinische Wochenschrift.* October 14, 1934;60:1550–1553.

44. Stauder K-H. Die tödliche Katatonie. *Archiv für Psychiatrie und Nervenkrankheiten.* 1934;102:614–634.

45. Arnold OH, Stepan H. Untersuchungen zur Frage der akuten tödlichen Katatonie. *Wiener Zeitschrift für Nervenheilkunde.* 1952;4:235–258, tab. 7, 240.

46. Vargha M, Kovács B. Über die Elektroshock-Behandlung der sogenannten akuten tödlichen Katatonie. *Psychiatrie, Neurologie und medizinische Psychologie.* 1953;5:173–175.

47. Tissot SA. *Traité des Nerfs.* Paris: Didot; 1779, vol. II (1), 383–384.

48. The medical historians, it must be said, have not distinguished themselves in this area, treating nostalgia as some kind of culturally induced hysteria rather than as a biological phenomenon. Jean Starobinski attributes the supposed decline of nostalgia to a decline in provincial particularism and reproaches medicine for having conducted la chasse aux bacilles rather than studying such psychological phenomena. Le Concept de Nostalgie, *Diogène.* 1966;54:92–115. George Rosen concludes that nostalgia disappeared from the

clinical scene during the last decades of the 19th century. Rosen G. Nostalgia: a "forgotten psychological disorder." *Psychological Medicine.* 1975;5:340–354, 351. Lisa O'Sullivan discusses the political and intellectual uses of the diagnosis and finds that it disintegrated as a medical condition; see The time and place of nostalgia: re-situating a French disease. *J Hist Med Allied Sci.* 2012;67:626–649. Stanley Jackson as well treats it as a simple cultural rise-and-fall story, saying nothing about acute delirium, manic delirium, and other diagnoses taking the baton from nostalgia. Jackson SW. *Melancholia and Depression: From Hippocratic Times to Modern Times.* New Haven: Yale University Press; 1986, 373–380; his discussion, nonetheless, is a model biography of a diagnosis, not of a disease. An extreme example of this kind of cultural reductionism of biological phenomena is Fuentenebro de Diego F et al. Nostalgia: a conceptual history. *History of Psychiatry.* 2014;25:404–411, which speaks of the 'creation' of a disease (p. 410). The larger point is that nostalgia as a clinical phenomenon did not disappear, though the term did. Rather, it was replaced by other concepts such as acute delirium.

49. We have not seen the Hofer dissertation but rely on Siegfried Gröf's excellent scholarly account, Diagnose: Heimweh. In T Lange et al. eds., *Kunst und Wissenschaft um 1800.* Würzburg: Königshausen; 2000, 89–106, 91. Gröf correctly gives the publication date as 1688, not 1678, as one often sees in the literature.

50. Nicolai EA. *Die Verbindung der Musik mit der Arzneygelahrheit [sic].* Halle: Hemmerde; 1745, 25–26.

51. On the early nostalgia literature, see Shorter E. *What Psychiatry Left Out.* New York: Routledge; 2015, 54–56.

52. Percy P-F, Laurent C. Nostalgie. In *Dictionaire [sic] des Sciences Médicales,* vol. 36. Paris: Panckoucke; 1819, 265–281, 268, 274.

53. Pinel P. Nostalgie. In *Encyclopédie Méthodique. Médecine,* vol. 10. Paris: Agasse; 1821, 661–663, 662.

54. Morel B-A. *Traité Théorique et Pratique des Maladies Mentales* (1852), vol. I, 298.

55. Morel B-A. *Traité des Maladies Mentales.* Paris: Masson; 1860, 240, 396.

56. Chaslin P. *Éléments de Sémiologie et Clinique Mentales.* Paris: Asselin; 1912, 53.

57. Scherrer P. La débâcle de 1940: receuil des malades mentaux à l'Hôpital Psychiatrique d'Auxerre. *AMP.* 1984;142:266–270.

58. Reil JC. *Rhapsodien über die Anwendung der psychischen Curmethode* (1803). Reprint Amsterdam: Bonset; 1968, 292.

59. Gruhle HW. *Psychiatrie für Aerzte* (1918), 2nd ed. Berlin: Springer; 1922, 18.

60. von Feuchtersleben E. *Lehrbuch der ärztlichen Seelenkunde.* Vienna: Gerold; 1845, 314–317.

61. Griesinger W. *Die Pathologie und Therapie der psychischen Krankheiten,* 2nd ed. Stuttgart: Krabbe; 1861, 302.

62. Schüle H. *Handbuch der Geisteskrankheiten.* Leipzig: Vogel; 1878, 506.

63. Fürstner C. Discussion, 13. Versammlung der südwestdeutschen Irrenärzte. *AZP.* 1881;38:90–91; the meeting was in 1880.

64. See Shorter, *What Psychiatry Left Out* (2015), 41–43.

65. Häfner H et al. Akute lebensbedrohliche Katatonie. *Nervenarzt.* 1982;53:385–394.

Chapter 9

1. Walter WG. *Curve of the Snowflake.* New York: W.W. Norton; 1956.

2. Klein DF, Fink M. Psychiatric reaction patterns to imipramine. *Am J Psychiatry.* 1962; 119:432–438;

3. Klein DF, Fink M. Behavioral reaction patterns with phenothiazines. *Arch Gen Psychiatry.* 1962; 7:449–459.

4. Fink M, Klein DF, Kramer J. Clinical efficacy of chlorpromazine-procyclidine combination, imipramine and placebo in depressive disorders. *Psychopharmacolgia (Berl.). 1965*; 7: 27–36.

5. These studies were accompanied by quantitative analyses of the EEG before and with each treatment. The agents differed in their influence on the frequencies, amplitudes, and patterns, leading to a classification based on the induced changes in the EEG measured using quantitative digital computer programs that predicted the effects of each agent on thought, mood, anxiety, and physiology. The patterns for CPZ, IMI, and PLO were distinct and distinguished the drug effects. The science of pharmaco-electroencephalography offers measurable effects that predict the clinical potential of new agents when studied in man. Fink M. Pharmacoelectroencephalography: a note on its history. *Neuropsychobiol.* 1984; 12: 173–178. Fink M. Remembering the lost neuroscience of pharmaco-EEG. *Acta Pyschiatr Scand.* 2010; 121:161–173.

6. Hearst ED, Munoz RA, Tuason VB. Catatonia: its diagnostic validity. *Dis Nerv Syst.* 1971; 32:453–456.

7. Delay J, Pichot P. Lempérière T. Un neuroleptique majeur non phenothiazine et non reserpinique, l'haloperidol, dans le traitement des psychoses. *AMP.* 1960; 118: 145–152.

8. Meltzer HY. Rigidity, hyperpyrexia and coma following fluphenazine enanthate. *Psychopharmacologia.* 1973; 29:337–346.

9. Weinberger DR, Kelly MJ. Catatonia and malignant syndrome: a possible complication of neuroleptic administration. *J Nerv Ment Dis.* 1977; 165:263–268.

10. Caroff SN. The neuroleptic malignant syndrome. *J Clin Psychiatry.* 1980; 41:79–83.

11. Hermesh H, Sirota P, Eviatar J. Recurrent neuroleptic malignant syndrome due to haloperidol and amantadine. *Biol Psychiatry.* 1989; 25:962–965.

12. Lazarus A, Mann SC, Caroff SN. *The Neuroleptic Malignant Syndrome and Related Conditions.* Washington DC: American Psychiatric Press, Inc.; 1989.

13. Greenberg LB, Gujavarty K. The neuroleptic malignant syndrome: review and report of three cases. *Comprehens Psychiatry.* 1985; 26:63–70.

14. Barron Lerner's review of the Libby Zion case is at http://www.washingtonpost.com/ wp-dyn/content/article/2006/11/24/AR2006112400985.html. In retrospect, Ms. Zion suffered first from the toxic serotonin syndrome (TSS), worsened by haloperidol to NMS. TSS is a form of NMS. Fink M. Toxic serotonin syndrome or neuroleptic malignant syndrome? *Pharmacopsychiatry.* 1996; 29: 159–161.

15. Keck PE et al. Risk factors for neuroleptic malignant syndrome. *AGP.* 1989; 46:914–918.

16. Rosebush PI et al. Catatonic syndrome in a general psychiatric population: frequency, clinical presentation, and response to lorazepam. *J Clin Psychiatry.* 1990; 51:357–362.

17. Spivak B et al. Neuroleptic malignant syndrome during abrupt reduction of neuroleptic treatment. *APS.* 1990; 81:168–169.

18. Osman AA, Khurasani MH. Lethal catatonia and neuroleptic malignant syndrome. A dopamine receptor shut-down hypothesis. *BJP.* 1994; 165: 548–550.

19. Berardi D et al.Clinical and pharmacologic risk factors for neuroleptic malignant syndrome: a case-control study. *Biol Psychiatry.* 1998; 44:748–754.

20. Shalev A, Hermesh H, Munitz H. Mortality from neuroleptic malignant syndrome. *J Clin Psychiatry.* 1989; 50: 18–25.

21. Lavie CJ, Ventura HO, Walker G. Neuroleptic malignant syndrome: three episodes with different drugs. *Southern Med J.* 1986; 79:1571–1573.

22. Lazarus A, Mann SC, Caroff SN. *The Neuroleptic Malignant Syndrome and Related Conditions* (1989).

23. Fink M, Taylor MA. *Catatonia: A Clinician's Guide to Diagnosis and Treatment.* New York: Cambridge University Press; 2003.

24. Lazarus A, Mann SC, Caroff SN. *The Neuroleptic Malignant Syndrome and Related Conditions* (1989).

25. Fink M, Taylor MA. *Catatonia* (2003).

26. An interesting example of this frenzy occurred in the summer of 1392, in French Brittany. It was insufferably hot when the Valois King Charles VI took his troops on a military campaign. Struggling in long marches, constantly fearing attack, a warning by a ragged vagrant frightened the King. Ill with fever, the King became confused, suddenly pictured his guards as the enemy, rampaged and slaughtered four, broke his sword, and collapsed. Now mute, staring, immobile, and fluctuating in stupor, he abandoned his campaign and was slowly nursed back to health. Fink M. Seeing the King's frenzy as catatonia. *APS.* 2015; 132(6): 500–501. Appiani FJ. Delirious mania of Charles VI of France during the fouteenth century. *APS* 2015; 132(6): 499–502.

27. Scheidegger W. Katatone Todesfälle in der Psychiatrischen Klinik von Zürich von 1900 bis 1928. *Zeitschrift für die gesamte Neurologie und Psychiatrie.* 1929; 120: 587–649.

28. Scheid KF. *Febrile Episoden bei schizophenen Psychosen. Eine klinische und pathologische Studie.* Leipzig: Thieme; 1937.

29. Billig O, Freeman WT. Fatal catatonia. *Am J Psychiatry.* 1943; 100:633–638.

30. Geller W, Mappes C. Deadly catatonia. *Arch Psychiatr Nervenkr.* 1952; 189:147–161.

31. Huber G. Zur nosologischen Differenzierung lebensbedrohlicher katatoner Psychosen. *Schweiz Arch Neurol Psychiat.* 1954: 216–222.

32. Pauleikhoff B. Die Katatonie (1868–1968). *Fortschritte der Neurologie-Psychiatrie und ihrer Grenzgebiete.* 1969; 37:461–496.

33. Borreguero AD. Catatonia mortal. Diencefalo, Electrochoque. *Revista Clínica Española.* 1947. 27: 161–176. Arnold OH, Stepan H. Untersuchungen zur Frage der akuten tödlichen Katatonie. *Wiener Zeitschrift für Nervenheilkunde.* 1952; 4: 235–258

34. Fink M. *Electroconvulsive Treatment: Guide for Patients and their Families.* New York: Oxford Univ Press; 2009.

35. Guze S. The occurrence of psychiatric illness in systemic lupus erythematosus. *Am J Psychiatry.* 1967; 123:1562–1570.

36. Fink, Taylor. *Catatonia* (2003).

37. Today, we would have induced treatments daily and resolved the syndrome more rapidly. Fink M. Delirious mania. *Bipolar Dis.*1999; 1: 54–60.

38. Fricchione GL et al. Electroconvulsive therapy and cyclophosphamide in combination for severe neuropsychiatric lupus with catatonia. *Am J Med.*1990; 88: 442–443.

39. Casamassima F et al. Neuroleptic malignant syndrome: further lessons from a case report. *Psychosomatics.* 2010 Jul–Aug;51(4):349–395.

40. Ali S et al. Encephalitis and catatonia treated with ECT. *Cogn Behav Neurol.* 2008 Mar;21(1):46–51

41. Mann SC et al. Lethal catatonia. *Am J Psychiatry.* 1986; 143:1374–1381; Mann SC et al. Electroconvulsive therapy of the lethal catatonia syndrome. *Convulsive Ther.* 1990; 6:239–47.

42. Rosebush P, Stewart T. A prospective analysis of 24 episodes of neuroleptic malignant syndrome. *Am J Psychiatry.* 1989; 146:717–725; Rosebush et al. Catatonic syndrome in a general psychiatric population (1990), 357–362.

43. Rummans T, Bassingthwaighte ME. Severe medical and neurologic complications associated with near-lethal catatonia treated with electroconvulsive therapy. *Convulsive Ther.* 1991; 7:121–24.

44. Fricchione GL. Neuroleptic catatonia and its relationship to psychogenic catatonia. *Biol Psychiatry.* 1985; 20:304–313.

45. White DAC, Robins AH. Catatonia: harbinger of the neuroleptic malignant syndrome. *Br J Psychiatry.* 1991; 158:419–421.

46. White DAC. Catatonia and the neuroleptic malignant syndrome—a single entity? *Br J Psychiatry.* 1992; 161:558–560.

47. Greenberg L, Gujavarty K. The neuroleptic malignant syndrome. *Comprehens Psychiatry* (1985), 26(1): 63–70.

48. Hermesh H, Aizenberg D, Weizman A. A successful electroconvulsive treatment of neuroleptic malignant syndrome. *Acta Psychiatr Scand.* 1987; 75: 237–239.

49. Fricchione GL, Kaufman LD, Gruber BL, Fink M. Electroconvulsive therapy and cyclophosphamide in combination for severe neuropsychiatric lupus with catatonia. *Am J Med* (1990), 442–443.

50. Rummans T, Bassingthwaighte ME. Severe medical and neurologic complications associated with near-lethal catatonia treated with electroconvulsive therapy. *Convulsive Ther.* (1991), 121–124.

51. Hawkins JM, Archer KJ, Strakowski SM, Keck PE. Somatic treatment of catatonia. *Intl J Psychiatry Med.* 1995; 25:345–369.

52. Davis JM, Janicak PG, Sakkas P, Gilmore C, Wang Z. Electroconvulsive therapy in the treatment of the neuroleptic malignant syndrome. *Convulsive Ther.* 1991; 7: 111–120.

53. Mann SC, Caroff SN, Bleier HR, Antelo E, Un H. Electroconvulsive therapy of the lethal catatonia syndrome *Convulsive Ther.* (1990), 239–247.

54. Hermesh H, Aizenberg D, Weizman A. A successful electroconvulsive treatment of neuroleptic malignant syndrome. *APS* (1987);75: 237–239.

55. Davis et al. Electroconvulsive therapy in the treatment of the neuroleptic malignant syndrome. *Convulsive Ther* (1991), 111–120.

56. Schott K, Bartels M, Heimann H, Buchkremer G. Ergebnisse der Elektrokrampf-therapie unter restriktiver Indikation. Eine retrospektive Studie über 15 Jahre. [Results of electroconvulsive therapy in restrictive indications. A retrospective study of 15 years.] *Nervenarzt.* 1992; 63:422–425.

57. Troller JN, Sachdev PS. Electroconvulsive treatment of neuroleptic malignant syndrome: a review and report of cases. *Aust NZ J Psychiatry.* 1999; 33:650–659.

58. Fricchione GL, Cassem NH, Hooberman D, Hobson D. Intravenous lorazepam in neuroleptic-induced catatonia. *J Clin Psychopharm.* 1983; 3:338–342.

59. Rosebush P, Stewart T. A prospective analysis of 24 episodes of neuroleptic malignant syndrome. *Am J Psychiatry* (1989), 717–725.

60. Rosebush PI, Hildebrand AM, Furlong BG, Mazurek MF. Catatonic syndrome in a general psychiatric population: Frequency, clinical presentation, and response to lorazepam. *J Clin Psychiatry* 1990; 51: 357–362..

61. Rummans T, Bassingthwaighte ME. Severe medical and neurologic complications associated with near-lethal catatonia treated with electroconvulsive therapy. *Convulsive Ther* 1991; 7:121–124..

62. Philbrick KL, Rummans TA. Malignant catatonia. *J Neuropsychiatry Clin Neurosci.* 1994; 6:1–13.

63. Bush G, Fink M, Petrides G, Dowling F, Francis A. Catatonia: II. Treatment with lorazepam and electroconvulsive therapy. *Acta Psychiatr. Scand.* 1996; 93;137–143..

64. A 23-item catatonia rating scale became identified as the Bush-Francis Catatonia Rating Scale.

65. Rosebush PI, Mazurek MF. Catatonia and its treatment. *Schizophr Bull.* 2010; 36(2):239–242.

66. For a discussion of the role of fear in the etiology of catatonia see Fink M. Rediscovering catatonia: the biography of a treatable syndrome. *Acta Psychiatr Scand.* 2013; 127: Supplement 441;1–50, and Fink M, Shorter E. Does persisting fear sustain catatonia? *Acta Psychiatr Scand.* 2017 Nov; 136(5):441–444..

67. Castillo E, Rubin RT, Holsboer-Trachsler E. Clinical differentiation between lethal catatonia and neuroleptic malignant syndrome. *Am J Psychiatry* 1989;146:324–328; Caroff SN, Mann SC. Neuroleptic malignant syndrome. *Med Clin North Am* 1993;77:185–202; Peralta V, Cuesta MJ, Serrano JF, Mata I. The Kahlbaum syndrome: A study of its clinical validity, nosological status, and relationship with schizophrenia and mood disorders. *Comprehens Psychiatry* 1997;38:61–67.

68. Carroll BT, Taylor BE. The nondichotomy between lethal catatonia and neuroleptic malignant syndrome. *J Clin Psychopharmacol.* 1997; 17:235–236.

69. Chandler JD. Psychogenic catatonia with elevated creatine kinase and autonomic hyperactivity. *Can J Psychiatry.* 1991; 36:530–532.

70. Fricchione G, Mann SC, Caroff SN. Catatonia, lethal catatonia and neuroleptic malignant syndrome. *Psychiatr Ann.* 2000; 30:347–355.

71. Koch M, Chandragiri S, Rizvi S, Petrides G, Francis A. Catatonic signs in neuroleptic malignant syndrome. *Comprehens Psychiatry.* 2000; 41:73–75.

72. Lazarus A, Mann SC, Caroff SN. *The Neuroleptic Malignant Syndrome and Related Conditions.* Washington D.C.: American Psychiatric Press, Inc., 1989..

73. Mann SC, Caroff SN, Keck PE, Lazarus A. *Neuroleptic Malignant Syndrome and Related Conditions.* Washington DC: American Psychiatric Press; 2003.

74. Fink M. Missed neuroleptic malignant syndrome. *BMJ.* 1992; 304:1246; Neuroleptic malignant syndrome and catatonia. One entity or two? *Biol Psychiatry.* 1996; 39: 1–4; Lethal catatonia, neuroleptic malignant syndrome, and catatonia: a spectrum of disorders. Reply. *J Clin Psychopharmacol.* 1997; 17: 237; Fricchione GL, Bush G, Fozdar M, Francis A, Fink M. Recognition and treatment of the catatonic syndrome. *Jrl Intensive Care Med.* 1997; 12:135–147.

75. The main respondents were Stanley Caroff, Andrew Francis, Gregory Fricchione, and Stephan Mann.

76. Malignant Hyperthermia Association of the United States, http://www.nmsis.org.

Chapter 10

1. Ellery R. *Schizophrenia: The Cinderella of Psychiatry.* Sydney: Australasian Medical Publishers; 1941, 52.

2. Gazdag G. Diagnosing and treating catatonia: an update. *Current Psychiatric Res.* 2013; 9:1–2.

3. Müller A. *Die Irren-Anstalt in dem königlichen Julius-Hospitale zu Würzburg.* Würzburg: Stahel; 1824, 78–79.

4. It is this alternation that answers Gabor Ungvari's question, what makes an agitation 'catatonic?' Ungvari GS et al. Nosology. In SN Caroff et al. eds., *Catatonia: From Psychopathology to Neurobiology.* Washington DC: American Psychiatric Press; 2004, 33–43, 35.

5. Schüle H. *Klinische Psychiatrie,* 3rd ed. Leipzig: Vogel; 1886, 209–210.

6. Kraepelin E. *Psychiatrie,* 5th ed. Leipzig: Barth; 1896, 454.

7. Kraepelin E. *Psychiatrie,* 8th ed, vol. 3. Leipzig: Barth; 1913, 810, 828.

8. Hack Tuke D. *A Dictionary of Psychological Medicine.* Philadelphia: Blakiston; 1892, vol. II, 724–725.

9. Devine H. The clinical significance of katatonic symptoms. *J Ment Sci.* 1914;60:278–291, 278.

10. Morel B-A. *Traité Théorique et Pratique des Maladies Mentales.* Nancy: Grimblot; 1853, vol. II, 281

11. Guiraud P, Saunet L. Pathogénie des symptômes du délire aigu. *AMP.* 1938;96: 574–580, 574.

12. Leonhard K. Zur Unterteilung und Erbbiologie der Schizophrenien. *AZP.* 1943;122: 39–86, 45.

13. Leonhard K. *Die Aufteilung der endogenen Psychosen.* East-Berlin: Akademie Verlag; 1957, 244.

14. Fish FJ. *Schizophrenia.* Bristol: Wright; 1962, 52, 63–64, 95.

15. See, for example, Beld JT, Philbrick K, Rummans T. Periodic catatonia. In SN Caroff et al. eds., *Catatonia from Psychopathology to Neurobiology.* Washington DC: American Psychiatric Press; 2004, 93–104.

16. Pauleikhoff B. Die Katatonie (1868–1968), *Fortschritte der Neurologie und Psychiatrie.* 1969;37:461–496, 475.

17. Anonymous to authors, January 15, 2015.

18. Wijemanne S, Jankovic J. Movement disorders in catatonia. *J Neurol Neurosurg Psych.* 2015;86:825–832, 827.

19. See, for example, Fein S, McGrath MG. Problems in diagnosing bipolar disorder in catatonic patients. *J Clin Psych.* 1990;51:203–205.

20. Brosius CM. Die Katatonie. *AZP.* 1877;35:770–802, 778–784; Kraepelin, *Psychiatrie,* 8th ed. (1913), vol. III, 956–960.

21. Ungvari G et al. The catatonic conundrum: evidence of psychomotor phenomena as a symptom dimension in psychotic disorders. *Schizophrenia Bulletin.* 2010;36: 231–238,

22. Morrison JR. Changes in subtype diagnosis of schizophrenia. 1920–1966, *AJP.* 1974;131:674–677.

23. Morrison JR. Catatonia: diagnosis and management. *Hosp Community Psych.* 1975;26: 91–94, 91.

24. Mahendra B. Where have all the catatonics gone? *Psychological Med.* 1981;11:669–670.

25. Berrios GE. *The History of Mental Symptoms.* Cambridge: Cambridge University Press; 1996, 380.

26. Ungvari GS, Caroff SN, Gerevich J. The catatonia conundrum: evidence of psychomotor phenomena as a symptom dimension in psychotic disorders. *Schizophr Bull* (2010), 231–238, 234.

27. Templer DI et al. The decline of catatonic schizophrenia. *J Orthomolecular Psychiatry.* 1981;10:156–158.

28. Rosebush PI, Mazurek MF. Catatonia: re-awakening to a forgotten disorder. *Movement Dis.* 1999;14:395–397.

29. van der Heijden FMMA et al. Catatonia: disappeared or under-diagnosed? *Psychopathology.* 2005;38:3–8, 5. Confusingly, the first and second periods both contain DSM-III-R.

30. Ainsworth P. A case of 'lethal catatonia' in a 14-year-old girl. *BJP.* 1987;150:110–112.

31. de Jong H, Baruk H. *La Catatonie Experimentale par la Bulbocapnine.* Paris: Masson; 1930.

32. See some of the critical comments on De Jong by the informants of Aubrey Lewis, who toured European neuroscience research centers in the late 1930s on behalf of the Rockefeller Foundation. Angel K et al. eds., *European Psychiatry on the Eve of War: Aubrey Lewis, the Maudsley Hospital and the Rockefeller Foundation in the 1930s.* London: Wellcome Trust Centre for the History of Medicine at UCL; 2003; *Medical History* (suppl. nr. 22):412–415

33. Müller A. *Periodische Katatonien.* Zurich: Medical dissertation; 1900.

34. Lorenz WF. Some observations on catatonia. *Psych Q.* 1930;4:95–102, 95.

35. Herman M et al. Nonschizophrenic catatonic states. *N Y State Med J.* 1942;42:624–627, 624.

36. Huber G. Zur Frage der mit Hirnatrophie einhergehenden Schizophrenie. *Archiv für Psychiatrie und Zeitschrift Neurologie.* 1953;190:429–448.

37. Schneider K. Kraepelin und die gegenwärtige Psychiatrie. *Fortschritte der Neurologie und Psychiatrie.* 1956;24:1–7, 6.

38. Bennett IF, Kinross-Wright V. Discussion. In JO Cole, RW Gerard, eds., *Psychopharmacology: Problems in Evaluation.* Washington DC: National Academy of Sciences; 1959, 415; the conference was held in 1956.

39. See Hoff H. Discussion. In M Rinkel, HE Himwich, eds., *Insulin Treatment in Psychiatry.* New York: Philosophical Library; 1959, 196–197.

40. Kline N. Discussion. *American Psychiatric Association, Pharmacologic Products Recently Introduced in the Treatment of Psychiatric Disorders; Research Reports* 1. Washington DC: APA; 1955, 146–147;

41. Clausen JA. Discussion. In J Zubin, ed., *Field Studies in the Mental Disorders.* New York: Grune & Stratton; 1961, 207; the conference was held in 1959.

42. Jaffe N. Catatonia and hepatic dysfunction. *Dis Nerv Sys.* 1967;28:606–608, 606.

43. Kendell JE et al. *Psychiatric Diagnosis in New York and London: A Comparative Study of Mental Hospital Admissions.* London: Oxford University Press; 1972.

44. Anon. United States–United Kingdom, cross-national project. *Schizophrenia Bull.* 1974;1:80–102, 95.

45. Morrison JR. Catatonia: retarded and excited types. *AGP.* 1973;28:39–41.

46. Morrison JR, Catatonia: diagnosis and treatment. *Hosp Community Psychiatry.* 1975; 26:91–94.

47. Gelenberg AJ. The catatonic syndrome. *Lancet.* June 19, 1976;1:1339–1341,

48. van Praag H. Über den unmöglichen Begriff Schizophrenie. *Psychiat Prax.* 1978;5:73–87, 74.

49. Abrams R, Taylor MA. Catatonia: a prospective clinical study. *AGP.* 1976;33:579–581, 579.

50. Abrams R, Taylor MA. Catatonia: prediction of response to somatic treatments. *Am J Psychiatry.* 1977;134:78–80.

51. Abrams R, Taylor MA, Stolurow KAC. Catatonia and mania: patterns of cerebral dysfunction. *Biol Psychiatry.* 1979;14:111–117.

52. Caroff SC, Mann SC, Campbell EC, Sullivan KA. Epidemiology. In S Caroff et al. eds., *Catatonia: From Psychopathology to Neurobiology.* Washington DC: American Psychiatric Press; 2004, 15–31, 22.

53. Barnes MP, Saunders M, Walls TJ et al. The syndrome of Karl Ludwig Kahlbaum. *J Neurol Neurosurg Psychiatry.* 1986;49:991–996.

54. Lohr JB, Wisniewski AA. *Movement Disorders: A Neuropsychiatric Approach.* New York: Guilford; 1987, 227.

Chapter 11

1. Max Fink to Edward Shorter, personal communication, April 26, 2016.

2. War Department. Nomenclature of psychiatric disorders and reactions, technical bulletin, medical 203. *J Clin Psychol.* 1946;2:289–296.

3. Abnormalities in cortisol metabolism mark melancholic depression, resolve with effective treatment, and return with relapse. Interest in this and other endocrine abnormalities was rejected by the American Psychiatric Association committee headed by Alexander Glassman. APA Task Force on Laboratory Tests in Psychiatry. The dexamethasone suppression test: an overview of its current status in psychiatry. *AJP.* 1987;144:1253–1262. Also: Shorter E, Fink M. *Endocrine Psychiatry.* New York: Oxford University Press; 2010.

4. Morrison JR. Catatonia: retarded and excited types. *Arch Gen Psychiatry.* 1973;28:39–41; Karl Kahlbaum and catatonia. *Comprehens Psychiatry.* 1974;15:315–316; Catatonia: diagnosis and treatment. *Hosp Community Psychiatry.* 1975;26:91–94; Catatonia: prediction of outcome. *Comprehens Psychiatry.* 1974;15:317–324.

5. Abrams R, Taylor MA. Catatonia, a prospective clinical study. *Arch Gen Psychiatry.* 1976;33:579–581; Catatonia: prediction of response to somatic treatments. *Am J Psychiatry.* 1977;134:78–80; Abrams R, Taylor MA, Stolurow KAC. Catatonia and mania: patterns of cerebral dysfunction. *Biol Psychiatry.* 1979;14:111–117.

6. Gelenberg AJ. The catatonic syndrome. *Lancet.* 1976;1:1339–1341; Gelenberg AJ, Mandel MR. Catatonic reactions to high potency neuroleptic drugs. *Arch Gen Psychiatry.* 1977;34:947–950.

7. Lohr JB, Wisniewski AA. *Movement Disorders: A Neuropsychiatric Approach.* New York: Guilford Press; 1987.

8. Taylor MA. Catatonia: a review of a behavioral neurologic syndrome. *Neuropsychiatry Neuropsychol Behav Neurol.* 1990;3:48–72.

9. Fink M, Taylor MA. Catatonia: a separate category for DSM-IV? *Integrative Psychiatry.* 1991;7:2–10.

10. Following cluster analysis of catatonia signs, two clusters were proposed to categorize catatonia: one of immobility, mutism, or stupor associated with one of catalepsy, automatic obedience, or posturing, and a second that was characterized by the other catatonia signs. Abrams R, Taylor MA, Stolurow KAC. Catatonia and mania: patterns of cerebral dysfunction. *Biol Psychiatry.* 1979;14:111–117.

11. Pichot P. Commentary. *Integrative Psychiatry.* 1991;7:6–7.

12. Spitzer R. Commentary. *Integrative Psychiatry.* 1991;7:7–8.

13. Spitzer RL et al. Preliminary report of the reliability of research diagnostic criteria applied in psychiatric case records. In A Sudilovsky et al. eds., *Predictability in Psychopharmacology.* New York: Raven Press; 1975, 1–47, 13.

14. Letter from DFK to MF, March 22, 1991. MF Archives Folder RG 64.17

15. Letter from AJR to MF, March 22, 1991. MF Archives Folder RG 64.17

16. American Psychiatric Association. *Diagnostic and statistical manual of mental disorders.* 4th ed. Washington, DC, 1994.

17. Another change was the addition of a catatonia features specifier for patients who met criteria for the principal mood disorders. This application carried no numeric designation and has served no clinical or research purpose.

18. Searches of PubMed for citations to catatonia for each year. June 19, 2017. Max Fink.

19. Lohr JB, Wisniewski AA. *Movement Disorders: A Neuropsychiatric Approach.* New York: Guilford Press; 1987.

20. Taylor MA. Catatonia: a review of a behavioral neurologic syndrome. *Neuropsychiatry Neuropsychol Behav Neurol.* 1990;3:48–72;Rosebush PI et al. Catatonic syndrome in a general psychiatric population: Frequency, clinical presentation, and response to lorazepam. *J Clin Psychiatry.* 1990;51:357–362;Rogers D. *Motor Disorder in Psychiatry: Towards a Neurological Psychiatry.* Chichester UK: John Wiley & Sons; 1992;Northoff G et al. Catatonia as a psychomotor syndrome: a rating scale and extrapyramidal motor symptoms. *Movement Disorders.* 1999;14:404–416;Bräunig P et al. The catatonia rating scale I: development, reliability, and use. *Comprehens Psychiatry.* 2000;41:147–158.

21. See Chapter 4, Kraepelin.

22. After reviewing the reports of Kahlbaum (1873), Morrison (1973, 1975), Gelenberg (1976), Taylor and Abrams (1977), Taylor (1990), Rogers (1985), Lohr and Wisniewski (1987), and Rosebush et al. (1990), the Stony Brook scholars identified 23 behaviors that constitute the main signs of catatonia. The authors developed a standardized 14-item screening instrument and a 23-item rating scale to identify patients with catatonia. Bush G et al. Catatonia: I: Rating scale and standardized examination. *Acta Psychiatr. Scand.* 1996;93;129–136.

23. Sienaert P, Rooseleer J, De Fruyt J. Measuring catatonia: a systematic review of rating scales. *J Affect Disord.* 2011;135(1–3):1–9.

24. Pataki J, Zervas IM, Jandorf L. Catatonia in a university inpatient service (1985–1990). *Convulsive Ther.* 1992;8(3) 163–173. At the time, patients were being treated with weakened forms of ECT, notably right unilateral electrode placement at modest energies based on seizure threshold criteria. Later studies reported that such treatments yielded 40% less effective treatments than using bitemporal electrodes. See Fink M, Taylor MA. Electroconvulsive therapy: evidence and challenges. *JAMA.* 2007;298:330–332.

25. Bush G et al. Catatonia: I: rating scale and standardized examination. *Acta psychiatr. Scand.* 1996;93;129–136.

26. Rosebush PI et al. Catatonic syndrome in a general psychiatric population: frequency, clinical presentation, and response to lorazepam. *J Clin Psychiatry.* 1990;51:357–362.

27. Ungvari GS, Leung CM, Lee TS. Benzodiazepines and the psychopathology of catatonia. *Pharmacopsychiatry.* 1994;27:242–245.

28. Ungvari GS et al. Benzodiazepines in the treatment of catatonic syndrome. *Acta Psychiatr Scand.* 1994;89:285–288.

29. Chalasani P, Healy D, Morriss R. Presentation and frequency of catatonia in new admissions to two acute psychiatric admission units in India and Wales. *Psychol Med.* 2005 Nov;35(11):1667–1675.

30. Fink M, Taylor MA. *Catatonia: A Clinician's Guide to Diagnosis and Treatment.* New York: Cambridge University Press; 2003. Table 5.3.

31. Bush G, Petrides G, Francis A. Catatonia and other motor syndromes in a chronically hospitalized psychiatric population. *Schizophrenia Res.* 1997;27:83–92.

32. Bush G et al. Catatonia: II. treatment with lorazepam and electroconvulsive therapy. *Acta Psychiatr Scand.* 1996;93;137–143.

33. Fink M, Taylor MA. *Catatonia: A Clinician's Guide to Diagnosis and Treatment.* New York: Cambridge University Press; 2003.

34. Caroff S, et al., eds. *Catatonia. From Psychopathology to Neurobiology.* Washington DC: American Psychiatric Press; 2004.

35. Rosebush PI et al. Catatonic syndrome in a general psychiatric population: frequency, clinical presentation, and response to lorazepam. *J Clin Psychiatry.* 1990;51:357–362.

36. White DAC. Catatonia and the neuroleptic malignant syndrome—a single entity? *Br J Psychiatry.* 1992;161:558–560.

37. Philbrick KL, Rummans TA. Malignant catatonia. *J Neuropsychiatry Clin Neurosci.* 1994;6:1–13.

38. Fink M. Neuroleptic malignant syndrome. One entity or two. *Biol Psychiatry.* 1996;39:1–4.

39. Electrical dosing in ECT for elderly depressed patients seeks to minimize cognitive effects by using unilateral electrode placement and minimal energies to induce the seizure. Delayed outcomes and lesser recovery rates are tolerated. For catatonia, especially for its malignant forms, bilateral placement, high energies, and daily treatments are required for effective relief. Fink M, Kellner CH, McCall V. Optimizing ECT technique in treating catatonia. *J ECT.* 2016;32(3):149–150.

40. The chairman was William Carpenter, director of the Maryland Psychiatric Research Center in Baltimore. In the ensuing years of interaction, much of the discussion was through Stephan Heckers of Vanderbilt University, Rajiv Tandon of the University of Florida, and Juan R. Bustillo of the University of New Mexico, members of this work group.

41. Max Fink Archives, Stephan Heckers Correspondence. 2009.

42. Fink M, Shorter E, Taylor MA. Catatonia is not schizophrenia: Kraepelin's error and the need to recognize catatonia as an independent syndrome in medical nomenclature. *Schizophrenia Bull.* 2009;36(2):314–320.

43. Rosebush P, Mazurek M. Catatonia and its treatment. *Schizophrenia Bull.* 2009;36(2):239–242.

44. Ungvari GS, Caroff SN, Gerevich J. The catatonia conundrum: Evidence of psychomotor phenomena as a symptom dimension in psychotic disorders. *Schizophrenia Bull.* 2009;36(2):231–238.

45. Heckers S, Tandon R, Bustillo J. Catatonia in the DSM- shall we move or not? *Schizophrenia Bull.* 2009;36(2):205–207.

46. Fink M. Catatonia. In Widiger TA et al. eds. *DSM-IV Sourcebook,* volume 2. Washington DC: American Psychiatric Association;1996;181–192.

47. Rajiv Tandon of the Work Group explained to Michael Taylor that the additional difficulty of establishing catatonia as a unique entity was the absence of an unassigned DSM number. (PC to Max Fink, October 16, 2017).

48. Francis A et al. Catatonia in the *Diagnostic and statistical manual of mental disorders,* Fifth edition. *J ECT.* 2010;26:246–248.

49. Max Fink Archives. Catatonia in DSM-V- Response to Heckers Editorial. April 21, 2010.

50. Max Fink Archives. Catatonia in DSM-V- 2012 Scholars Responses.

51. Tandon R et al. Catatonia in DSM-5. *Schizophr Res.* 2013;150 (1):26–30.

52. Tandon R et al. Definition and description of schizophrenia in the DSM-5. *Schizophr Res.* 2013 Oct;150 (1):3–10.

53. Fink M, Taylor MA. The many varieties of catatonia. *Eur Arch Psychiatry Clin Neurosci.* 2001.251: Suppl. 1:8–13.

54. Fink M. Rediscovering catatonia *Acta Psychiatr Scand.* 2013;127(suppl 447):1–50.

55. Jacobowski NL, Heckers S, Bobo WV. Delirious mania: detection, diagnosis, and clinical management in the acute setting. *J Psychiatr Pract.* 2013 Jan;19(1):15–28.

56. Bobo WV, Murphy MJ, Heckers SH. Recurring episodes of Bell's mania after cerebrovascular accident. *Psychosomatics.* 2009 May-Jun;50(3):285–288.

57. Wilson JE et al. The diagnostic criteria and structure of catatonia. *Schiz Res* (2015). http://dx.doi.org/10.1016/J.schres.2014.12.036.

58. Fink M, Fricchione G, Rummans T, Shorter E. Catatonia is a systemic medical disorder. *Acta Psychiatr Scand.* 133(1):250–251.

Chapter 12

1. Grinell F. *The Scientific Attitude,* 2nd ed. New York: Guilford Press; 1992.

2. Fink M, Taylor MA. *Catatonia: A Clinician's Guide to Diagnosis and Treatment.* New York: Cambridge University Press; 2003.

3. Bush G et al. Catatonia: I: rating scale and standardized examination. *Acta Psychiatr Scand.* 1996;93;129–136.

4. Mahendra B. Editorial: Where have all the catatonics gone? *Psychol Med.* 1981;11:669–671.

5. Fricchione GL et al. Intravenous lorazepam in neuroleptic-induced catatonia. *J Clin Psychopharm.* 1983;3:338–342.

6. Bush G et al. Catatonia: I: Rating scale and standardized examination. *Acta Psychiatr. Scand.* 1996;93;129–136.

7. Bush G et al. Catatonia: II. Treatment with lorazepam and electroconvulsive therapy. *Acta Psychiatr. Scand.* 1996;93;137–143.

8. Sienaert P et al. A clinical review of the treatment of catatonia. *Front Psychiatry.* 2014 Dec 9;5:181.

9. Taylor, MA, Atre Vaidya N. *Descriptive Psychopathology: The Signs and Symptoms of Behavioral Disorders.* Cambridge: Cambridge University Press; 2008.

10. Taylor MA, Shorter E, Vaidya NA, Fink M. The failure of the schizophrenia concept and the argument for its replacement by hebephrenia: applying the medical model for disease recognition. *Acta Psychiatr Scand.* 2010;122:173–183.

11. Fink M. DSM-V: applying the medical model. *Psychiatric Times.* June 9, 2009;26(6), http://www.psychiatrictimes.com/display/article/10168/1420772.

12. Robins E, Guze SB. Establishment of diagnostic validity in psychiatric illness, its application to schizophrenia. *Am J Psychiatry.* 1970;126:983–987

13. Fink M, Taylor MA. *Catatonia: A Clinician's Guide to Diagnosis and Treatment.* New York: Cambridge University Press; 2003.

14. Taylor MA, Fink M. Catatonia in psychiatric classification: a home of its own. *Am J Psychiatry.* 2003;160:1233–1241.

15. Fink M. Rediscovering catatonia: the biography of a treatable syndrome. *Acta Psychiatr Scand.* 2013;Suppl 127:1–50.

16. Medline reviews for anti-NMDAR encephalitis and for Dalmau J. were made on various dates, the latest on July 20, 2017.

17. Sabin TD, Jednacz JA, Staats PN. Case records of the Massachusetts General Hospital. #26, 2008. A 26-year-old woman with headaches and behavioral changes. *N Engl J Med.* 2008;359:842–853.

18. Chapman MR, Vause HE. Anti-NMDA receptor encephalitis: diagnosis, psychiatric presentation, and treatment. *Am J Psychiatry.* 2011;168:245–251.

19. Dhossche D, Fink M, Shorter E, Wachtel LE. Anti-NMDA receptor encephalitis versus pediatric catatonia. *Am J Psychiatry.* 2011;168:749–750.

20. Dalmau J et al. Anti-NMDA-receptor encephalitis: case series and the analysis of the effects of antibodies. *Lancet Neurol.* 2008;7:1091–1098.

21. Kung DH, Qiu C, Kass JS. Psychiatric manifestations of anti-NMDA receptor encephalitis in a man without tumor. *Psychosomatics.* 2011;52:82–85.

22. Dalmau J. Clinical experience and laboratory investigation in patients with anti-NMDAR encephalitis. *Lancet Neurol.* 2011;63–74.

23. Lennox BR, Coles AJ, Vincent A. Antibody-mediated encephalitis: a treatable cause of schizophrenia. *Br J Psychiatry.* 2012;200:92–94.

24. Fink M. Rediscovering catatonia: the biography of a treatable syndrome. *Acta Psychiatr Scand.* 2013;127(suppl 441).

25. Gough JL et al. Electroconvulsive therapy and/or plasmapheresis in autoimmuneencephalitis? *World J Clin Cases.* 2016 August 16;4(8):223–228.

26. Rajahram GS et al. Anti N-Methyl-D-Aspartate receptor encephalitis: an under-recognised cause of encephalitis. *Med J Malaysia.* 2015 Dec;70(6):363–364.

27. Kanbayashi T et al. Anti-NMDA encephalitis in psychiatry; malignant catatonia, atypical psychosis and ECT. *Rinsho Shinkeigaku.* 2014;54(12):1103–1106. doi: 10.5692/clinicalneurol.54.1103. Japanese.

28. Shorter E, Wachtel L. Childhood catatonia, autism and psychosis past and present: is there an iron triangle? (clinical overview), *Acta Psychiatrica Scand.* July. 2013;128(1):21–33.

29. Kanner L. Autistic disturbances of affective contact. *Nerv Child.* 1943;2:217–250.

30. Asperger H. Die Autistischen Psychopathen im Kindesalter. *Archiv für Psychiatrie.* 1944;117:76–136.

31. Wachtel LE, Shorter E. Self-injurious behavior in children: a treatable catatonic syndrome. *Aust N Z J Psychiatry.* 2013;47(12):1113–1115.

32. Down JL *On Some of the Mental Affections of Childhood and Youth.* London: Churchill; 1887.

33. Ziehen T. *Die Geisteskrankheiten einschliesslich des Schwachsinns und die Psychopathischen Konstitutionen im Kindesalter (1915),* s.l., Reuther. 2nd ed.; 1926..

34. Tate BG, Baroff GS. Aversive control of self-injurious behavior in a psychotic boy. *Behav Res Ther.* 1966;4:281–287

35. Caryophylis G. Complexus symptomatique constitué par de l'aphagie (refus de manger), alalie (refus de parler), et astasie abasie guéri par la suggestion forcée. *Progrès médical.* 1892;20:241–243.

36. Trepsat L. Étude des troubles physiques dans la démence précoce hébéphrénique-catatonique. (Paris medical dissertation.) Paris: Michalon; 1905, 17–19.

37. Hollaender P. Démence précoce infantile (Dementia praecocissima) (Geneva medical dissertation.) Cahors: Coueslant; 1911, 13–17, 26–36.

38. Leonhard K. In E Robins ed., *The Classification of Endogenous Psychoses*. New York: Irvington Publications; 1979.

39. Mahendra B. Editorial: where have all the catatonics gone? *Psychol Med.* 1981;11:66.

40. Carr V et al. The use of ECT for mania in childhood bipolar disorder. *Br J Psychiatry.* 1983;143:411–415.

41. Black D, Wilcox J, Stewart M. The use of ECT in children: case-report. *J Clin Psychiatry.* 1985;46:98–99.

42. Cizadlo BC, Wheaton A. Case study: ECT treatment of a young girl with catatonia. *J Am Acad Child Adolesc Psychiatry.* 1995;34:332–335.

43. Wing L, Shah A. Catatonia in autistic spectrum disorders. *Br J Psychiatry.* 2000;176:357–362.

44. Billstedt E, Gilberg C, Gilberg C. Autism after adolescence: population based 13- to 22-year follow-up study of 120 individuals with autism diagnosed in childhood. *J Autism Dev Dis.* 2005;35:351–360.

45. Ghaziuddin N, Dhossche D, Marcotte K. Retrospective chart review of catatonia in child and adolescent psychiatric patients. *Acta Psychiatr Scand.* 125(1):33–38.

46. Wachtel L et al. Electroconvulsive therapy for catatonia in an autistic girl. *Am J Psychiatry.* 2008:329–333.

47. Chung A, Varghese J. Treatment of catatonia with electroconvulsive therapy in an 11 year-old girl. *ANZUS J Psychiatry.* 2008;42:251–253.

48. Wachtel L et al. ECT for lf-injury in an autistic boy. *Eur Child Adolesc Psychiatry.* 2009;18(7):458–463.

49. Wachtel L, Jaffe R, Kellner CH. Electroconvulsive therapy for psychotropic-refractory bipolar affective disorder and severe self-injury and aggression in an 11-year-old autistic boy. *Eur Child Adolesc Psychiatry.* 2011;20(3):147–152.

50. Siegel M et al. Electroconvulsive therapy in an adolescent with autism and bipolar I disorder. *J ECT.* 2012;28(4):252–255.

51. Dhossche DM et al. Tics as signs of catatonia: electroconvulsive therapy response in 2 men. *J ECT.* 2010;26(4):266–269.

52. Wachtel L, Griffin M, Reti I. Electroconvulsive therapy in a man with autism experiencing severe depression, catatonia and self-injury. *J ECT.* 2010;26(1):70–73.

53. Consoli A et al. Electroconvulsive therapy in adolescents with intellectual disability and severe self-injurious behavior and aggression: a retrospective study. *Eur Child Adolesc Psychiatry.* 2013;22(1):55–62.

54. Haq AU, Ghaziuddin N. Maintenance electroconvulsive therapy for aggression and self-injurious behavior in two adolescents with autism and catatonia. *J Neuropsychiatry Clin Neurosci.* 2014;26(1):64–72.

55. Thuppal M, Fink M. Electroconvulsive therapy and mental retardation. *JECT.* 1999;15:140–149.

56. Fink M. *Electroshock: Restoring the Mind.* New York: Oxford University Press; 1999. Patient Donald Paine, on page 77.

57. Lutz AS. *Each Day I Like It Better.* Nashville TN: Vanderbilt University Press; 2014.

58. Wachtel L, Dhossche D, Kellner C. When is electroconvulsive therapy appropriate for children and adolescents? *Med Hypotheses.* 2010;76(3):395–399.

59. Fink M. Rediscovering catatonia, the biography of a treatable syndrome. *Acta Psychiatr Scand.* 2013;127(suppl 441):1–50.

60. Wachtel LE, Shorter E. Self-injurious behaviour in children: a treatable catatonic syndrome. *Aust N Z J Psychiatry.* 2013;47(12):1113–1115.

61. Lask B et al. Children with pervasive refusal. *Arch Dis Child.* 1991;66:866–869

62. Christensen AM, Thielle T. Pervasive refusal syndrome in a 12-year-old boy. *Ugeskr Laeger.* 2011;173:1214–1215.

63. Graham PJ, Foreman DM. An ethical dilemma in child and adolescent psychiatry. *Psychiatric Bull.* 1995;19:84–86.

64. Fink M, Klein DF. An ethical dilemma in child psychiatry. *Psychiatric Bull.* 1995;19: 650–651.

65. McNicholas F, Prior C, Bates G. A case of pervasive refusal syndrome: a diagnostic conundrum. *Clin Child Psychol Psychiatry.* 2012;18(1):137–150.

66. Klee A. Akinetic mutism: review of the literature and report of a case. *J Nerv Ment Dis.* 1961;133:536–553.

67. Shorter E. What historians and clinicians can learn from the history of medicine: the example of fatal catatonia. *Med e Storia.* 2011;21/22:5–17.

68. Nicita F et al. Sudden benzodiazepine-induced resolution of post-operative pediatric cerebellar mutism syndrome: a clinical-SPECT study. *Acta Neurochir.* 2017; doi: 10.1007/s00701-016-3059-y.

69. Formisano R et al. Vegetative state, minimally conscious state, akinetic mutism and parkinsonism as a continuum of recovery from disorders of consciousness. *Funct Neurol.* 2011;26:15–24.

70. Fink M. *Electroconvulsive Therapy: Guide for Patients and Their Families.* New York: Oxford University Press; 2009.

Chapter 13

1. Romano J. On the nature of schizophrenia: changes in the observer as well as the observed (1932–77). *Schizophrenia Bull.* 1977;3:532–559, 534.

2. O'Neill W. A case of catalepsy. *Lancet.* June 23, 1877;1:905–907.

3. Shorter E. *Before Prozac: The Troubled History of Mood Disorders in Psychiatry.* New York: Oxford University Press; 2009, 17.

4. Kahlbaum K. *Die Katatonie.* Berlin: Hirschwald; 1874, 104; he found it ineffective as well in the catatonia of melancholia, yet reported partial success in at least one case of nonmelancholic catatonia (p. 95).

5. Berger H. Zur Pathogenese des katatonischen Stupors, *Münchener Medizinische Wochenschrift.* April 15, 1921;68:448–450, 449.

6. Gullotta S. Sulla interruzione della sindrome catatonica. *Rivista di Patologia Nervosa.* 1932;40:241–257, la scatatonizzazione (p. 243); first chemical treatment of catatonic stupor (p. 241).

7. Jacobi A. Die psychische Wirkung des Cocains in ihrer Bedeutung für die Psychopathologie. *Archiv für Psychiatrie und Nervenkrankheiten.* 1927;79:383–406, 405.

8. For the history of psychiatry and neurology in Wisconsin, see Hansotia P et al. The history of neurology in Wisconsin: the early years, 1907–1957. *Wisc Med J.* 2004;103:37–41.

9. Loevenhart AS et al. Stimulation of the respiration by sodium cyanid and its clinical application. *Arch Int Med.* 1918;21:109–129, see case no. 10, 128.

10. Loevenhart AS, Lorenz WF, Waters RM. Cerebral stimulation. *JAMA*. March 16, 1929;92:880–883, 883.

11. Langenstrass KH, Friedman-Buchman E. Stupor in zirkulären und schizophrenen Psychosen: Versuch einer aktiven Behandlung. *Zeitschrift für die gesamte Neurologie und Psychiatrie*. 1931;135:83–94.

12. Langenstrass K. Cerebral stimulation in catatonia. *Clin Med Surg*. 1931;38:335–336.

13. Hinsie LE, Shatzky J. *Psychiatric Dictionary*. London: Oxford University Press; 1940.

14. LE Hinsie et al. The treatment of dementia praecox by continuous oxygen administration in chambers and oxygen and carbon dioxide inhalations. *Psych Q*. 1934;8:34–71. 42.

15. Herman M et al. Nonschizophrenic catatonic states. *N Y State Med J*. 1942;42:624–627, 626.

16. See, for example, D'Elseaux FC et al. Use of carbon dioxide mixtures in stupors occurring in psychoses. *[AMA] Arch Neurol Psychiatry*. 1933;29:213–230, 224.

17. Meerloo AM. Zur Pathologie und Psychopathologie der Schlafmittelkuren. *Zeitschrift für die gesamte Neurologie und Psychiatrie*. 1930;127:168–187, 168.

18. Claude H, Baruk H. L'épreuve du somnifène dans la catatonie. *L'Encéphale*. 1928;8:724–730.

19. Bleckwenn WJ. Discussion. In CP Wagner, pharmacologic action of barbiturates. *JAMA*. December 2, 1933;10:1787–1792.

20. Bleckwenn WJ. Production of sleep and rest in psychotic cases. *[AMA] Arch Neurol Psychiatry*. 1930;24:365–372.

21. Lorenz WF. Some observations on catatonia. *Psych Q*. 1930;4:93–102, 98–99.

22. Bleckwenn WJ. The use of sodium amytal in catatonia. In GH Kirby et al. eds., *Schizophrenia (Dementia Praecox): An Investigation of the Most Recent Advances; the Proceedings of the Association, New York, December 27th and 28th, 1929* (Baltimore: Williams & Wilkins; 1931; Association for Research in Nervous and Mental Diseases, Research Publications, 10, 224–229.

23. Bleckwenn WJ. Catatonia cases after IV sodium Amytal Injection [motion picture], in National Library of Medicine, ID 8501040A.

24. Bleckwenn WJ. Narcosis as therapy in neuropsychiatric conditions. *JAMA*. October 18, 1930;95:1168–1171, 1169. In a paper to the State Medical Society of Wisconsin in September 1930, Bleckwenn described the technique of Amytal treatment in detail; see Sodium Amytal in certain nervous and mental conditions. *Wisc Med J*. 1930;29:693–696.

25. Berrington WP. A psycho-pharmacological study of schizophrenia, with particular reference to the mode of action of cardiazol, sodium Amytal and alcohol in schizophrenic stupor. *J Ment Sci*. 1939;85:406–488.

26. Lindemann E. The psychopathological effect of sodium Amytal, *J Soc Exp Study Biol Med*. 1931;28:864–866.

27. Lindemann E. Psychological changes in normal and abnormal individuals under the influence of sodium Amytal. *AJP*. 1932;88:1083–1091, 1086.

28. Freeman W. Discussion. In CP Wagner, Pharmacologic action of barbiturates. *JAMA*. December 2, 1933;101:1787–1792, 1792.

29. Hoch PH. The present status of narco-diagnosis and therapy. *JNMD*. 1946;103:248–259, 256.

30. Kety S. Interview. In M Shepherd, ed., *Psychiatrists on Psychiatry*. Cambridge: Cambridge University Press; 1982, 83–97, 85.

31. McCall WV et al. Controlled investigation of the amobarbital interview for catatonic mutism. *AJP*. 1992;149:202–206.

32. McCall WV. The response to an amobarbital interview as a predictor of therapeutic outcome in patients with catatonic mutism. *Convulsive Ther.* 1992;8:174–178, 177.

33. Fink J. Interview. In TA Ban, ed., *An Oral History of Neuropsychopharmacology: The First Fifty Years.* Brentwood TN: ACNP; 2011, ix, 93.

34. Wilkinson G. An account of the good effects of electricity in a case of violent spasmodic affection. *Medical Facts and Observations.* 1793;3:52–61.

35. Meduna L. Autobiography. *Convulsive Ther.* 1985;1:43–57;121–138.

36. Gazdag G et al. László Meduna's pilot studies with camphor inductions of seizures: the first 11 patients. *J ECT.* 2009;25:3–11.

37. Meduna L. *Die Konvulsionstherapie der Schizophrenie.* Halle: Carl Marhold; 1937.

38. For the Meduna story, see Shorter E, Healy D. *Shock Therapy: A History of the Electroconvulsive Treatment of Mental Illness.* Brunswick NJ: Rutgers University Press; 2007, 21–30. His autobiography is published in *Convulsive Ther.* 1985;1:43–57, 121–138.

39. See Shorter and Healy, *Shock Therapy* (2007), 31–48.

40. Kalinowsky LB et al. Results with electric convulsive therapy in 200 cases of schizophrenia. *Psych Q.* 1943;17:144–153, 149.

41. Hamilton DM, Wall JH. The hospital treatment of dementia praecox. *AJP.* 1948;105:346–352, 352.

42. Wells DA. Electroconvulsive treatment for schizophrenia. A ten-year survey in a university hospital psychiatric department. *Comprehens Psychiatry.* 1973;14:291–298, 294.

43. Morrison JR. Catatonia: results of treatment. In DF Ricks et al., eds., *Life History Research in Psychopathology,* vol. 3. Minneapolis: University of Minnesota Press; 1974, 336–349, 340.

44. Rohland BM et al. ECT in the treatment of the catatonic syndrome. *J Affect Dis.* 1993;29:255–261.

45. Dominguez Borreguerro A. Catatonia mortal. Diencefalo. Electrochoque. *Revista Clínica Española.* 1947;27:161–176, 176.

46. Arnold OH. Untersuchungen zur Frage der akuten tödlichen Katatonien. *Wiener Zeitschrift für Nervenheilkunde.* 1949;2:386–401, 392. Arnold was not the first to emphasize the importance of early treatment in catatonia. In 1941, Anton von Braunmühl at the Eglfing-Haar asylum in Bavaria documented for the period 1936–41 that, of the 54 patients with agitated catatonia receiving combined insulin coma-Cardiazol seizure treatments, 64.3 percent of those who had been ill less than a year recovered from the current episode; of those ill over one year, 32.7 percent. Similar figures prevailed for the stuporous catatonics. von Braunmühl A. Fünf Jahre Shock- und Krampfbehandlung in Eglfing-Haar. *Archiv für Psychiatrie und Nervenkrankheiten.* 1941;114:410–440, 425.

47. von Braunmühl A. Der Elektrokrampf in der Psychiatrie. *Münchener Medizinische Wochenschrift.* May 10, 1940;87:511–514, 514. Braunmühl devised a block method for the combination of insulin coma and Cardiazol seizures in Die kombinierte Shock-Krampfbehandlung der Schizophrenie am Beispiel der "Blockmethode." *Zeitschrift für die gesamte Neurologie und Psychiatrie.* 1938;164:69–92.

48. Arnold OH, Stepan H. Untersuchungen zur Frage der akuten tödlichen Katatonie. *Wiener Zeitschrift für Nervenheilkunde.* 1952;4:235–257, 243.

49. For information on Arnold's life, we are grateful to Dr. Eberhard Gabriel and Dr. Gertrude Langer-Ostrawsky at the Nieder-Österreichisches Landesarchiv, and Mag Thomas Maisel at the Wiener Universitäts-Archiv.

50. Lingjaerde O. Delirium acutum. *Nordisk Med.* 1954;28:742–746;; Die Behandlung der akuten malignen Delirien. *Deutsche Medizinische Wochenschrift.* January 27, 1961;86: 160–162; Contributions to the study of the schizophrenias and the acute, malignant deliria. *J Oslo City Hospitals.* 1963;14:43–83.

51. Tolsma FJ. Acute "pernicious" psychose [*sic*]. *Psych Neurol Neurochir.* 1967;70:10–32, 31.

52. Häfner H et al. Akute lebensbedröhliche Katatonie. *Nervenarzt.* 1982;53:385–394, 392.

53. Sauer H et al. Folgen unterlassener Elektrokrampftherapie. *Nervenarzt.* 1985;56: 150–152, 151.

Chapter 14

1. These lines were added as an introduction by Ludwig van Beethoven to Friedrich Schiller's *Ode to Joy* as text for his Symphony No. 9.

2. Rosebush P, Mazurek MF. Serum iron and neuroleptic malignant syndrome. *Lancet* 1991;338:149–151.

3. Raja M et al. Neuroleptic malignant syndrome and catatonia. A report of three cases. *Eur Arch Psychiatry Clin Neuroscience* 1994;243:299–303.

4. Lee JW. Serum iron in catatonia and neuroleptic malignant syndrome. *Biol Psychiatry* 1998;44: 499–507.

5. Peralta V et al. Serum iron in catatonic and non-catatonic psychotic patients. *Biol Psychiatry* 1999;45: 788–790.

6. Fink M, Taylor MA. *Catatonia: A Clinician's Guide to Diagnosis and Treatment.* New York: Cambridge University Press, 2003.

7. Fink M, Kellner CH, McCall V. Optimizing ECT technique in treating catatonia. *J ECT* 2016;32(3):149–150.

8. Fink M et al. Catatonia is a systemic medical syndrome. *Acta Psychiatr Scand.* 2016 Mar;133(3):250–251.

9. Taylor MA. *Hippocrates Cried.* New York: Oxford University Press, 2013; Shorter E. *What Psychiatry Left Out.* New York: Routledge, 2015.

10. Moskowitz A. 2004. "Scared stiff": catatonia as an evolutionary-based fear response. *Psycholog Rev* 111:984–1002.

11. Fink M. Rediscovering catatonia: the biography of a treatable syndrome. *Acta Psychiatr Scand* 2013;127:Suppl 441;1–52.

12. Taylor MA. Catatonia: A review of a behavioral neurologic syndrome. *Neuropsychiatry Neuropsychol Behav Neurol* 1990;3:48–72.

13. Ellul P, Choucha W. Neurobiological approach of catatonia and treatment perspectives. *Frontiers Psychiatry* 2015;6(12): Article 182:1–4.

14. In the early days of digital computing, when increasingly large IBM devices were being created, the belief that analyses of big datasets would assure answers to many questions was a popular selling point. IBM scientists encouraged the warning motto of GIGO—"garbage in, garbage out." That warning is as appropriate today in studies of *DSM*-defined populations.

15. Taylor MA, Fink M. *Melancholia: The Diagnosis, Pathophysiology and Treatment of Depressive Illness.* Cambridge: Cambridge University Press, 2006.

16. Fink M, Taylor MA. *Catatonia: A Clinician's Guide to Diagnosis and Treatment.* Cambridge: Cambridge University Press, 2003.

17. Shorter E, Fink M. *Endocrine Psychiatry: Solving the Riddle of Melancholia.* New York: Oxford University Press, 2010.

INDEX

Abrams, Richard 124
académie française, 110
acute delirium, 62, 96, 97, 119, 152
acute dementia, 15, 16–17
acute fatal catatonia, 103
acute hallucinatory confusion, 72
acute idiopathic fulminating psychosis, 102
adolescent insanity, 3–4, 43, 50, 167. *See also*
    hebephrenia
agitation, alternation with stupor, 4, 19–20,
akinetic mutism, 141–42
Albrecht, Paul, 70–71
Allenberg asylum (East Prussia), 94–95
alternation
    agitation with stupor, 4, 19–20, 118
    case study, 117–18
    in catatonia, 19–20, 117–20
    Kraepelin's view on, 118
    Leonhard's view on, 119
    Morel's view on, 119
    mutism and, 95
    Neisser's view on, 118–19
    Schüle's view on, 118
    self-injurious behavior and, 95
    Tuke's view of, 118–19
amantadine, 113
ambitendency of the will, in schizophrenia,
    59–60, 61
ambivalence, 59
American Medical Association, 146
American Medico-Psychological
    Association, 125
American Psychiatric Association (APA), 5,
    125–26. *See also Diagnostic and Statistical
    Manual of Mental Disorders* series
amobarbital. *See* sodium Amytal
    (amobarbital)
Amytal. *See* sodium Amytal (amobarbital)

anatomical localization, 43
Andriezen, William Lloyd, 74–75
animal electricity, 9
Annales Médico-Psychologiques journal, 16
anticatatonic treatments, 110
anticholinergics, 110
anti-*N*-methyl-D-aspartate receptor
    encephalitis, 136–37, 156, 191
antipsychotics, 110
antischizophrenic treatments, 110
apparent death, 22–24
Archives of Neurology and Psychiatry
    (AMA), 146
Arieti, Silvano, 76–77
Arndt, Rudolph Gottfried, 27, 84
Arnold, Ottokar ("Otto"), 152, 195
Aschaffenburg, Gustav, 60, 65–66, 67
Asperger, Hans, 138
Association for Research in Nervous and
    Mental Diseases, 146
Auenbrugger, Joseph Leopold, 95
autism/autism spectrum disorders, 59, 136
    Bleuler on, 59, 61
    catatonia with, 139–40
    SIB in children with, 14–15, 138–40
    signs/symptoms, 138
automatic obedience, 33, 46, 49–50, 52,
    61, 82, 117, 135
automatism, 95
L'Automatisme Psychologique (Janet), 86

babbling, 13
Bacon, Francis, 23
Baillarger, Jules, 16, 37
Bakirköy Hospital (Istanbul), 2
Bantu peoples (South Africa), 24
barbiturates, 4–5, 65, 110. *See also*
    benzodiazepines; sodium Amytal